OSTEOMYELITIS

Edited by **Mauricio S. Baptista**
and **João Paulo Tardivo**

Osteomyelitis
Edited by Mauricio S. Baptista and João Paulo Tardivo

Published by InTech
Janeza Trdine 9, 51000 Rijeka, Croatia

Publishing Process Manager Bojan Rafaj

Technical Editor Teodora Smiljanic

Cover Designer InTech Design Team

Additional hard copies can be obtained from orders@intechopen.com

Osteomyelitis, Edited by Mauricio S. Baptista and João Paulo Tardivo
p. cm.
ISBN 978-953-51-0399-8

For EU product safety concerns:
IN TECH d.o.o., Prolaz Marije Krucifikse Kozulić 3, 51000 Rijeka, Croatia,
info@intechopen.com or visit our website at intechopen.com.

Meet the editors

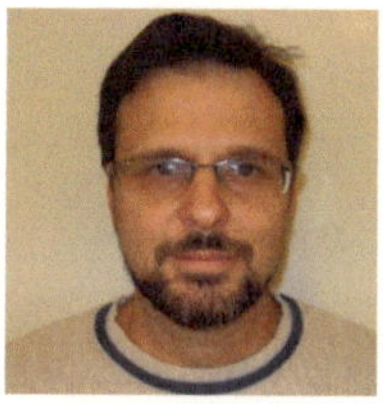

Mauricio S. Baptista graduated in Pharmacy and Biochemistry, University of São Paulo in 1990, obtained a Master in Biological Sciences (Biochemistry) at the University of São Paulo in 1992 and a Ph.D. in Chemistry at Marquette University, USA in 1996. He did post-doctorate at UW-Madison School of Pharmacy, USA in 1997 and was a visiting professor at the Université Joseph Fourier (Grenoble-France) in 2006. Has been a faculty in the Department of Biochemistry, University of Sao Paulo since 1998 where he is currently a professor of Biochemistry. Has scientific interest in the following subjects: photochemistry/photobiology, photodynamic therapy, redox processes, cell death, cell membranes and interfaces. Has published over 90 papers in international journals and has more than 1300 citations.

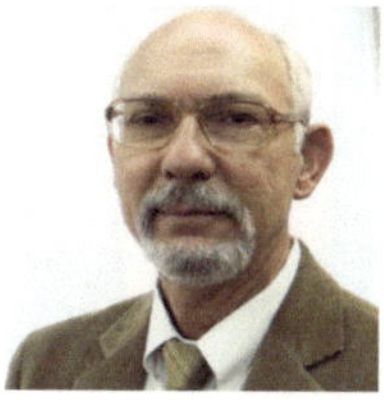

João Paulo Tardivo is assistant professor of angiology and vascular surgery and director of the Center for the Treatment of Diabetic Foot in the Faculdade de Medicina do ABC, where he obtained his Master in Health Sciences in 2004 and is currently working to obtain his PhD. He graduated in medicine from the Medical School of ABC in 1976 and obtained his specialization in Vascular Surgery in 1979 in the Hospital Gastroclinica-São Paulo. Working in vascular surgery since 1979, began his studies with medical lasers in 1987. In mid-1999 began to be interested in Photodynamic Therapy in Dermatology and superficial tumors and since 2009 has doing research in the use of Photodynamic Therapy to treat Diabetic Foot.

Contents

Preface

We hope this book will help interested readers to have a general perspective of osteomyelitis as well as to know recent advances in this field. What caught much attention is the diversity of osteomyelitis types, i.e., in skull bones, in childhood, in diabetes, non-bacterial, post-trauma, and the range of diagnosis and treatment tools that are available. In the first chapter Mayank Roy and co-workers explore the basic fundamentals of the pathophysiology and pathogenesis of this disease. In what follows the book brings a section of diagnosis and specific types of osteomyelitis. Singh Baljinder and co-workers compare the merits and disadvantages of several diagnosis techniques starting from the relatively poor results obtained with the conventional imaging modalities and how nuclear medicine, especially bone scintillography in combination with some labeling protocols (gallium, for example), can make a difference in terms of sensitivity and specificity of the diagnosis. Myoung Soo Kim addresses skull osteomyelitis describing its history, and the development of diagnosis, treatment and preventive methods. Paivi MH Miettunen reports on the rare but not less important chronic non-bacterial osteitis, which is an impressive mimic of infectious osteomyelitis. The last section of the book assembles chapters focusing in new treatment modalities. Starting with the chapter by Tardivo and Baptista, which describes how light and photoactivable drugs (photosensitizers) can be combined to treat and cure difficult cases of osteomyelitis. The chapter of Samuel Sumont describes the use of acrylic bone cement loaded with antibiotics as a strategy to perform local and efficient delivery of antibiotics making a good impact in the management of osteomyelitis. In the last chapter Tadeusz Wellisz discuss the importance of blood management during bone surgery specifically comparing the use of wax and some synthetic materials, which could be used to control bleeding and to also deliver local antibiotics.

Mauricio S. Baptista
Department of Biochemistry, University of Sao Paulo
João Paulo Tardivo
Center for the Treatment of Diabetic Foot in the Faculdade de Medicina do ABC
Brazil

Part 1

Etiology and Pathogenesis

1

Pathophysiology and Pathogenesis of Osteomyelitis

Mayank Roy[1], Jeremy S. Somerson[1], Kevin G. Kerr[2] and Jonathan L. Conroy[2]
[1]University of Texas Health Science Centre, San Antonio, Texas
[2]Harrogate District Hospital, North Yorkshire
[1]USA
[2]UK

1. Introduction

The term osteomyelitis encompasses a broad group of infectious diseases characterized by infection of the bone and/or bone marrow. The pathogenesis of these diseases can follow acute, subacute or chronic courses and involves a range of contributory host and pathogen factors. A commonly used aetiological classification distinguishes between three types of osteomyelitis: acute or chronic haematogenous disease seeded by organisms in the bloodstream, local spread from a contiguous source of infection and secondary osteomyelitis related to vascular insufficiency.

1.1 Acute haematogenous osteomyelitis

Acute haematogenous osteomyelitis refers to infection of bone resulting from bacteria in the bloodstream. This is seen most often in children, with initial infection thought to occur in the richly vascularised metaphyseal region (Gutierrez, 2005). Children are thought to experience frequent episodes of bacteraemia, often with no apparent symptoms, leading to seeding and development of osteomyelitis (Conrad, 2010). The pathogenesis of this process has been theoretically described. Inoculation of the metaphyseal vessels occurs at the transition point from the arteriolar vessels to the venous sinusoids, slowing blood flow and increasing vascular turbulence (Jansson et al., 2009). These sites of turbulence may be predisposed to bacterial infection by providing an opportunity for local invasion (Fig. 1).

Although rarely seen in developed countries, haematogenous osteomyelitis may take on a chronic course within bone if left untreated. Sequelae of this devastating condition may include chronic sinuses with exposed bone, loss of structural integrity and growth disturbances (Beckles et al., 2010).

Local trauma to bone in the setting of bacteraemia may also be a contributing factor. Animal studies have shown significantly increased rates of haematogenous osteomyelitis when direct injury to bone was combined with intravenous bacterial seeding. (Kabak et al., 1999; Morrissy & Haynes, 1989). A recent series of 450 cases of acute haematogenous osteomyelitis found the rate of preceding blunt trauma to be 63% (Labbe et al., 2010). Further research is needed to elucidate the role of trauma in this condition.

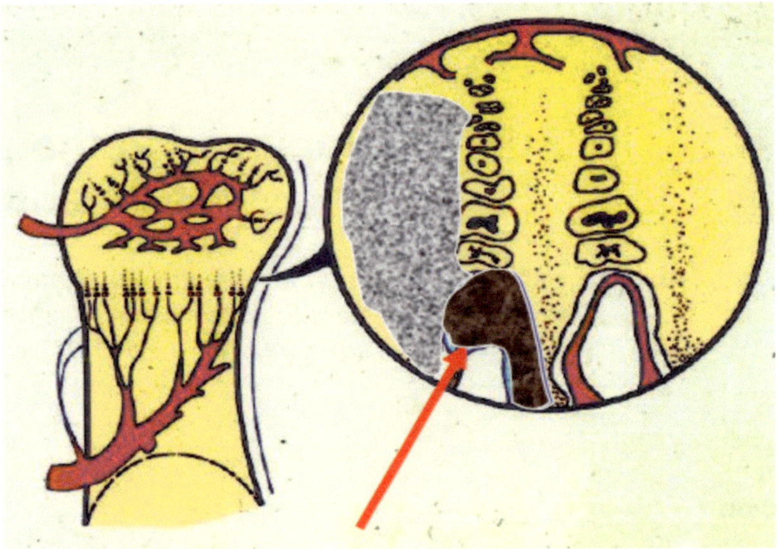

Fig. 1. Schematic drawing showing the vascular supply to the physis. The callout represents a detailed view of the physis. The red arrow indicates an area of transition. These transitional zones show increased turbulence and allow for local invasion. (Image used with permission from Dr. Kaye Wilkins)

1.2 Vertebral osteomyelitis

Osteomyelitis involving the spine is also most commonly caused by haematogenous seeding of bacteria into the vertebrae (Tay et al., 2002). The pathophysiology of this condition reflects the unique vascular structures of the spine. The venous anatomy of the spine, originally investigated for its role in cancer metastasis, allows retrograde flow from the pelvic venous plexus due a lack of valvular structures, providing an opportunity for haematogenous deposition of bacteria (Batson, 1967). Fine arteriolar structures surrounding the vertebral end plate may also represent a location at which bacteria can become trapped (Wiley & Trueta, 1959). Infections are predominantly localized to the lumbar and thoracic spine, with significantly less frequent involvement of the cervical spine (Beronius et al., 2001). In children, a markedly different disease process has been observed in infections of the spine. Blood vessels in the paediatric spine pass through the physeal cartilage and terminate within the intervertebral disc, allowing for seeding of infection from the osseous vasculature (Tay, et al., 2002). This results in a direct extension of infection into the disc that is not seen in adult patients (Fig. 2). For this reason, this condition is referred to by some authors as paediatric discitis rather than osteomyelitis.

1.3 Osteomyelitis secondary to contiguous infection

In adult patients, the majority of osteomyelitis cases are due to inoculation from contiguous infection. Sources can include direct contamination at a site of injury, iatrogenic contamination at the time of an invasive procedure, or invasive infection from surrounding soft tissue. The epidemiology of contiguous infection osteomyelitis is biphasic, with young patients suffering trauma and related surgery and older patients suffering decubitus ulcers

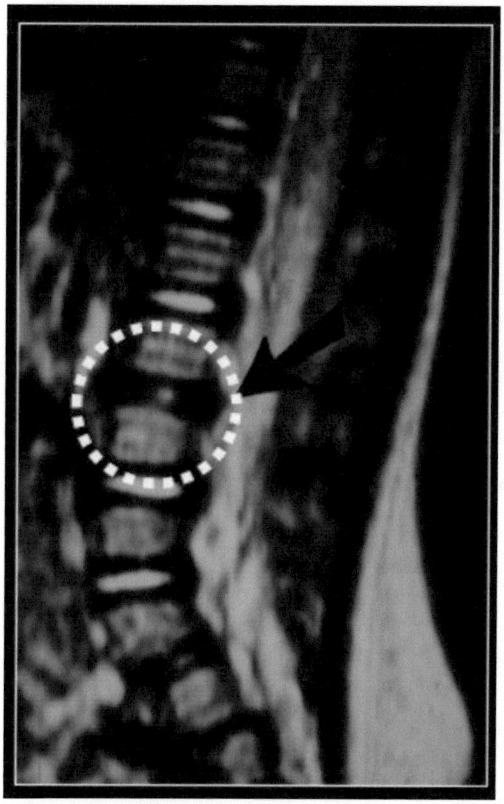

Fig. 2. MRI scan showing disc space infection. The lack of normal disc signal at the circled segment (black arrow) represents infection. This type of spinal infection is seen more commonly in children. (Image used with permission from Dr. Kaye Wilkins).

(Mader et al., 1999). Chronic infection often results, with clinical courses complicated by loss of bone structural integrity and soft tissue envelope disturbance.

The progression of disease in localized osteomyelitis is characterized by a cycle of microbial invasion, vascular disruption, necrosis and sequestration. The host inflammatory response, discussed in detail below, results in obstruction of small vessels due to coagulopathy and oedema. As a result of this, cortical bone undergoes necrosis and is detached from surrounding live bone, creating an area known as a sequestrum. This provides a fertile environment for further bacterial invasion and progression continues. Simultaneously, induction of bone begins at the intact periosteum, forming a layer of viable osseous tissue around the site of infection known as involucrum. This mechanism is thought to result from an inflammatory reaction of the periosteum.

Osteomyelitis of the diabetic foot represents a common form of localized infection. Aetiological factors have been thought to include peripheral neuropathy with associated superficial ulceration and peripheral vascular disease. However, a large recent study of risk factors for osteomyelitis in 1666 diabetic patients found no association of osteomyelitis with either peripheral neuropathy or vascular disease (Lavery et al., 2009). History and physical examination findings associated with increased relative risk for osteomyelitis in this study included a previous history of foot ulceration prior to enrolment, the presence of multiple foot wounds or wounds that penetrated deep to bone or joint. This supports prior literature suggesting that clinical ability to probe bone directly in a diabetic ulcer is diagnostic of underlying osteomyelitis (Grayson et al., 1995).

2. Host factors

The pathogenesis of osteomyelitis is a complex process involving interactions between a host and an infectious agent. The host's inflammatory response to a pathogen can further the physical spread of disease by clearing space in bone. Predisposing genetic differences in immune function are increasingly seen as an aetiological factor in some cases of osteomyelitis. Acquired factors such as diseases causing immune or vascular compromise and implantation of foreign materials are frequently involved in the disease process as well.

2.1 Inflammatory response to infection

The unique demarcated environment of osteomyelitis results in a high-grade local inflammatory host response with systemic effects ranging from minimal to severe. The initial host response to infection of bone is characterized by a local increase in proinflammatory cytokines. Involvement of human monocyte cells in this process has been well-described. When presented with *Staphylococcus aureus* cells or bacterial cell wall components such as peptidoglycan (PepG) or lipopolysaccharide (LPS), monocytes secrete large amounts of interleukin 1-beta (IL-1beta), IL-6, IL-8, tumour necrosis factor alpha (TNF-alpha) and macrophage inflammatory protein 1-alpha (MIP-1alpha) (Fullilove et al., 2000; Klosterhalfen et al., 1996; Wang et al., 2000). This has been confirmed in an *in vivo* animal model demonstrating up-regulation of cytokines following intravenous infusion of PepG and LPS (Ruud et al., 2007).

Matrix metalloproteases, a zinc-dependent group of endopeptidases, have been proposed as a key element of bone loss in osteomyelitis. These enzymes are secreted by mesenchymal stromal cells and osteoblasts and work to degrade the extracellular matrix (ECM) in various ways. MMPs have also been shown to activate osteoclast function, leading directly to cell-mediated bone resorption (Ortega et al., 2003). Future therapeutic interventions may target these inflammatory pathways to influence progression of disease.

2.2 Genetics

The role of genetics in the pathogenesis of osteomyelitis is a field of growing research interest. This has partly been driven by new technologies that quickly and affordably perform DNA sequencing of targeted areas. Multiple genetic differences have been identified between patients with osteomyelitis and control subjects, indicating possible hereditary susceptibilities. A recent study identified polymorphisms resulting in upregulation of MMPs with significantly higher frequency in patients with osteomyelitis than in healthy controls (Angel Hugo Montes et al., 2010). The mutation may cause an increase in osteoblast MMP1 production, which has been linked to osteodestructive activity in metastasis (Lu et al., 2009) and inflammatory arthropathy (Neidhart et al., 2009). The IL-1α (-889 TT) genotype has also been found to be more common in patients with osteomyelitis. (VÃctor Asensi et al., 2003; Tsezou et al., 2008). Mutations in the G(-248)A

Genetic change	Related molecules	Potential mechanism
MMP1 (- 1607 1G/2G)	MMP1	Increased osteoblast MMP1 production in 2G allele carriers
IL-1α (-889 CC/TT)	IL-1α	Increased IL-1α circulating levels in carriers of -889 polymorphism (Hulkkonen et al., 2000)
IL-4 (-1098 GG/TT and -590 CC/TT)	IL-4	Increased frequency in osteomyelitis patients; unknown mechanism
IL-6 (-174 GG/CC)	IL-6	Increased frequency in osteomyelitis patients; unknown mechanism
G(-248)A promoter	Bax protein	Lower neutrophil apoptosis rate and longer neutrophil life span in A allele carriers
NOS3 (27-bp repeat, intron 4)	endothelial NOS3 synthase	Increased NO production in the presence of bacteria (Victor Asensi et al., 2007)
TLR4 (Asp299Gly)	Toll-like receptor, NF-kappaB	Decreased IL-6 and TNF-alpha levels; phosphorylation of NF-kappaB inhibitor in polymorphism carriers (A. H. Montes et al., 2006)
HLA-DRB1*100101	HLA class II alleles	Increased susceptibility of HLA genotype carriers to sickle cell osteomyelitis (Al-Ola et al., 2008)

Table 1. Selected genetic factors related to osteomyelitis

polymorphism at the promoter region of the bax gene was observed significantly more frequently in osteomyelitis patients (Ocaña et al., 2007).

2.3 Osteomyelitis secondary to host disease

Patients with diseases of the immune system are at increased risk for osteomyelitis. For patients with human immunodeficiency virus (HIV) infection, musculoskeletal infection can represent a devastating complication. Mortality rates for osteomyelitis in HIV-infected patients of >20% have been reported, although published data involve patients treated prior to the use of highly active antiretroviral therapy (HAART) (Vassilopoulos et al., 1997). Future research addressing the outcomes of musculoskeletal infections in HIV-infected patients with modern treatment regimens is needed to provide a clearer picture of this disease process.

The pathophysiology of osteomyelitis in the HIV-infected patient is multifactorial, with vascular disruption suggested as a contributing aetiological factor. In a small series taken from a single infectious disease practice in the United States, the incidence of avascular necrosis in an HIV-positive population has been reported to be 45 times that seen in the general population (Brown & Crane, 2001). This could play a role in initial bacterial colonization. Infections with *S. aureus* remain the most common type seen in HIV-positive patients. However, atypical infections with agents such as *Mycobacterium tuberculosis* or *Bartonelle henselae* are also frequently reported (Tehranzadeh et al., 2004).

Other disease processes have also been associated with opportunistic infectious agents due to specific deficits in host function. Multiple cases of *Aspergillus* osteomyelitis have been reported in sufferers of chronic granulomatous disease (Dotis & Roilides, 2011). Fungal invasion of bone is facilitated in these patients due to defective phagocyte function. In patients suffering from sickle cell disease, microvascular changes lead to predisposition for bone infection. While authors disagree as to whether Salmonella or Staphlyococcus osteomyelitis represents the most common form of bone infection seen in the sickle cell population, published literature uniformly supports a higher rate of Salmonella osteomyelitis than in the general population (Hernigou et al., 2010; Smith, 1996). The pathogenesis of Salmonella osteomyelitis in sickle cell patients may be related to gastrointestinal mini-infarction and resultant bacteraemic episodes. Bone infarction due to impaired microcirculation and impaired opsonisation has also been suggested to play a role (Wilson & Thomas, 1979). Clinical understanding of predisposition and altered pathophysiology of osteomyelitis in patients with these underlying illnesses is required for prompt diagnosis and appropriate treatment.

2.4 Implanted materials and osteomyelitis

Surgically implanted devices in and around bone represent a risk factor for the development of osteomyelitis. Due to the high global rate of total hip and knee replacement, endoprostheses represent an increasingly common source of infection, although infections of other implants such as orthopaedic internal fixation devices are also commonly seen. Stainless steel, titanium, and titanium alloys are the most commonly used materials for osteosynthesis implants, although biodegradable polymers such as poly(L-lactide) are regularly used in non-load bearing fractures, eg, some areas of maxillofacial surgery. The differences between stainless steel and titanium are well documented (Arens et al., 1996; Melcher et al., 1994), with stainless steel implants being associated with significantly greater infection rates than titanium implants. A possible reason for this is the fact that soft tissue adheres firmly to titanium-implant surfaces (Gristina, 1987; Perren, 1991), whilst a known reaction to steel implants is the formation of a fibrous capsule, enclosing a liquid filled void (Gristina, 1987). Bacteria can spread and multiply freely in this unvascularized space, which is also less accessible to the host defence mechanisms. Electro-polishing titanium and titanium alloys has been shown to be more cytocompatible to fibroblasts in static culture conditions than standard surfaces (Meredith et al., 2005). Coatings based on human protein such as albumin or human serum have been shown to reduce *S. aureus* and *S. epidermidis* adhesion to the surface (Kinnari et al., 2005). Poly(l-lysine)-*grafted*-poly(ethylene glycol) (PLL- *g*-PEG) coatings have been extensively studied for use in biomedical applications, and are highly effective in reducing the adsorption of blood serum, blood plasma and single proteins, such as fibrinogen and albumin (Tosatti et al., 2003). It is also known that fibroblast and osteoblast cell adhesion and spreading on metal oxide surfaces coated with PLL-*g*-PEG is strongly reduced in comparison to uncoated oxide surfaces (VandeVondele et al., 2003).There has also been interest in coating osteosynthesis implants (stainless steel, titanium, or titanium alloy) with a thin layer of antibiotic-loaded biocompatible, biodegradable polymer, such as polylactic-co-glycolic acid (PLGA) (Price et al., 1996), and poly(D,L-lactide) (PDLLA) (Gollwitzer et al., 2003). The ideology behind this is that the antibiotic is slowly eluted locally at high concentration from the polymer coating as it degrades. Various antibiotics have been studied, including gentamicin (Gollwitzer, et al., 2003), ciprofloxacin (Makinen et al., 2005) and vancomycin (Adams et al., 2009). However, the main concern with all of these antibiotics is the development of bacterial resistance. To prevent this, the amount of antibiotic eluted from the implant must remain above the minimal inhibitory concentration (MIC) value of the selected antibiotic for the time the implant is in the body. A novel idea to prevent bacterial colonization on external fixation devices and wires was described by Forster et al (Forster et al., 2004), who fitted gentamicin-coated polyurethane sleeves over the pins and wires of the external fixation device. The sleeves substantially reduced the incidence of pin tract infections caused by *S. epidermidis*, and elution tests revealed that the concentration of gentamicin in the pin tract remained above the 4 μg/ml MIC breakpoint for gentamicin for up to 26 weeks. To date no surface modification or coating fully prevents bacterial adhesion, however, many of the methods discussed have decreased the numbers of adherent bacteria significantly. An important factor to help the fight against infection is the development of biocompatible surfaces or coatings that allow fibroblast and osteoblast cells to adhere and proliferate, leading to soft- and hard-tissue integration and vascularization, while preventing bacterial adhesion. This tissue-covered implant surface then confronts bacteria with an integrated viable tissue layer with a functional host defence mechanism, and may therefore be the best solution we have so far in conquering bacterial adhesion (Harris & Richards, 2006).

The majority of these infections can be traced to intraoperative contamination rather than haematogenous spread (Gillespie, 1990). Because of this, absolute sterility of the operating theatre and implants must be ensured during implantation. The pathogenesis of implant-related infections of bone is related to interactions between the device and local granulocytes, which impairs host clearance of microbes (Zimmerli & Sendi, 2011). Treatment of these infections is complicated by the propensity of infectious agents to form biofilms on implanted surfaces, as discussed in detail below.

3. Pathogen factors

The initial event in the localization of infection appears to be adhesion of the bacteria to the extracellular matrix (ECM). Various factors govern this adhesion process. Once a bacteria reaches the biomaterial surface by haematogenous route they acquire a conditioning film of ECM proteins. Osteoblast play an active role in the internalization of the bacteria. Subsequently a multi-layered biofilm is made by the bacteria, which protects it from phagoctytosis and antibiotics.

3.1 Extracellular matrix attachment and adhesins

The ECM is a biologically active layer composed of a complex mixture of macromolecules, such as fibronectin, fibrinogen, albumin, vitronectin, and collagen. Host cell adhesion, migration, proliferation, and differentiation are all influenced by the composition and structural organization of the surrounding ECM. Interaction between host cells and the ECM is known to be mediated by specific receptors such as integrins, which are composed of α and ß units and link many ECM proteins to the eukaryotic cellular cytoskeleton (Ruoslahti, 1991). The ECM not only serves as a substrate for host cells, but also for colonizing bacteria. If an infection is to develop, pathogenic bacteria must cling to the tissue in order to overcome removal by physical forces. As well as using non-specific hydrophobic and electrostatic forces to interact with their hosts, bacteria have surface proteins with specific affinity for components of the ECM and for plasma proteins. These proteins are often called ECM-binding proteins (ECMBPs) or MSCRAMMs (microbial surface components recognizing adhesive matrix molecules). The *S. aureus* proteins responsible for binding to fibronectin (fibronectin binding protein; *fnbp*), collagen (collagen binding protein; *cna*) and fibrinogen (clumping factor; *cifA* and *cifB*) are the best-studied ECMBPs (Flock, 1999). Peacock et al. showed that seven putative virulence genes in *S. aureus*, including the adhesin genes *fnbA* and *cna*, the toxin genes *sej*, *eta* and *hlg*, and *icaA*, which are involved in biofilm production, were found to be associated with invasive isolates (Peacock et al., 2002). Some studies have shown that immunization with *cna* can protect against septic death (Nilsson et al., 1998; Smeltzer & Gillaspy, 2000). Smeltzer concluded in his study that the inclusion of immunogens derived from conserved adhesins (e.g., *fnbpA* and *clfA*) would be required to achieve maximum effectiveness. However, failure to include *cna* would result in an immune response that would not necessarily limit the ability of a *cna*-positive strain to colonize musculoskeletal tissues (Smeltzer & Gillaspy, 2000). Besides collagen binding, *S. aureus* cells isolated from patients with osteomyelitis bind to bone sialoprotein suggesting that sialoprotein binding may also serve to localize the infection to bone tissue (Ryden et al., 1989).

Capsular polysaccharides expressed on the bacterial cell surface are a major virulence factor known to promote evasion of or interference with the host immune system. Binding of *S. aureus* to bone collagen is clearly associated with the protein 'adhesin' and is inhibited by the presence of a capsule on the bacterium. The latter has been demonstrated by experiments utilizing *S. aureus* strains Cowan and Wood. Strain Cowan (originally isolated from a patient with septic arthritis) lacks a capsule and demonstrates extensive binding to purified type I collagen. Strain Wood is encapsulated and demonstrated very poor binding ability to purified type I collagen in the same study (Buxton et al., 1990).

3.2 Attachment to biomaterial surfaces

S. aureus is a common cause of metal-biomaterial, bone-joint, and soft-tissue infections (Petty et al., 1985), while *S. epidermidis* is more common with polymer-associated implant infections (von Eiff et al., 2002). It has been shown that both fibrinogen (Brokke et al., 1991) and fibronectin (Fischer et al., 1996) deposited *in vivo* onto the implant surface mediate bacterial adherence. Bacteria compete with host cells for attachment to the implant surface, a phenomenon that has been referred to as 'the race for the surface' (Gristina, 1987) (Fig. 3). Once a biomaterial has been implanted, they acquire a conditioning film of ECM proteins (Baier et al., 1984).

3.3 Role of osteoblasts

The skeleton is a dynamic organ system, in a state of perpetual turnover which is continually remodelled by the actions of two cell types (Henderson & Nair, 2003). Osteoblasts are responsible for the deposition of bone matrix; they are found on bone surfaces and are derived from mesenchymal osteoprogenitor cells. These cells secrete osteoid, a mixture of bone matrix proteins primarily made up of type I collagen (over 90%), proteoglycans such as decorin and biglycan, glycoproteins such as fibronectin, osteonectin and tenascin-C, osteopontin, osteocalcin and bone sialoprotein, oriented along stress lines (Mackie, 2003).The opposing action of bone matrix removal is performed by osteoclasts, multinucleate cells that are derived from the macrophage-monocyte lineage. These cells express large quantities of a vacuolar-type H(+)-ATPase on their cell surface, along with chloride channel 7 (ClC 7) enabling localized hydrochloric acid secretion into a closed

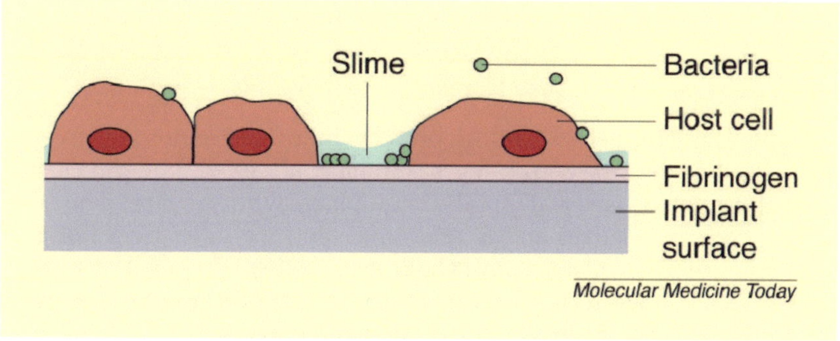

Fig. 3. Adherence of contaminating bacteria to implant surfaces competes with attachment of host cells. The implant surface soon becomes covered with plasma proteins, mainly fibrinogen, to which both host cells and bacteria can bind. In this 'race for the surface', bacteria are often the winners. Secondary to adherence to fibrinogen, staphylococci (mainly *S. epidermidis*) produce slime, further promoting adherence. Early intervention by blocking primary bacterial adherence would favour eukaryotic cells in the race. The slimy polysaccharide prevents phagocytosis and protects the bacteria from antibiotics. Reprinted from Flock, J.I., *Extracellular-matrix-binding proteins as targets for the prevention of Staphylococcus aureus infections.* Mol Med Today, 1999. 5(12): p. 532-7 with permission from Elsevier.

compartment, known as the resorption lacuna, and subsequent solubilization of bone mineral (Blair et al., 1989). The balance of activity between these two cell types is crucial to maintaining the proper homeostasis of bone turnover, and any shift in the relative levels of osteoblast and osteoclast activity can result in bone pathology (Henderson & Nair, 2003). Infection with a pathogen such as *S. aureus* is capable of stimulating such a shift, mediated in part by induction of an inflammatory response. There is an intimate interaction between the two cell types, with osteoblasts interpreting the majority of extracellular signals and subsequently modulating osteoclast differentiation and function (Henderson & Nair, 2003; Matsuo & Irie, 2008). Interaction between the RANK (receptor activator for nuclear factor κB) receptor, expressed by osteoclast precursors, and its cognate ligand, RANKL, expressed by osteoblasts is essential for osteoclastogenesis (Matsuo & Irie, 2008). Osteoprotegrin (OPG) is an endogenous inhibitor of RANKL signaling, functioning as a decoy receptor that binds to RANKL and prevents its association with RANK (Wada et al., 2006).

S. aureus permanently colonizes the anterior nares of the nostrils of about 20% of the population and is transiently associated with the rest (Foster, 2009). Colonisation is a risk factor for developing infection. Until recently *S. aureus* was regarded as an extracellular pathogen. However it is clear that the organism can adhere to and become internalized by a variety of host cells (Garzoni & Kelley, 2009), including osteoblasts (Ahmed et al., 2001), and that this is likely to be important in disease pathogenesis. *S. aureus* expresses several components that are capable of interacting with osteoblasts. Hudson demonstrated initial association of *S. aureus* strains with osteoblasts was independent of the presence of matrix collagen produced by the osteoblasts (Hudson et al., 1995). Internalization of bacteria required live osteoblasts, but not live *S. aureus*, indicating osteoblasts are active in ingesting the organisms. The bacteria were not killed by the osteoblasts, since viable bacteria were cultured several hours after ingestion. From a clinical standpoint, it has become clear that patients can have recurrent attacks of osteomyelitis after completion of therapy even when causative organisms cannot be isolated (Craigen et al., 1992). The observation that *S. aureus* can be internalized by osteoblasts may be relevant to this clinical problem.

Uptake is promoted by fibronectin binding proteins that capture fibronectin and use it as a bridge between bacteria and the a5b1 integrin (Sinha et al., 1999). Integrin clustering results in signaling that leads to bacterial uptake into phagocytic vesicles. The mechanism of invasion differs between *S. aureus* and *S. epidermidis* and the latter does not gain entry via the fibronectin-integrin $\alpha5\beta1$ mechanism (Khalil et al., 2007). The level of expression of the alternative sigma factor, σB, affects *fnbA* expression and the fibronectin binding ability of *S. aureus* strains correlates with the level of internalization of bacteria by osteoblasts suggesting that σB-mediated up-regulation of FnBP expression may facilitate invasion (Nair et al., 2003). Once internalized bacteria can escape the phagosome and cause necrosis (Wright & Nair, 2010). Slow growing variants (called small colony variants) often emerge allowing the bacteria and the infection to persist (von Eiff, Bettin et al., 1997). These bacteria are mutant forms of Staphylococcus that may have an adaptive advantage enabling persistent bone colonisation. Small colony variants can be associated with both refractory and relapsing infections that are poorly responsive to standard treatment regimens. Their decreased metabolic activity and decreased a-toxin production may enable them to survive intracellularly and to exhibit decreased susceptibility to antibiotics (von Eiff, Heilmann et al., 1997). Because of their slow growth, atypical colonial morphology, and other altered phenotypes, these organisms may be missed or incorrectly identified by clinical laboratories (Proctor et al., 1995).

Protein A (SpA) is an important virulence factor of *S. aureus*. It binds to a variety of ligands including the Fc region of IgG (Cedergren et al., 1993), Willebrand factor (O'Seaghdha et al., 2006), tumour necrosis factor receptor-1 (TNFR-1) (Gomez et al., 2006), the Fab-heavy chains of the Vh3 subclass (Viau & Zouali, 2005) and the epidermal growth factor receptor (EGFR) (Gomez et al., 2007). By binding the Fc portion of SpA ligand TNFa has been implicated in a wide spectrum of bone diseases including osteoporosis and rheumatoid arthritis (Chen & Goeddel, 2002). Several reports have demonstrated that *S. aureus* can induce apoptosis in osteoblasts (Alexander et al., 2003). Osteoblasts express high levels of TNFR-1. *S. aureus* SpA binds to osteoblasts, possibly through an interaction with the death receptor TNFR-1 which induces host cell expression of tumour necrosis factor apoptosis inducing ligand (TRAIL) produced by *S. aureus*-infected osteoblasts induces caspase-8 activation and apoptosis in cultured osteoblasts (Alexander, et al., 2003) (Fig. 4).

TRAIL can induce apoptosis in human osteoclasts via TRAIL receptor 2, and also inhibits osteoclast differentiation (Colucci et al., 2007). It is therefore possible that apoptosis of bone cells infected with *S. aureus*, and potentially of neighbouring uninfected cells may contribute to bone loss in osteomyelitis (Henderson and Nair, 2003). *S. aureus* infection of osteoblasts led to a significant increase in RANKL expression in their membrane (Somayaji et al., 2008). RANKL displayed on the membrane of osteoblasts stimulates differentiation in osteoclasts and is a key induction molecule involved in bone resorption leading to bone destruction (Boyce & Xing, 2008). In essence binding of major *S. aureus* virulence protein, SpA with osteoblasts results in the generation of multiple signals leading to inhibition of osteoblast proliferation, induction of osteoblast apoptosis, inhibition of mineralization and release of mediators capable of inducing bone resorption via osteoclast activation (Claro et al., 2011)(Fig. 4).

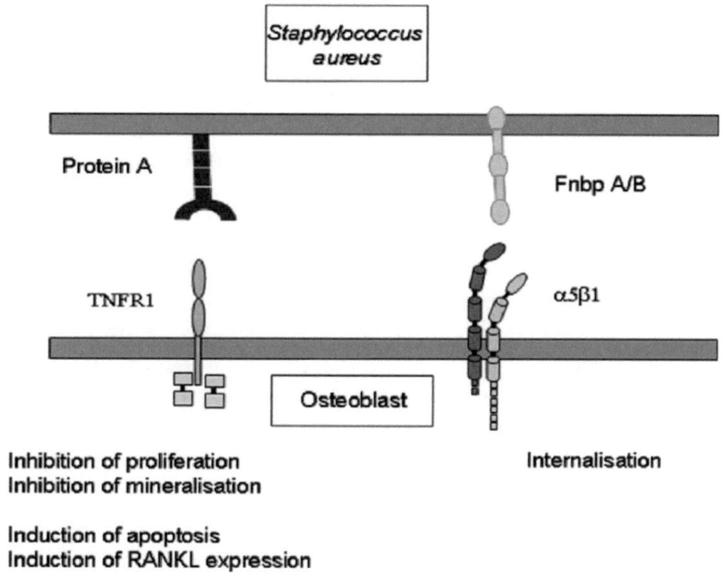

Fig. 4. Proposed mechanism of *Staphylococcus aureus* – osteoblast interaction. Claro, T., et al., *Staphylococcus aureus protein A binds to osteoblasts and triggers signals that weaken bone in osteomyelitis*. PLoS One, 2011. 6(4): p. e18748

3.4 Biofilm formation

A biofilm is defined as a microbially derived sessile community, typified by cells that are attached to a substratum, interface, or to each other, are embedded in a matrix of extracellular polymeric substance, and exhibit an altered phenotype with regard to growth, gene expression, and protein production (Donlan & Costerton, 2002). Biofilm depth can vary, from a single cell layer to a thick community of cells surrounded by a thick polymeric milieu. Structural analyses have shown that these thick biofilms possess a complex architecture in which microcolonies can exist in distinct pillar or mushroom-shaped structures (Costerton et al., 1995), through which an intricate channel network runs. These channels provide access to environmental nutrients even in the deepest areas of the biofilm.

By adopting this sessile mode of life, biofilm-embedded microorganisms benefit from a number of advantages over their planktonic counterparts:

1. The capability of the extracellular matrix to seize and concentrate a number of environmental nutrients, such as carbon, nitrogen, and phosphate (Beveridge et al., 1997).
2. The facilitation of resistance to a number of removal tactics, such as elimination by antimicrobial agents, shear stress, host phagocytic clearance, and host oxygen radical and protease defences. This innate resistance to antimicrobial factors is mediated through very low metabolic levels and radically down-regulated rates of cell division of the deeply entrenched micro-organisms.
3. The potential for dispersion via detachment. Microcolonies may detach under the direction of mechanical fluid shear or through a genetically programmed response that mediates the detachment process (Boyd & Chakrabarty, 1994). Under the direction of fluid flow, this microcolony travels to other regions of the host system to attach and

promote biofilm formation in previously uninfected areas. In addition, detachment and seeding of virgin surfaces may be accomplished by the migration of single, motile cells from the cores of attached microcolonies (Sauer et al., 2002). Therefore, this advantage allows an enduring bacterial source population that is resilient against antimicrobial agents and the host immune response, while simultaneously enabling continuous shedding to encourage bacterial spread.

Formation of biofilm is a two-stage process in which bacteria first attach to a substrate (e.g., bone) and then attach to each other as the biofilm grows and matures. The two-stage process is consistent with the scenario described for *S. epidermidis*, which is a common cause of infections involving in-dwelling medical devices. In this case, the initial attachment appears to be dependent on the production of one or more protein adhesins, whereas the subsequent aggregation of bacteria into a biofilm is dependent on the production of exopolysaccharide adhesins (Heilmann et al., 1996). It is known that once a biofilm has formed, the bacteria within the biofilm are protected from phagocytosis and antibiotics (Hoyle & Costerton, 1991), and a mouse bacteraemia model found that the biofilm enhanced *S. aureus* virulence factors, such as the α-toxin (Caiazza & O'Toole, 2003; Thakker et al., 1998). A final detachment (or dispersal) phase involves the detachment of single cells or cell clusters by various mechanisms and is believed to be crucial for the dissemination of the bacteria, in the case of pathogens to new infection sites in the human body.

Staphylococcus spp. can produce a multilayered biofilm embedded within a glycocalyx, or slime layer. The glycocalyx develops on devitalized tissue and bone, or on medically implanted devices, to produce an infection (Akiyama et al., 1993). Early studies described the solid component of the glycocalyx as primarily composed of teichoic acids (80%) and staphylococcal and host proteins (Hussain et al., 1993). In recent years, the polysaccharide intercellular adhesin (PIA) has been found in many *S. aureus* strains (Cramton et al., 1999), and is required for biofilm formation and bacterium-bacterium adhesion (Fig. 6). PIA is produced in vitro from UDP-N-acetylglucosamine via products of the intercellular adhesion (ica) locus (Cramton, et al., 1999). The genes and products of the ica locus [icaR (regulatory) and icaADBC (biosynthetic) genes] have been demonstrated to be necessary for biofilm formation and virulence, and are up-regulated in response to anaerobic growth, such as the conditions seen in the biofilm environment (Cramton et al., 2001). Another important component of the staphylococcal biofilm is extracellular DNA (eDNA). The discovery that this substance is an important component of biofilms was recently made in *P. aeruginosa* (Whitchurch et al., 2002). Rice et al. very recently showed that eDNA is important for biofilm formation and adherence in *S. aureus*, and that this DNA release seems to be, at least in part, mediated through the cidA murein hydrolase (Rice et al., 2007). This gene has been shown to be a holin homologue involved in cell lysis, and it is thought that this gene allows *S. aureus* biofilm cells to lyse and release DNA into the extracellular milieu.

Many factors seem to play a role in regulation of biofilm. The agr quorum sensing (QS) system, a central regulator of virulence, has been shown to down-regulate genes of cell wall-associated adherence factors (Chan et al., 2004). This would lead to lesser adherence and thus, indirectly, decreased initial biofilm formation. As well, the agr system has been shown to up-regulate the expression of detergent-like peptides that seem to increase biofilm detachment (Kong et al., 2006), and mutation of the system leads to increased biofilm growth. Another regulatory system, Target of RAP (TRAP), has been implicated in biofilm

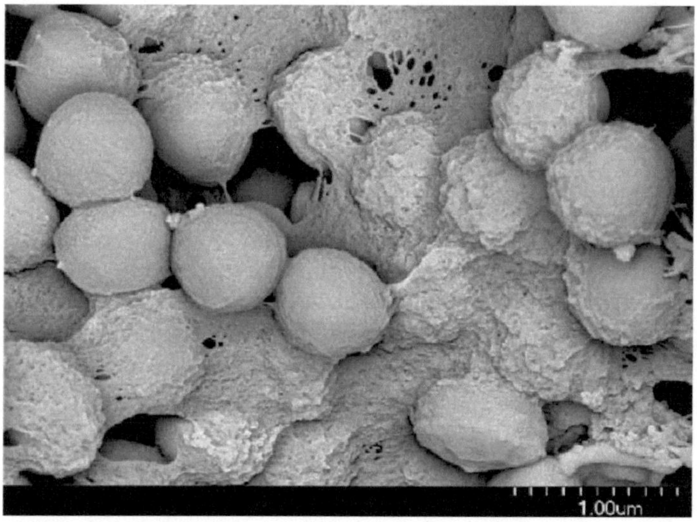

Fig. 5. SEM of a staphylococcal biofilm. Note the multiple layer of bacteria covered with a polysaccharide matrix. Reprinted from Cramton, S.E., et al., *The intercellular adhesion (ica) locus is present in Staphylococcus aureus and is required for biofilm formation.* Infect Immun, 1999. 67(10): p. 5427-33 with permission from Elsevier.

formation, with its secreted factor [RNAIII activating peptide (RAP)] increasing biofilm growth and its antagonistic peptide [RNAIII inhibitory peptide (RIP)] inhibiting it (Korem et al., 2005). TRAP is believed to work through the Agr system, activating RNAIII production (the effector of the Agr response) when RAP levels are high (Balaban et al., 2007).

Biofilms are recalcitrant to clearance by antimicrobials because of their altered metabolic and lessened diffusion of the antibiotic into the biofilm. Some of the recent strategies suggested are anti-PIA antibodies and use of RIP heptapeptide, which is proposed to inhibit RNAIII-activated virulence factors (Giacometti et al., 2003; Maira-Litran et al., 2005; McKenney et al., 1999). Surgical interventions remain the most effective means of treatment of biofilm-associated infections. In osteomyelitis infections, this means debridement of all infected bone.

4. Aetiology of osteomyelitis

The spectrum of agents associated with osteomyelitis is an ever-widening one, partly because of accumulating evidence to suggest that microorganisms previously considered as specimen contaminants are capable of causing infection (Haidar et al., 2010; Wong et al., 2010) and partly because of the increasing application of newer diagnostic modalities, such as DNA amplification. These methodologies are more sensitive than conventional microbiological techniques in identifying conventional, emerging and new pathogens in clinical material (Bang et al., 2008; Ceroni et al., 2010; Cremniter et al., 2008). Although *Staphylococcus aureus* remains the pre-eminent cause of infection, the wide and increasing range of aetiological agents associated with osteomyelitis presents a challenge to the clinician in terms of selection of empiric antimicrobial therapy; nevertheless particular clinical features as well as patient-specific risk factors and underlying conditions can be used to guide treatment.

As noted above, osteomyelitis can be broadly classified according to source of infection: spread from a contiguous site or following haematogenous seeding. The latter is more likely to be associated with monomicrobial infection while the former is often polymicrobial in origin including obligately anaerobic bacteria Osteomyelitis in individuals with vascular insufficiency including patients with diabetes mellitus is also frequently polymicrobial (Powlson & Coll, 2010).

There are also aetiological associations with patient age. In neonates, for example, the bacteria most frequently associated with acute haematogenous osteomyelitis are those which cause neonatal sepsis, notably Lancefield group B streptococci (*Streptococcus agalactiae*) and *Escherichia coli* as well as *S. aureus* (Dessi et al., 2008). In older children, *S. aureus* infection predominates and in some countries, such as the US, community-acquired methicillin-resistant strains (CA-MRSA) are increasingly recognized (Vander Have et al., 2009). *Kingella kingae* has also emerged in recent years as an important cause of osteomyelitis in children (Dubnov-Raz et al., 2008). In contrast, *Haemophilus influenzae* infections, once common in patients aged under five years, have markedly declined as a result of vaccination against Pittman type b strains of this bacterium (Howard et al., 1999). In adults, as with younger patients, *S. aureus* is the most frequent agent of infection.

Risk factor/feature	**Microorganism**
Geographic location	*Mycobacterium tuberculosis* *Brucella* species (Colmenero et al., 2008) Dimorphic fungi e.g. Coccidiodes immitis (Holley et al., 2002)
Intravenous drug use	*Staphylococcus aureus* *Pseudomonas aeruginosa* (Miskew et al., 1983) *Candida albicans* (Lafont et al., 1994) *Eikenella corrodens* ("needle lickers' osteomyelitis") (Swisher et al., 1994)
Post-human or animal bite	*Staphylococcus aureus* *Pasteurella multocida* (Jarvis et al., 1981) *Eikenella corrodens* (Schmidt & Heckman, 1983) Obligate anaerobes (Brook, 2008)
Vertebral osteomyelitis	*Staphylococcus aureus* Coagulase-negative staphylococci *Propionibacterium acnes* (post-spinal surgery) (Kowalski, Berbari, Huddleston, Steckelberg, Mandrekar et al., 2007; Kowalski, Berbari, Huddleston, Steckelberg, & Osmon, 2007) *Escherichia coli* (McHenry et al., 2002) *Pseudomonas aeruginosa* (Patzakis et al., 1991)
Prosthetic devices	*Staphylococcus aureus* Coagulase-negative staphylococci *Propionibacterium acnes* (Lew & Waldvogel, 2004)
Puncture wounds of the foot	*Pseudomonas aeruginosa* ("sneaker osteomyelitis") (Dixon & Sydnor, 1993)

Table 2. Aetiological association

Osteomyelitis in patients with immunocompromise, both congenital and acquired, can be caused by an extremely wide range of conventional and opportunistic pathogens including fungi (See section 2.3). Examples of other aetiological associations are shown in Table 2.

5. References

Adams, C. S., Antoci, V., Jr., Harrison, G., Patal, P., Freeman, T. A., Shapiro, I. M., et al. (2009). Controlled release of vancomycin from thin sol-gel films on implant surfaces successfully controls osteomyelitis. *Journal of Orthopaedic Research: Official Publication of the Orthopaedic Research Society*, Vol. 27, No. 6, pp. (701-709)

Ahmed, S., Meghji, S., Williams, R. J., Henderson, B., Brock, J. H., & Nair, S. P. (2001). Staphylococcus aureus fibronectin binding proteins are essential for internalization by osteoblasts but do not account for differences in intracellular levels of bacteria. *Infect Immun*, Vol. 69, No. 5, pp. (2872-2877), 0019-9567

Akiyama, H., Torigoe, R., & Arata, J. (1993). Interaction of Staphylococcus aureus cells and silk threads in vitro and in mouse skin. *J Dermatol Sci*, Vol. 6, No. 3, pp. (247-257), 0923-1811

Al-Ola, K., Mahdi, N., Al-Subaie, A. M., Ali, M. E., Al-Absi, I. K., & Almawi, W. Y. (2008). Evidence for HLA class II susceptible and protective haplotypes for osteomyelitis in pediatric patients with sickle cell anemia. *Tissue Antigens*, Vol. 71, No. 5, pp. (453-457),

Alexander, E. H., Rivera, F. A., Marriott, I., Anguita, J., Bost, K. L., & Hudson, M. C. (2003). Staphylococcus aureus - induced tumor necrosis factor - related apoptosis - inducing ligand expression mediates apoptosis and caspase-8 activation in infected osteoblasts. *BMC Microbiol*, Vol. 3, No., pp. (5), 1471-2180

Arens, S., Schlegel, U., Printzen, G., Ziegler, W. J., Perren, S. M., & Hansis, M. (1996). Influence of materials for fixation implants on local infection. An experimental study of steel versus titanium DCP in rabbits. *J Bone Joint Surg Br*, Vol. 78, No. 4, pp. (647-651), 0301-620X

Asensi, V., Alvarez, V., Valle, E., Meana, A., Fierer, J., Coto, E., et al. (2003). IL-1 alpha (-889) promoter polymorphism is a risk factor for osteomyelitis. *American Journal of Medical Genetics. Part A*, Vol. 119A, No. 2, pp. (132-136)

Asensi, V., Montes, A. H., Valle, E., Ocaña, M. G., Astudillo, A., Alvarez, V., et al. (2007). The NOS3 (27-bp repeat, intron 4) polymorphism is associated with susceptibility to osteomyelitis. *Nitric Oxide: Biology and Chemistry / Official Journal of the Nitric Oxide Society*, Vol. 16, No. 1, pp. (44-53)

Baier, R. E., Meyer, A. E., Natiella, J. R., Natiella, R. R., & Carter, J. M. (1984). Surface properties determine bioadhesive outcomes: methods and results. *J Biomed Mater Res*, Vol. 18, No. 4, pp. (327-355), 0021-9304

Balaban, N., Cirioni, O., Giacometti, A., Ghiselli, R., Braunstein, J. B., Silvestri, C., et al. (2007). Treatment of Staphylococcus aureus biofilm infection by the quorum-sensing inhibitor RIP. *Antimicrob Agents Chemother*, Vol. 51, No. 6, pp. (2226-2229), 0066-4804

Bang, D., Herlin, T., Stegger, M., Andersen, A. B., Torkko, P., Tortoli, E., et al. (2008). Mycobacterium arosiense sp. nov., a slowly growing, scotochromogenic species causing osteomyelitis in an immunocompromised child. *Int J Syst Evol Microbiol*, Vol. 58, No. Pt 10, pp. (2398-2402), 1466-5026

Batson, O. V. (1967). The vertebral system of veins as a means for cancer dissemination. *Progress in Clinical Cancer,* Vol. 3, No., pp. (1-18)

Beckles, V. L. L., Jones, H. W., & Harrison, W. J. (2010). Chronic haematogenous osteomyelitis in children: a retrospective review of 167 patients in Malawi. *The Journal of Bone and Joint Surgery. British Volume,* Vol. 92, No. 8, pp. (1138-1143)

Beronius, M., Bergman, B., & Andersson, R. (2001). Vertebral Osteomyelitis in Goteborg, Sweden: A Retrospective Study of Patients During 1990-95. *Scandinavian Journal of Infectious Diseases,* Vol. 33, No. 7, pp. (527-532)

Beveridge, T. J., Makin, S. A., Kadurugamuwa, J. L., & Li, Z. (1997). Interactions between biofilms and the environment. *FEMS Microbiol Rev,* Vol. 20, No. 3-4, pp. (291-303), 0168-6445

Blair, H. C., Teitelbaum, S. L., Ghiselli, R., & Gluck, S. (1989). Osteoclastic bone resorption by a polarized vacuolar proton pump. *Science,* Vol. 245, No. 4920, pp. (855-857), 0036-8075

Boyce, B. F., & Xing, L. (2008). Functions of RANKL/RANK/OPG in bone modeling and remodeling. *Arch Biochem Biophys,* Vol. 473, No. 2, pp. (139-146), 1096-0384

Boyd, A., & Chakrabarty, A. M. (1994). Role of alginate lyase in cell detachment of Pseudomonas aeruginosa. *Appl Environ Microbiol,* Vol. 60, No. 7, pp. (2355-2359), 0099-2240

Brokke, P., Dankert, J., Carballo, J., & Feijen, J. (1991). Adherence of coagulase-negative staphylococci onto polyethylene catheters in vitro and in vivo: a study on the influence of various plasma proteins. *J Biomater Appl,* Vol. 5, No. 3, pp. (204-226), 0885-3282

Brook, I. (2008). Microbiology and management of joint and bone infections due to anaerobic bacteria. *J Orthop Sci,* Vol. 13, No. 2, pp. (160-169), 0949-2658

Brown, P., & Crane, L. (2001). Avascular necrosis of bone in patients with human immunodeficiency virus infection: report of 6 cases and review of the literature. *Clinical Infectious Diseases: An Official Publication of the Infectious Diseases Society of America,* Vol. 32, No. 8, pp. (1221-1226)

Buxton, T. B., Rissing, J. P., Horner, J. A., Plowman, K. M., Scott, D. F., Sprinkle, T. J., et al. (1990). Binding of a Staphylococcus aureus bone pathogen to type I collagen. *Microb Pathog,* Vol. 8, No. 6, pp. (441-448), 0882-4010

Caiazza, N. C., & O'Toole, G. A. (2003). Alpha-toxin is required for biofilm formation by Staphylococcus aureus. *J Bacteriol,* Vol. 185, No. 10, pp. (3214-3217), 0021-9193

Cedergren, L., Andersson, R., Jansson, B., Uhlen, M., & Nilsson, B. (1993). Mutational analysis of the interaction between staphylococcal protein A and human IgG1. *Protein Eng,* Vol. 6, No. 4, pp. (441-448), 0269-2139

Ceroni, D., Cherkaoui, A., Ferey, S., Kaelin, A., & Schrenzel, J. (2010). Kingella kingae osteoarticular infections in young children: clinical features and contribution of a new specific real-time PCR assay to the diagnosis. *J Pediatr Orthop,* Vol. 30, No. 3, pp. (301-304), 1539-2570

Chan, C., Burrows, L. L., & Deber, C. M. (2004). Helix induction in antimicrobial peptides by alginate in biofilms. *J Biol Chem,* Vol. 279, No. 37, pp. (38749-38754), 0021-9258

Chen, G., & Goeddel, D. V. (2002). TNF-R1 signaling: a beautiful pathway. *Science,* Vol. 296, No. 5573, pp. (1634-1635), 1095-9203

Claro, T., Widaa, A., O'Seaghdha, M., Miajlovic, H., Foster, T. J., O'Brien, F. J., et al. (2011). Staphylococcus aureus protein A binds to osteoblasts and triggers signals that weaken bone in osteomyelitis. *PLoS One,* Vol. 6, No. 4, pp. (e18748), 1932-6203

Colmenero, J. D., Ruiz-Mesa, J. D., Plata, A., Bermudez, P., Martin-Rico, P., Queipo-Ortuno, M. I., et al. (2008). Clinical findings, therapeutic approach, and outcome of brucellar vertebral osteomyelitis. *Clin Infect Dis,* Vol. 46, No. 3, pp. (426-433), 1537-6591

Colucci, S., Brunetti, G., Cantatore, F. P., Oranger, A., Mori, G., Pignataro, P., et al. (2007). The death receptor DR5 is involved in TRAIL-mediated human osteoclast apoptosis. *Apoptosis,* Vol. 12, No. 9, pp. (1623-1632), 1360-8185

Conrad, D. A. (2010). Acute Hematogenous Osteomyelitis. *Pediatrics in Review,* Vol. 31, No. 11, pp. (464-471),

Costerton, J. W., Lewandowski, Z., Caldwell, D. E., Korber, D. R., & Lappin-Scott, H. M. (1995). Microbial biofilms. *Annu Rev Microbiol,* Vol. 49, No., pp. (711-745), 0066-4227

Craigen, M. A., Watters, J., & Hackett, J. S. (1992). The changing epidemiology of osteomyelitis in children. *J Bone Joint Surg Br,* Vol. 74, No. 4, pp. (541-545), 0301-620X

Cramton, S. E., Gerke, C., Schnell, N. F., Nichols, W. W., & Gotz, F. (1999). The intercellular adhesion (ica) locus is present in Staphylococcus aureus and is required for biofilm formation. *Infect Immun,* Vol. 67, No. 10, pp. (5427-5433), 0019-9567

Cramton, S. E., Ulrich, M., Gotz, F., & Doring, G. (2001). Anaerobic conditions induce expression of polysaccharide intercellular adhesin in Staphylococcus aureus and Staphylococcus epidermidis. *Infect Immun,* Vol. 69, No. 6, pp. (4079-4085), 0019-9567

Cremniter, J., Bauer, T., Lortat-Jacob, A., Vodovar, D., Le Parc, J. M., Emile, J. F., et al. (2008). Prosthetic hip infection caused by Tropheryma whipplei. *J Clin Microbiol,* Vol. 46, No. 4, pp. (1556-1557), 1098-660X

Dessi, A., Crisafulli, M., Accossu, S., Setzu, V., & Fanos, V. (2008). Osteo-articular infections in newborns: diagnosis and treatment. *J Chemother,* Vol. 20, No. 5, pp. (542-550), 1973-9478

Dixon, R. S., & Sydnor, C. H. t. (1993). Puncture wound pseudomonal osteomyelitis of the foot. *J Foot Ankle Surg,* Vol. 32, No. 4, pp. (434-442), 1067-2516

Donlan, R. M., & Costerton, J. W. (2002). Biofilms: survival mechanisms of clinically relevant microorganisms. *Clin Microbiol Rev,* Vol. 15, No. 2, pp. (167-193), 0893-8512

Dotis, J., & Roilides, E. (2011). Osteomyelitis due to Aspergillus species in chronic granulomatous disease: an update of the literature. *Mycoses,* [Epub ahead of print]

Dubnov-Raz, G., Scheuerman, O., Chodick, G., Finkelstein, Y., Samra, Z., & Garty, B. Z. (2008). Invasive Kingella kingae infections in children: clinical and laboratory characteristics. *Pediatrics,* Vol. 122, No. 6, pp. (1305-1309), 1098-4275

Fischer, B., Vaudaux, P., Magnin, M., el Mestikawy, Y., Proctor, R. A., Lew, D. P., et al. (1996). Novel animal model for studying the molecular mechanisms of bacterial adhesion to bone-implanted metallic devices: role of fibronectin in Staphylococcus aureus adhesion. *J Orthop Res,* Vol. 14, No. 6, pp. (914-920), 0736-0266

Flock, J. I. (1999). Extracellular-matrix-binding proteins as targets for the prevention of Staphylococcus aureus infections. *Mol Med Today,* Vol. 5, No. 12, pp. (532-537), 1357-4310

Forster, H., Marotta, J. S., Heseltine, K., Milner, R., & Jani, S. (2004). Bactericidal activity of antimicrobial coated polyurethane sleeves for external fixation pins. *J Orthop Res,* Vol. 22, No. 3, pp. (671-677), 0736-0266

Foster, T. J. (2009). Colonization and infection of the human host by staphylococci: adhesion, survival and immune evasion. *Vet Dermatol,* Vol. 20, No. 5-6, pp. (456-470), 1365-3164

Fullilove, S., Jellis, J., Hughes, S. P., Remick, D. G., & Friedland, J. S. (2000). Local and systemic concentrations of tumour necrosis factor-alpha, interleukin-6 and interleukin-8 in bacterial osteomyelitis. *Transactions of the Royal Society of Tropical Medicine and Hygiene,* Vol. 94, No. 2, pp. (221-224),

Garzoni, C., & Kelley, W. L. (2009). Staphylococcus aureus: new evidence for intracellular persistence. *Trends Microbiol,* Vol. 17, No. 2, pp. (59-65), 0966-842X

Giacometti, A., Cirioni, O., Gov, Y., Ghiselli, R., Del Prete, M. S., Mocchegiani, F., et al. (2003). RNA III inhibiting peptide inhibits in vivo biofilm formation by drug-resistant Staphylococcus aureus. *Antimicrob Agents Chemother,* Vol. 47, No. 6, pp. (1979-1983), 0066-4804

Gillespie, W. J. (1990). Infection in total joint replacement. *Infectious Disease Clinics of North America,* Vol. 4, No. 3, pp. (465-484),

Gollwitzer, H., Ibrahim, K., Meyer, H., Mittelmeier, W., Busch, R., & Stemberger, A. (2003). Antibacterial poly(D,L-lactic acid) coating of medical implants using a biodegradable drug delivery technology. *J Antimicrob Chemother,* Vol. 51, No. 3, pp. (585-591), 0305-7453

Gomez, M. I., O'Seaghdha, M., Magargee, M., Foster, T. J., & Prince, A. S. (2006). Staphylococcus aureus protein A activates TNFR1 signaling through conserved IgG binding domains. *J Biol Chem,* Vol. 281, No. 29, pp. (20190-20196), 0021-9258

Gomez, M. I., Seaghdha, M. O., & Prince, A. S. (2007). Staphylococcus aureus protein A activates TACE through EGFR-dependent signaling. *EMBO J,* Vol. 26, No. 3, pp. (701-709), 0261-4189

Grayson, M. L., Gibbons, G. W., Balogh, K., Levin, E., & Karchmer, A. W. (1995). Probing to bone in infected pedal ulcers. A clinical sign of underlying osteomyelitis in diabetic patients. *JAMA: The Journal of the American Medical Association,* Vol. 273, No. 9, pp. (721-723),

Gristina, A. G. (1987). Biomaterial-centered infection: microbial adhesion versus tissue integration. *Science,* Vol. 237, No. 4822, pp. (1588-1595), 0036-8075

Gutierrez, K. (2005). Bone and Joint Infections in Children. *Pediatric Clinics of North America,* Vol. 52, No. 3, pp. (779-794),

Haidar, R., Najjar, M., Der Boghossian, A., & Tabbarah, Z. (2010). Propionibacterium acnes causing delayed postoperative spine infection: review. *Scand J Infect Dis,* Vol. 42, No. 6-7, pp. (405-411), 1651-1980

Harris, L. G., & Richards, R. G. (2006). Staphylococci and implant surfaces: a review. *Injury,* Vol. 37 Suppl 2, No., pp. (S3-14), 0020-1383

Heilmann, C., Schweitzer, O., Gerke, C., Vanittanakom, N., Mack, D., & Gotz, F. (1996). Molecular basis of intercellular adhesion in the biofilm-forming Staphylococcus epidermidis. *Mol Microbiol,* Vol. 20, No. 5, pp. (1083-1091), 0950-382X

Henderson, B., & Nair, S. P. (2003). Hard labour: bacterial infection of the skeleton. *Trends Microbiol,* Vol. 11, No. 12, pp. (570-577), 0966-842X

Hernigou, P., Daltro, G., Flouzat-Lachaniette, C.-H., Roussignol, X., & Poignard, A. (2010). Septic arthritis in adults with sickle cell disease often is associated with osteomyelitis or osteonecrosis. *Clinical Orthopaedics and Related Research,* Vol. 468, No. 6, pp. (1676-1681)

Holley, K., Muldoon, M., & Tasker, S. (2002). Coccidioides immitis osteomyelitis: a case series review. *Orthopedics,* Vol. 25, No. 8, pp. (827-831, 831-822), 0147-7447

Howard, A. W., Viskontas, D., & Sabbagh, C. (1999). Reduction in osteomyelitis and septic arthritis related to Haemophilus influenzae type B vaccination. *J Pediatr Orthop,* Vol. 19, No. 6, pp. (705-709), 0271-6798

Hoyle, B. D., & Costerton, J. W. (1991). Bacterial resistance to antibiotics: the role of biofilms. *Prog Drug Res,* Vol. 37, No., pp. (91-105), 0071-786X

Hudson, M. C., Ramp, W. K., Nicholson, N. C., Williams, A. S., & Nousiainen, M. T. (1995). Internalization of Staphylococcus aureus by cultured osteoblasts. *Microb Pathog,* Vol. 19, No. 6, pp. (409-419), 0882-4010

Hulkkonen, J., Laippala, P., & Hurme, M. (2000). A rare allele combination of the interleukin-1 gene complex is associated with high interleukin-1 beta plasma levels in healthy individuals. *European Cytokine Network,* Vol. 11, No. 2, pp. (251-255),

Hussain, M., Wilcox, M. H., & White, P. J. (1993). The slime of coagulase-negative staphylococci: biochemistry and relation to adherence. *FEMS Microbiol Rev,* Vol. 10, No. 3-4, pp. (191-207), 0168-6445

Jansson, A., Jansson, V., & von Liebe, A. (2009). [Pediatric osteomyelitis]. *Der OrthopÃ¤de,* Vol. 38, No. 3, pp. (283-294)

Jarvis, W. R., Banko, S., Snyder, E., & Baltimore, R. S. (1981). Pasteurella multocida. Osteomyelitis following dog bites. *Am J Dis Child,* Vol. 135, No. 7, pp. (625-627), 0002-922X

Kabak, S., Tuncel, M., Halici, M., Tutuş, A., Baktir, A., & Yildirim, C. (1999). Role of trauma on acute haematogenic osteomyelitis aetiology. *European Journal of Emergency Medicine: Official Journal of the European Society for Emergency Medicine,* Vol. 6, No. 3, pp. (219-222),

Khalil, H., Williams, R. J., Stenbeck, G., Henderson, B., Meghji, S., & Nair, S. P. (2007). Invasion of bone cells by Staphylococcus epidermidis. *Microbes Infect,* Vol. 9, No. 4, pp. (460-465), 1286-4579

Kinnari, T. J., Peltonen, L. I., Kuusela, P., Kivilahti, J., Kononen, M., & Jero, J. (2005). Bacterial adherence to titanium surface coated with human serum albumin. *Otol Neurotol,* Vol. 26, No. 3, pp. (380-384), 1531-7129

Klosterhalfen, B., Peters, K. M., Tons, C., Hauptmann, S., Klein, C. L., & Kirkpatrick, C. J. (1996). Local and systemic inflammatory mediator release in patients with acute and chronic posttraumatic osteomyelitis. *The Journal of Trauma,* Vol. 40, No. 3, pp. (372-378),

Kong, K. F., Vuong, C., & Otto, M. (2006). Staphylococcus quorum sensing in biofilm formation and infection. *Int J Med Microbiol,* Vol. 296, No. 2-3, pp. (133-139), 1438-4221

Korem, M., Gov, Y., Kiran, M. D., & Balaban, N. (2005). Transcriptional profiling of target of RNAIII-activating protein, a master regulator of staphylococcal virulence. *Infect Immun,* Vol. 73, No. 10, pp. (6220-6228), 0019-9567

Kowalski, T. J., Berbari, E. F., Huddleston, P. M., Steckelberg, J. M., Mandrekar, J. N., & Osmon, D. R. (2007). The management and outcome of spinal implant infections: contemporary retrospective cohort study. *Clin Infect Dis,* Vol. 44, No. 7, pp. (913-920), 1537-6591

Kowalski, T. J., Berbari, E. F., Huddleston, P. M., Steckelberg, J. M., & Osmon, D. R. (2007). Propionibacterium acnes vertebral osteomyelitis: seek and ye shall find? *Clin Orthop Relat Res,* Vol. 461, No., pp. (25-30), 0009-921X

Labbe, J. L., Peres, O., Leclair, O., Goulon, R., Scemama, P., Jourdel, F., et al. (2010). Acute osteomyelitis in children: The pathogenesis revisited? *Orthopaedics & Traumatology: Surgery & Research,* Vol. 96, No. 3, pp. (268-275)

Lafont, A., Olive, A., Gelman, M., Roca-Burniols, J., Cots, R., & Carbonell, J. (1994). Candida albicans spondylodiscitis and vertebral osteomyelitis in patients with intravenous heroin drug addiction. Report of 3 new cases. *J Rheumatol,* Vol. 21, No. 5, pp. (953-956), 0315-162X

Lavery, L. A., Peters, E. J. G., Armstrong, D. G., Wendel, C. S., Murdoch, D. P., & Lipsky, B. A. (2009). Risk factors for developing osteomyelitis in patients with diabetic foot wounds. *Diabetes Research and Clinical Practice,* Vol. 83, No. 3, pp. (347-352)

Lew, D. P., & Waldvogel, F. A. (2004). Osteomyelitis. *The Lancet,* Vol. 364, No. 9431, pp. (369-379),

Lu, X., Wang, Q., Hu, G., Van Poznak, C., Fleisher, M., Reiss, M., et al. (2009). ADAMTS1 and MMP1 proteolytically engage EGF-like ligands in an osteolytic signaling cascade for bone metastasis. Vol. 23, No. 16, pp. (1882-1894)

Mackie, E. J. (2003). Osteoblasts: novel roles in orchestration of skeletal architecture. *Int J Biochem Cell Biol,* Vol. 35, No. 9, pp. (1301-1305), 1357-2725

Mader, J. T., Shirtliff, M., & Calhoun, J. H. (1999). The host and the skeletal infection: classification and pathogenesis of acute bacterial bone and joint sepsis. *Best Practice & Research Clinical Rheumatology,* Vol. 13, No. 1, pp. (1-20),

Maira-Litran, T., Kropec, A., Goldmann, D. A., & Pier, G. B. (2005). Comparative opsonic and protective activities of Staphylococcus aureus conjugate vaccines containing native or deacetylated Staphylococcal Poly-N-acetyl-beta-(1-6)-glucosamine. *Infect Immun,* Vol. 73, No. 10, pp. (6752-6762), 0019-9567

Makinen, T. J., Veiranto, M., Knuuti, J., Jalava, J., Tormala, P., & Aro, H. T. (2005). Efficacy of bioabsorbable antibiotic containing bone screw in the prevention of biomaterial-related infection due to Staphylococcus aureus. *Bone,* Vol. 36, No. 2, pp. (292-299), 8756-3282

Matsuo, K., & Irie, N. (2008). Osteoclast-osteoblast communication. *Arch Biochem Biophys,* Vol. 473, No. 2, pp. (201-209), 1096-0384

McHenry, M. C., Easley, K. A., & Locker, G. A. (2002). Vertebral osteomyelitis: long-term outcome for 253 patients from 7 Cleveland-area hospitals. *Clin Infect Dis,* Vol. 34, No. 10, pp. (1342-1350), 1537-6591

McKenney, D., Pouliot, K. L., Wang, Y., Murthy, V., Ulrich, M., Doring, G., et al. (1999). Broadly protective vaccine for Staphylococcus aureus based on an in vivo-expressed antigen. *Science,* Vol. 284, No. 5419, pp. (1523-1527), 0036-8075

Melcher, G. A., Claudi, B., Schlegel, U., Perren, S. M., Printzen, G., & Munzinger, J. (1994). Influence of type of medullary nail on the development of local infection. An experimental study of solid and slotted nails in rabbits. *J Bone Joint Surg Br,* Vol. 76, No. 6, pp. (955-959), 0301-620X

Meredith, D. O., Eschbach, L., Wood, M. A., Riehle, M. O., Curtis, A. S., & Richards, R. G. (2005). Human fibroblast reactions to standard and electropolished titanium and Ti-6Al-7Nb, and electropolished stainless steel. *J Biomed Mater Res A,* Vol. 75, No. 3, pp. (541-555), 1549-3296

Miskew, D. B., Lorenz, M. A., Pearson, R. L., & Pankovich, A. M. (1983). Pseudomonas aeruginosa bone and joint infection in drug abusers. *J Bone Joint Surg Am,* Vol. 65, No. 6, pp. (829-832), 0021-9355

Montes, A. H., Asensi, V., Alvarez, V., Valle, E., Ocaña, M. G., Meana, A., et al. (2006). The Toll-like receptor 4 (Asp299Gly) polymorphism is a risk factor for Gram-negative and haematogenous osteomyelitis. *Clinical and Experimental Immunology,* Vol. 143, No. 3, pp. (404-413)

Montes, A. H., Valle-Garay, E., Alvarez, V., Pevida, M., García Pérez, E., Paz, J., et al. (2010). A functional polymorphism in MMP1 could influence osteomyelitis development. *Journal of Bone and Mineral Research: The Official Journal of the American Society for Bone and Mineral Research,* Vol. 25, No. 4, pp. (912-919)

Morrissy, R. T., & Haynes, D. W. (1989). Acute hematogenous osteomyelitis: a model with trauma as an etiology. *Journal of Pediatric Orthopedics,* Vol. 9, No. 4, pp. (447-456)

Nair, S. P., Bischoff, M., Senn, M. M., & Berger-Bachi, B. (2003). The sigma B regulon influences internalization of Staphylococcus aureus by osteoblasts. *Infect Immun,* Vol. 71, No. 7, pp. (4167-4170), 0019-9567

Neidhart, M., Baraliakos, X., Seemayer, C., Zelder, C., Gay, R. E., Michel, B. A., et al. (2009). Expression of cathepsin K and matrix metalloproteinase 1 indicate persistent osteodestructive activity in long-standing ankylosing spondylitis. *Annals of the Rheumatic Diseases,* Vol. 68, No. 8, pp. (1334-1339),

Nilsson, I. M., Patti, J. M., Bremell, T., Hook, M., & Tarkowski, A. (1998). Vaccination with a recombinant fragment of collagen adhesin provides protection against Staphylococcus aureus-mediated septic death. *J Clin Invest,* Vol. 101, No. 12, pp. (2640-2649), 0021-9738

O'Seaghdha, M., van Schooten, C. J., Kerrigan, S. W., Emsley, J., Silverman, G. J., Cox, D., et al. (2006). Staphylococcus aureus protein A binding to von Willebrand factor A1 domain is mediated by conserved IgG binding regions. *FEBS J,* Vol. 273, No. 21, pp. (4831-4841), 1742-464X

Ocaña, M. G., Valle-Garay, E., Montes, A. H., Meana, A., Cartón, J. A., Fierer, J., et al. (2007). Bax gene G(-248)A promoter polymorphism is associated with increased lifespan of the neutrophils of patients with osteomyelitis. *Genetics in Medicine: Official Journal of the American College of Medical Genetics,* Vol. 9, No. 4, pp. (249-255)

Ortega, N., Behonick, D., Stickens, D., & Werb, Z. (2003). How Proteases Regulate Bone Morphogenesis. *Annals of the New York Academy of Sciences,* Vol. 995, No. 1, pp. (109-116)

Patzakis, M. J., Rao, S., Wilkins, J., Moore, T. M., & Harvey, P. J. (1991). Analysis of 61 cases of vertebral osteomyelitis. *Clin Orthop Relat Res,* Vol., No. 264, pp. (178-183), 0009-921X

Peacock, S. J., Moore, C. E., Justice, A., Kantzanou, M., Story, L., Mackie, K., et al. (2002). Virulent combinations of adhesin and toxin genes in natural populations of Staphylococcus aureus. *Infect Immun,* Vol. 70, No. 9, pp. (4987-4996), 0019-9567

Perren, S. M. (1991). The concept of biological plating using the limited contact-dynamic compression plate (LC-DCP). Scientific background, design and application. *Injury,* Vol. 22 Suppl 1, No., pp. (1-41), 0020-1383

Petty, W., Spanier, S., Shuster, J. J., & Silverthorne, C. (1985). The influence of skeletal implants on incidence of infection. Experiments in a canine model. *J Bone Joint Surg Am,* Vol. 67, No. 8, pp. (1236-1244), 0021-9355

Powlson, A. S., & Coll, A. P. (2010). The treatment of diabetic foot infections. *J Antimicrob Chemother,* Vol. 65 Suppl 3, No., pp. (iii3-9), 1460-2091

Price, J. S., Tencer, A. F., Arm, D. M., & Bohach, G. A. (1996). Controlled release of antibiotics from coated orthopedic implants. *J Biomed Mater Res,* Vol. 30, No. 3, pp. (281-286), 0021-9304

Proctor, R. A., van Langevelde, P., Kristjansson, M., Maslow, J. N., & Arbeit, R. D. (1995). Persistent and relapsing infections associated with small-colony variants of Staphylococcus aureus. *Clin Infect Dis,* Vol. 20, No. 1, pp. (95-102), 1058-4838

Rice, K. C., Mann, E. E., Endres, J. L., Weiss, E. C., Cassat, J. E., Smeltzer, M. S., et al. (2007). The cidA murein hydrolase regulator contributes to DNA release and biofilm development in Staphylococcus aureus. *Proc Natl Acad Sci U S A,* Vol. 104, No. 19, pp. (8113-8118), 0027-8424

Ruoslahti, E. (1991). Integrins. *J Clin Invest,* Vol. 87, No. 1, pp. (1-5), 0021-9738

Ruud, T. E., Gundersen, Y., Wang, J. E., Foster, S. J., Thiemermann, C., & Aasen, A. O. (2007). Activation of cytokine synthesis by systemic infusions of lipopolysaccharide and peptidoglycan in a porcine model in vivo and in vitro. *Surgical Infections,* Vol. 8, No. 5, pp. (495-503)

Ryden, C., Yacoub, A. I., Maxe, I., Heinegard, D., Oldberg, A., Franzen, A., et al. (1989). Specific binding of bone sialoprotein to Staphylococcus aureus isolated from patients with osteomyelitis. *Eur J Biochem,* Vol. 184, No. 2, pp. (331-336), 0014-2956

Sauer, K., Camper, A. K., Ehrlich, G. D., Costerton, J. W., & Davies, D. G. (2002). Pseudomonas aeruginosa displays multiple phenotypes during development as a biofilm. *J Bacteriol,* Vol. 184, No. 4, pp. (1140-1154), 0021-9193

Schmidt, D. R., & Heckman, J. D. (1983). Eikenella corrodens in human bite infections of the hand. *J Trauma,* Vol. 23, No. 6, pp. (478-482), 0022-5282

Sinha, B., Francois, P. P., Nusse, O., Foti, M., Hartford, O. M., Vaudaux, P., et al. (1999). Fibronectin-binding protein acts as Staphylococcus aureus invasin via fibronectin bridging to integrin alpha5beta1. *Cell Microbiol,* Vol. 1, No. 2, pp. (101-117), 1462-5814

Smeltzer, M. S., & Gillaspy, A. F. (2000). Molecular pathogenesis of staphylcoccal osteomyelitis. *Poult Sci,* Vol. 79, No. 7, pp. (1042-1049), 0032-5791

Smith, J. A. (1996). Bone disorders in sickle cell disease. *Hematology/Oncology Clinics of North America,* Vol. 10, No. 6, pp. (1345-1356),

Somayaji, S. N., Ritchie, S., Sahraei, M., Marriott, I., & Hudson, M. C. (2008). Staphylococcus aureus induces expression of receptor activator of NF-kappaB ligand and prostaglandin E2 in infected murine osteoblasts. *Infect Immun,* Vol. 76, No. 11, pp. (5120-5126), 1098-5522

Swisher, L. A., Roberts, J. R., & Glynn, M. J. (1994). Needle licker's osteomyelitis. *Am J Emerg Med,* Vol. 12, No. 3, pp. (343-346), 0735-6757

Tay, B. K. B., Deckey, J., & Hu, S. S. (2002). Spinal Infections. *J Am Acad Orthop Surg,* Vol. 10, No. 3, pp. (188-197),

Tehranzadeh, J., Ter-Oganesyan, R. R., & Steinbach, L. S. (2004). Musculoskeletal disorders associated with HIV infection and AIDS. Part I: Infectious musculoskeletal conditions. *Skeletal Radiology,* Vol. 33, No. 5, pp. (249-259),

Thakker, M., Park, J. S., Carey, V., & Lee, J. C. (1998). Staphylococcus aureus serotype 5 capsular polysaccharide is antiphagocytic and enhances bacterial virulence in a murine bacteremia model. *Infect Immun,* Vol. 66, No. 11, pp. (5183-5189), 0019-9567

Tosatti, S., De Paul, S. M., Askendal, A., VandeVondele, S., Hubbell, J. A., Tengvall, P., et al. (2003). Peptide functionalized poly(L-lysine)-g-poly(ethylene glycol) on titanium: resistance to protein adsorption in full heparinized human blood plasma. *Biomaterials,* Vol. 24, No. 27, pp. (4949-4958), 0142-9612

Tsezou, A., Poultsides, L., Kostopoulou, F., Zintzaras, E., Satra, M., Kitsiou-Tzeli, S., et al. (2008). Influence of interleukin 1alpha (IL-1alpha), IL-4, and IL-6 polymorphisms on genetic susceptibility to chronic osteomyelitis. *Clinical and Vaccine Immunology: CVI,* Vol. 15, No. 12, pp. (1888-1890),

Vander Have, K. L., Karmazyn, B., Verma, M., Caird, M. S., Hensinger, R. N., Farley, F. A., et al. (2009). Community-associated methicillin-resistant Staphylococcus aureus in acute musculoskeletal infection in children: a game changer. *J Pediatr Orthop,* Vol. 29, No. 8, pp. (927-931), 1539-2570

VandeVondele, S., Voros, J., & Hubbell, J. A. (2003). RGD-grafted poly-L-lysine-graft-(polyethylene glycol) copolymers block non-specific protein adsorption while promoting cell adhesion. *Biotechnol Bioeng,* Vol. 82, No. 7, pp. (784-790), 0006-3592

Vassilopoulos, D., Chalasani, P., Jurado, R. L., Workowski, K., & Agudelo, C. A. (1997). Musculoskeletal infections in patients with human immunodeficiency virus infection. *Medicine,* Vol. 76, No. 4, pp. (284-294)

Viau, M., & Zouali, M. (2005). Effect of the B cell superantigen protein A from S. aureus on the early lupus disease of (NZBxNZW) F1 mice. *Mol Immunol,* Vol. 42, No. 7, pp. (849-855), 0161-5890

von Eiff, C., Bettin, D., Proctor, R. A., Rolauffs, B., Lindner, N., Winkelmann, W., et al. (1997). Recovery of small colony variants of Staphylococcus aureus following gentamicin bead placement for osteomyelitis. *Clin Infect Dis,* Vol. 25, No. 5, pp. (1250-1251), 1058-4838

von Eiff, C., Heilmann, C., Proctor, R. A., Woltz, C., Peters, G., & Gotz, F. (1997). A site-directed Staphylococcus aureus hemB mutant is a small-colony variant which persists intracellularly. *J Bacteriol,* Vol. 179, No. 15, pp. (4706-4712), 0021-9193

von Eiff, C., Peters, G., & Heilmann, C. (2002). Pathogenesis of infections due to coagulase-negative staphylococci. *Lancet Infect Dis,* Vol. 2, No. 11, pp. (677-685), 1473-3099

Wada, T., Nakashima, T., Hiroshi, N., & Penninger, J. M. (2006). RANKL-RANK signaling in osteoclastogenesis and bone disease. *Trends Mol Med,* Vol. 12, No. 1, pp. (17-25), 1471-4914

Wang, Z.-M., Liu, C., & Dziarski, R. (2000). Chemokines Are the Main Proinflammatory Mediators in Human Monocytes Activated by Staphylococcus aureus,

Peptidoglycan, and Endotoxin. *Journal of Biological Chemistry,* Vol. 275, No. 27, pp. (20260 -20267)

Whitchurch, C. B., Tolker-Nielsen, T., Ragas, P. C., & Mattick, J. S. (2002). Extracellular DNA required for bacterial biofilm formation. *Science,* Vol. 295, No. 5559, pp. (1487), 1095-9203

Wiley, A. M., & Trueta, J. (1959). The vascular anatomy of the spine and its relationship to pyogenic vertebral osteomyelitis. *The Journal of Bone and Joint Surgery. British Volume,* Vol. 41-B, No., pp. (796-809)

Wilson, W. A., & Thomas, E. J. (1979). Activation of the alternative pathway of human complement by haemoglobin. *Clinical and Experimental Immunology,* Vol. 36, No. 1, pp. (140-144)

Wong, J. S., Seaward, L. M., Ho, C. P., Anderson, T. P., Lau, E. O., Amodeo, M. R., et al. (2010). Corynebacterium accolens-associated pelvic osteomyelitis. *J Clin Microbiol,* Vol. 48, No. 2, pp. (654-655), 1098-660X

Wright, J. A., & Nair, S. P. (2010). Interaction of staphylococci with bone. *Int J Med Microbiol,* Vol. 300, No. 2-3, pp. (193-204), 1618-0607

Zimmerli, W., & Sendi, P. (2011). Pathogenesis of implant-associated infection: the role of the host. *Seminars in Immunopathology,* Vol. 33, No. 3, pp. (295-306)

Part 2

Diagnosis and Types of Osteomyelitis

2

Role of Nuclear Medicine in Infection Imaging

Baljinder Singh, Sarika C.N.B. Harisankar,
B.R. Mittal and Bhattacharya Anish
*Department of Nuclear Medicine, Postgraduate Institute of
Medical Education and Research (PGIMER)
India*

1. Introduction

Inflammation is a complex tissue reaction to injury that may be caused by physical, chemical, or immunological agents or even by radiation. Acute inflammation is the early or an immediate response to injury that lasts for a short duration (8-10 days), whereas the condition characterized as chronic inflammation is of longer duration, lasting for several weeks to even years.

A variety of conventional imaging modalities such as radiography, computed tomography and magnetic resonance imaging are available for evaluation of osteomyelitis. The diagnosis of acute osteomyelitis is relatively straight forward. Conventional imaging modalities perform poorly when there is a previous insult (fracture, trauma and infection) to the bone. The limitations of the conventional imaging modalities necessitate utilization of functional modalities. Nuclear medicine techniques are ideally suited for these patients.

Several different nuclear medicine techniques are utilized for the evaluation of osteomyelitis. Bone scintigraphy with diphosphonates is an easily available technique in the initial evaluation of osteomyelitis. It has high sensitivity but suffers from low specificity. However, in patients with chronic osteomyelitis and those with previous insult to the bone, the diagnostic performance of bone scintigraphy alone is limited. To overcome the low specificity of bone scintigraphy alone, bone scintigraphy combined with 67 Gallium, leukocytes and bone marrow imaging could improve the specificity. An approach of labeled antibiotics imaging preferentially picks up active bacterial infection in both soft tissue as well as bone. 18-F Fluorodeoxyglucose-positron emission tomography (FDG-PET) has become an encouraging imaging modality in musculoskeletal infection. This application has an incremental value in the assessment of both acute and chronic infection and has shown to be more accurate in detecting chronic osteomyelitis than conventional radionuclide imaging.

Functional imaging modalities are especially useful in patients with orthopedic hardware and those with diabetic foot infection. The above mentioned conditions are dealt separately because of the peculiar difficulties posed by them. Nuclear medicine and PET techniques are cornerstone in the evaluation of infected orthopedic hardware.

2. Inflammation and infection

Inflammation is a complex tissue reaction to injury that may be caused by physical, chemical, or immunological agents or even by radiation. If the injury is caused by or involves living microbes, the injury leads to infection. In general, the inflammatory response is characterized by local hyperemia (rubor, calor), edema or swelling (tumor), pain (dolor). Inflammation may be classified broadly as acute or chronic depending on the duration of inflammatory reaction and also on other pathological and clinical features.

Acute inflammation is the early or an immediate response to injury that lasts for a short duration (8-10 days), whereas the condition characterized as chronic inflammation is of longer duration, lasting for several weeks to even years. Acute inflammation is associated with many regional and systemic changes, such as vasodilation, increased vascular permeability, and formation of exudate. These events are followed by local cellular events [1]. Neutrophils are the predominant cells in acute inflammation. If the inciting agent persists chronic inflammation follows. Chronic inflammatory stage is characterized by reduction in the number of neutrophils and an increased infiltration of macrophages, lymphocytes, plasma cells, and fibroblasts.

2.1 Osteomyelitis

Osteomyelitis is an infection involving the cortical bone as well as the myeloid (bone marrow). The infection may be limited to the periosteum (periosteitis) without involvement of cortex and marrow but when the cortex is involved, it is called osteitis and osteomyelitis. Osteomyelitis may be classified based on several factors such as route of infection (hematogenous or nonhematogenous), underlying etiology (diabetic foot), age of onset (infantile). Staphylococcus aureus is the most common gram-positive bacterium involved [2]. One of the consequences of osteomyelitis is reactive new bone formation resulting in increased blood flow. Chronic osteomyelitis is characterized by less marked infiltration of inflammatory cells than seen in the acute state and may exhibit variable amount of necrotic tissue. Osteomyelitis in the diabetic foot is a unique clinical and pathologic problem. It is a common complication of diabetes and generally occurs as a result of the spread of infection from adjacent foot ulcers. Patients undergoing hip or knee arthroplasties may experience discomfort due to loosening with or without infection. The extent of reactive bone formation, however, depends on the nature of prosthetic material; the cementless porous coated prosthesis induces more reactive bone formation than the cemented prosthesis. Finally, infectious or septic arthritis refers to the invasion of synovial space by microorganisms and represent medical emergency.

3. Imaging techniques of osteomyelitis

3.1 Radiological techniques

Standard radiography, magnetic resonance imaging (MRI), and computed tomography (CT) commonly are used to detect skeletal infections. Radiographs provide morphological data about the region of interest. MRI has been used widely because of its excellent soft-tissue contrast and its sensitivity to tissue edema and hyperemia. MRI is valuable in the visualization of septic arthritis, spinal infection, and diabetic foot infections. However, these modalities are of limited value to detect early infection when morphological changes are absent. Similarly in patients with previous insult to the bones (previous infection, fracture, surgery replacement etc), morphological imaging methods have limited role. Artifacts caused by prosthetic joints or metallic implants in the spine or extremities can degrade images sufficiently to make diagnosis impossible in both CT and MRI. Therefore, nuclear medicine procedures are needed as a functional adjunct to complement morphologic imaging techniques [2].

3.2 Nuclear medicine techniques

A variety of radiopharmaceuticals are available for skeletal infection imaging [3] and several new tracer are being evaluated for use in imaging infection [4]. The characteristics of an ideal infection imaging agents are mentioned in Table 1. The physical characteristics, advantages and disadvantages of the commonly used radiopharmaceuticals are summarized in Table 2. The various Nuclear Medicine skeletal imaging techniques are as follows:

a. **Static imaging:** Static imaging of a part of the body is the one of the most commonly used technique in nuclear medicine. The technique is similar to radiography. Images are obtained using gamma camera for a fixed amount of time or for fixed counts. Images can be obtained in any of the views, though anterior, posterior and oblique views are the ones that are commonly performed.
b. **Dynamic imaging:** Dynamic imaging is rapid acquisition of several static images which can be later viewed in a cine format. It is especially useful in studying the changes in blood flow, uptake of the tracer in the bones etc. Dynamic imaging is frequently performed in the diagnosis of osteomyelitis. The significant increase in the bloodflow to the affected site can be easily identified using dynamic imaging.
c. **Whole body imaging:** Whole body imaging is routinely used for the evaluation of bone disorders, especially in the case of metastatic bone disease. This technique images the whole body and displays the entire skelton as a single image.
d. **Three phase imaging:** Three phase imaging is a combination of dynamic imaging followed by static imaging at fixed time intervals. It involves an initial dynamic imaging of the site of interest immediately after the intravenous injection of the radiotracer. These images help in identification of the increase in bloodflow, if any, to the site of interest. This is followed by static images of the region during the soft tissue phase (immediately after completion of the dynamic phase) and bone phase (3 hours after injection). Fourth phase imaging (static image at 24 hours) can also be done and shows modest increase in specificity for identifying osteomyelitis)
e. **Fusion imaging (Hybrid SPECT/CT):** The lack of anatomic detail in nuclear medicine images can be overcome by fusion imaging. Fusion imaging consists of a combined anatomic (usually CT scan) and a functional imaging (nuclear medicine imaging) in a single sitting in the same position. The two images are then fused together and used for interpretation. Addition of CT aids in anatomical localization, attenuation correction and also helps in increasing specificity by providing anatomical details. In the case of osteomyelitis, it is especially useful in differentiating soft tissue infection from bony infection.
f. **Positron emission tomography (PET):** PET is a functional imaging technique which utilizes annihilation radiation (two 511 keV gamma rays) for imaging. It has advantage of high sensitivity and higher spatial resolution compared to the general nuclear medicine procedures.

- Should be easily available, cheap and easy to prepare
- Should have high sensitivity and high specificity to detect infection
- Should differentiate between acute and chronic infection
- Should differentiate between infection and sterile inflammation
- Should be non-immunogenic and non-toxic
- Minimum radiation burden to the patient

Table 1. Characteristics of an ideal skeletal infection imaging agent.

RP	Mechanism of localisation	Advantages	Disadvantages
^{99m}Tc -MDP	Increased vascularity and permeability. Uptake in areas of new bone formation	Simple to perform Very high sensitivity	Low specificity
^{99m}Tc - HMPAO labeled leukocytes	Migration of WBCs into areas of infection	High specificity Reasonable sensitivity	Handling blood products Low sensitivity in chronic infection
^{99m}Tc-Ciprofloxacin	Increased vascular permeability ? Binding to bacteria	Simple preparation High sensitivity	Specificity not proven yet.
^{68}Ga- citrate	Vascular permeability Binds to transferrin, lactoferrin and siderophores	More specific than diphosphonates	Long half life. Radiation burden
^{111}In- Oxine labeled leukocytes	Migration of WBCs into areas of infection	High specificity	Long half life Prolonged imaging times Radiation burden is higher.
^{18}F- FDG	Uptake by GLUT receptors. Localises in areas of increased glycolysis	Simple with high sensitivity	Higher cost. Specificity yet to be proven
^{18}F- FDG labeled WBC	Migration of WBCs into areas of infection	High specificity	Handling blood products. Skilled person is necessary

Table 2. Radiopharmaceuticals for skeletal infection imaging

4. Radionuclide imaging of osteomyelitis

4.1 Acute osteomyelitis

Patients with acute osteomyelitis usually present with pain and swelling at the involved site with systemic features of infection. Among the radionuclide techniques, the three phase bone scan is the frequently used for evaluating acute osteomyelitis. The three phase bone scan reveals increased perfusion, soft tissue blood pooling and bony uptake in a typical case of acute osteomyelitis (Fig.1). In some patients, especially pediatric population, there may be a cold area (cold osteomyelitis) [5]. Spread of infection to the joint space can be detected, if

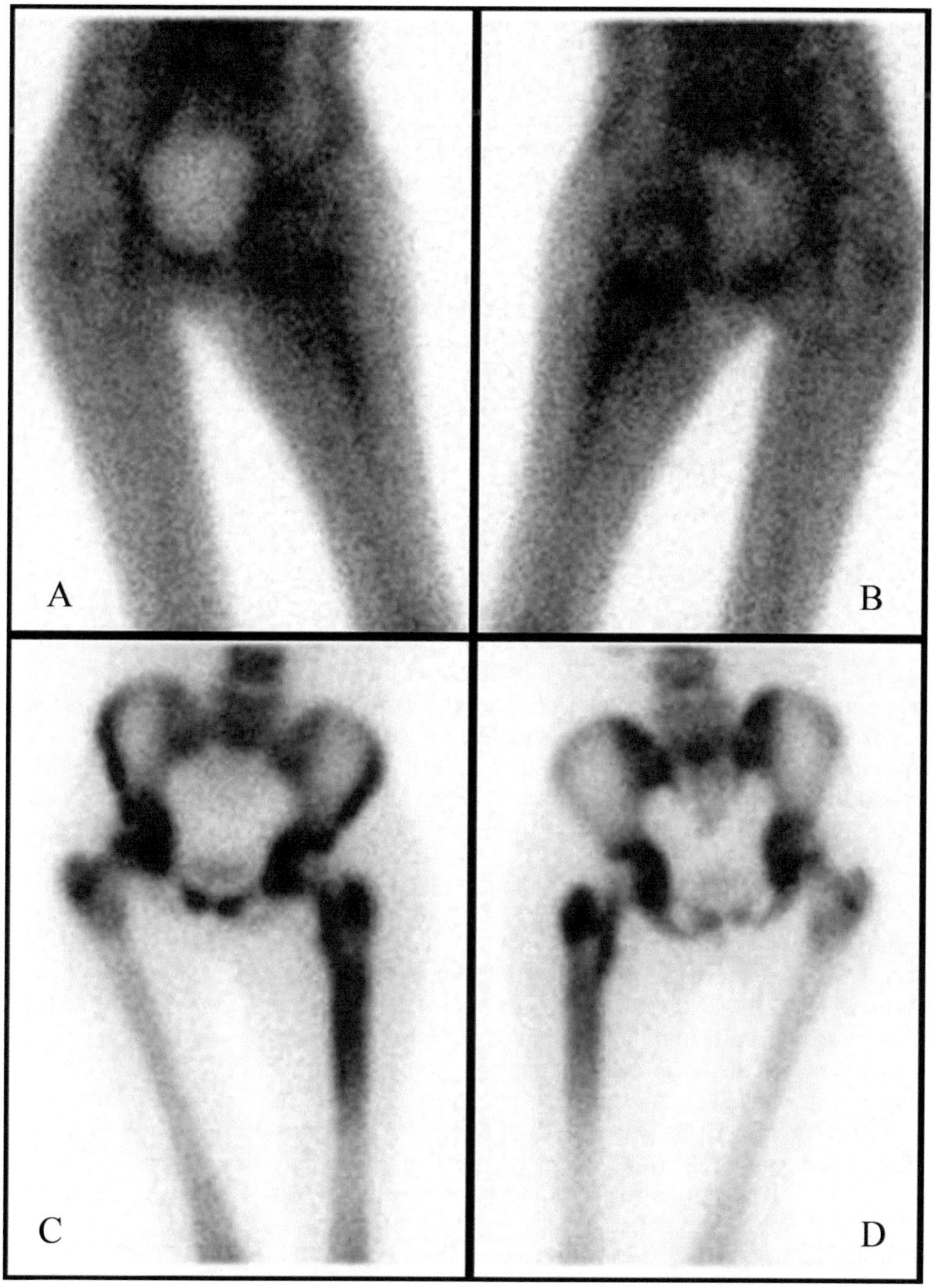

Fig. 1. Images of three phase bone scintigraphy of a patient with osteomyelitis of the left femur. Blood pool images in the anterior (A) and posterior (B) views show increased perfusion and soft tissue pooling of tracer around the proximal part of the left femur. Bone phase images in the anterior (C) and posterior (D) views also show increased tracer uptake in the proximal shaft of the left femur.

there is any. In the absence of previous insult to the bone, the clinical and radionuclide imaging features are adequate for the diagnosis of acute osteomyelitis. Though labeled leukocytes are highly specific for the diagnosis, they are usually not indicated. Labelled leukocytes imaging, because of the limited spatial resolution cannot differentiate between soft tissue and bone infection in the peripheral skeleton. Addition of hybrid imaging techniques like SPECT/CT helps in precise anatomical localization. Among the various conventional nuclear medicine procedures, ^{111}In-labeled leukocytes is one of the most specific imaging techniques and is useful in acute infection, in osteomyelitis of the diabetic foot, and in the neuropathic joint. Disadvantages in imaging with Indium labeled leukocytes include need for prolonged imaging, combining with bone marrow imaging, higher radiation burden, need for handling blood and limited limited availability . ^{99m}Tc- labeled leukocytes are a better alternative. Images are acquired at 1, 4 & 24-h. However, interpretation without bone marrow imaging is difficult.

4.2 Chronic osteomyelitis

Chronic and low grade infections are more difficult to diagnose with the routine imaging modalities. Bone / Gallium imaging is extremely useful in cases of vertebral osteomyelitis. FDG PET has a special role in the evaluation of chronic infection because the activated macrophages avidly take up FDG. A negative FDG PET can virtually rule out osteomyelitis [6]. FDG PET is also better than labeled leukocyte imaging for axial skeleton. FDG-PET and FDG-PET/CT have many advantages over conventional nuclear medicine imaging techniques: complete image acquisition within 1 hour, high sensitivity, high arget-to-background contrast, and high-resolution tomographic images. PET/CT also provides exact anatomic localization of FDG uptake and increases the specificity compared with PET alone. The logistics of the PET technique make its use easier in chronic than in acute inflammation.

4.3 Disc space infection

Diagnosis of disc space infection is a challenge. Radiography may be normal within the first 8 weeks. Contrast enhanced MRI shows high sensitivity in the early diagnosis of disc space infection. Degenerative lesions in the spine can potentially mimic infection on MRI. Three phase bone scintigraphy and labeled leukocytes have a limited role. Bone scintigraphy with ^{67}Gallium SPECT is the radionuclide imaging of choice. Recently, FDG-PET has been shown to have higher sensitivity and specificity than gallium SPECT. Paravertebral soft tissue involvement can also be detected by PET. FDG PET is also useful in excluding disc space infection when equivocal MRI findings are present. One study has shown FDG PET to be 100% sensitive and specific while MRI had sensitivity of only 50% [7].

4.4 Prosthesis Infection

Nearly 700,000 hip and knee arthroplasties are performed annually in the United States [8]. Although, the clinical results of these procedures in the vast majority of cases are excellent, these implants do fail. Failures caused by heterotopic ossification, fracture, and dislocation are now relatively rare and usually can be diagnosed radiographically [9]. Failure caused by aseptic loosening, however, has continued to increase in frequency.

More than one-quarter of all prostheses eventually demonstrate evidence of loosening, often necessitating revision arthroplasty [10]. The most frequent cause of aseptic loosening is an inflammatory reaction to one or more of the prosthetic components. Particulate debris, produced by component fragmentation, presumably attracts and activates tissue phagocytes normally present around the prosthesis. The heightened inflammatory response leads to osteolysis, causing loss of supporting osseous tissues and, eventually, loosening of the prosthesis.

Infection, although uncommon, is perhaps the most serious complication of joint arthroplasty surgery, ranging in frequency from about 1% to 2% for primary implants, to about 3% to 5% for revision implants. Approximately, one-third of prosthetic joint infections develop within 3 months, another one-third within 1 year, and the remainder more than 1 year after surgery. Histopathologically, the inflammatory reaction that accompanies the infected prosthesis can be similar to that present in aseptic loosening, with one important difference: neutrophils, which usually are absent in aseptic loosening, are invariably present in large numbers in infection [10,11]. The treatment of infected hardware often requires multiple admissions. An excisional arthroplasty, or removal of the prosthesis, is performed, followed by a protracted course of antimicrobial therapy. A revision arthroplasty eventually is performed. Aseptic loosening, in contrast, usually is managed with a single-stage exchange arthroplasty requiring only 1 hospital admission and 1 surgical intervention [10, 12]. Because their treatments are so different, distinguishing infection from aseptic loosening of a prosthesis is extremely important.

Unfortunately, differentiating aseptic loosening from infection can be challenging. Clinical signs of infection often are absent. Increased peripheral blood leukocytes, erythrocyte sedimentation rate, and C-reactive protein levels are neither sensitive nor specific for infection. Joint aspiration with Gram stain and culture is considered the definitive diagnostic test; its sensitivity, however, is variable, ranging from 28% to 92%. Its specificity is more consistent, ranging from 92% to 100% [13].Among the various imaging studies, plain radiographs are neither sensitive nor specific and cross-sectional imaging modalities, such as computed tomography and magnetic resonance imaging, can be limited by hardware induced artifacts. Radionuclide imaging is not affected by metallic hardware and is the current imaging modality of choice for evaluation of suspected joint replacement infection.

5. Scintigraphic techniques

5.1 Bone scintigraphy

Bone scintigraphy is an extremely sensitive investigation for detecting bone disorders. Its role in the evaluation of painful joint replacement has been extensively investigated. Magnuson and coworkers [14] reviewed 49 painful lower-extremity joint replacements and found that 3-phase bone scintigraphy was 100% sensitive, 18% specific, and 53% accurate for diagnosing infection.

Weiss and coworkers, [15] using focally increased uptake at the tip of the femoral component or in the region of the acetabular component as the criterion for an abnormal study, reported that bone scintigraphy was 100% sensitive and 77% specific for diagnosing infection or loosening of the total hip replacement.

Williamson and coworkers [16] found that focal periprosthetic uptake was associated with aseptic loosening, whereas diffuse uptake around the femoral and acetabular components was associated with infection.

Increased periprosthetic activity on bone images reflects increased bone mineral turnover, which can result from any of a number of conditions besides infection. This problem is further complicated by the numerous patterns of periprosthetic uptake associated with asymptomatic hip and knee replacements. Up to 10% of asymptomatic patients will have persistent periprosthetic uptake after 1 year of joint replacement. Assessment of the total knee replacement with bone scintigraphy also is problematic, with more than 60% of femoral components and nearly 90% of tibial components demonstrating persistent periprosthetic activity more than 12 months after implantation.

The overall accuracy of radionuclide bone imaging in the evaluation of the painful prosthetic joint is about 50-70%, too low to be clinically useful, except perhaps as a screening test, or in conjunction with other radionuclide studies like gallium or labeled leukocyte imaging.

5.2 Bone / gallium imaging

^{67} Gallium Citrate has the propensity to accumulate in sites of infection and inflammation. When combined with a sensitive investigation like bone scan, the specificity of gallium study will help in better identification of infected prostheses. Reing and coworkers [17] evaluated 79 joint replacements with both bone and gallium scintigraphy. Bone scintigraphy had 100% sensitivity in identifying infected prostheses, but also was abnormal in 50 uninfected prostheses, rendering it very nonspecific (15%). In contrast, gallium had 95% sensitivity and 100% specificity in identifying infected prostheses. These results suggest that performing gallium imaging in addition to bone scintigraphy greatly enhances the accuracy of the radionuclide diagnosis of the infected joint replacement.

Gallium accumulates in both septic and aseptic inflammation, as well as in the bone marrow, and in areas of increased bone mineral turnover in the absence of infection. In an effort to improve the accuracy of both bone and gallium imaging, the two studies are often interpreted together, according to standardized criteria (Table 3).

Test result	Bone /Gallium Finidngs
Positive	a. Distribution of the 2 tracers is spatially incongruent b. Distribution is spatially incongruent with intensity of gallium uptake is greater than diphosphonate
Negative	a. Gallium images are normal b. Distribution of tracers is spatially incongruent with intensity of gallium uptake is lesser than diphosphonate
Equivocal	a. Distribution of the 2 radiotracers is congruent, both spatially and in terms of intensity

Table 3. Interpretation of combined bone / gallium imaging in the diagnosis of infection

However, many studies have reported less satisfactory results with combined bone gallium imaging. Overall, combined bone/gallium imaging, with an accuracy of about 65-80%, offers only a modest improvement over bone scintigraphy alone.

5.3 Labelled leukocyte imaging and leukocyte / bone imaging

Theoretically, labeled leukocyte imaging should be well suited for diagnosing the infected joint replacement because white cells usually do not accumulate at sites of increased bone mineral turnover in the absence of infection. However, its efficacy in infected prostheses has been disappointing. Poor sensitivity of labeled leukocyte imaging for diagnosing prosthetic joint infection has been attributed to the chronic nature of the process. Combining leukocyte imaging with bone imaging has been shown to increase the specificity of the study marginally (Fig.2).

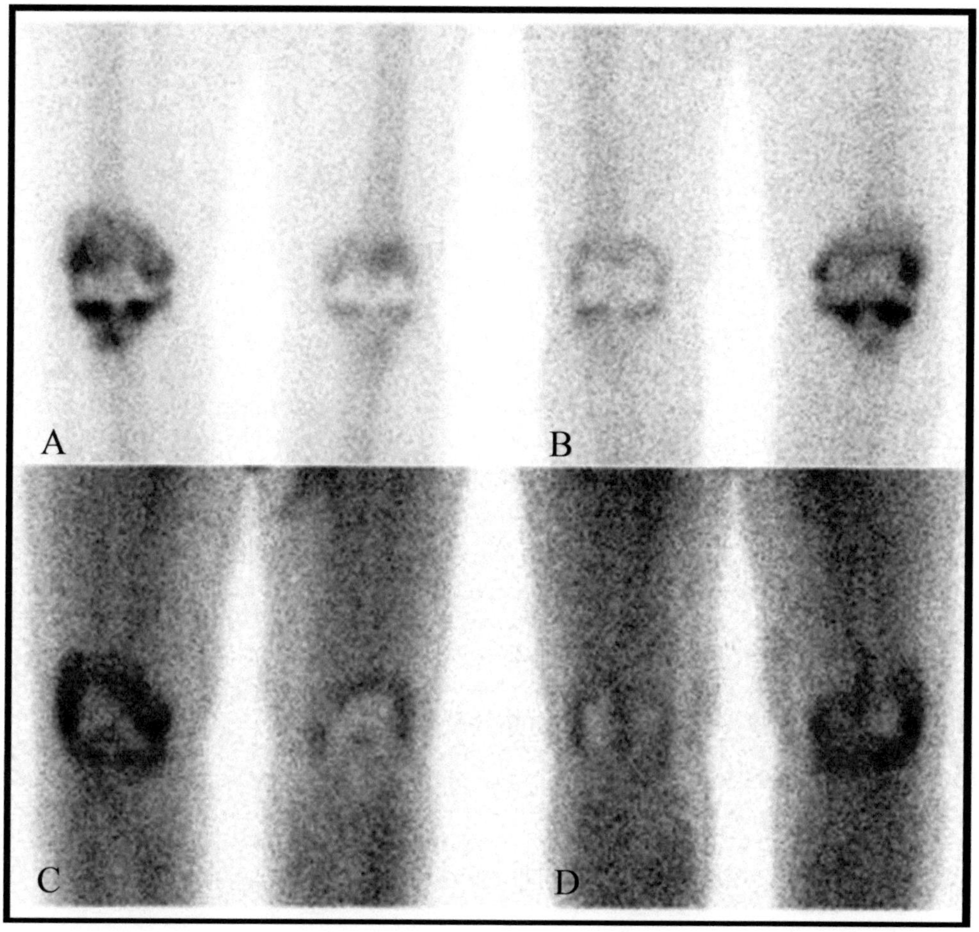

Fig. 2. Bone scintigraphic images of the knees in the anterior (A) and posterior (B) views showing increased tracer accumulation around the right knee joint. On labeled leukocyte imaging intense leukocyte accumulation around the right knee is noted in the anterior (C) and posterior (D) static images. Surgery confirmed infection around the knee prosthesis.

5.4 Leukocyte / bone marrow imaging

Labeled leukocyte and bone marrow images both reflect radiotracer accumulation in the reticuloendothelial cells, or fixed macrophages of the marrow. The distribution of bone marrow activity is similar on leukocyte and bone marrow images in normal individuals as well as in those with underlying marrow abnormalities, i.e, the images are spatially congruent. However, in osteomyelitis there is spatially incongruent uptake i.e. accumulation of leukocytes with a cold spot in bone marrow imaging.

The quoted sensitivity, specificity, and accuracy of leukocyte/ marrow imaging were 96%, 87%, and 91%, respectively. The test was significantly more accurate than bone (50%), bone/gallium (66%), and leukocyte/bone imaging (70%) in their population. These results confirm the sensitivity and specificity of leukocyte/marrow imaging for diagnosing prosthetic joint infection as well as its superiority over other radionuclide tests (Fig.3). However, meticulous labeling of blood, handling of blood products, potential for spread of infection and prolonged imaging are the main disadvantages in this technique.

5.5 FDG PET imaging

Positron emission tomography has the inherent advantages of high sensitivity, high resolution and ability to acquire tomographic images. The procedure is simple, rapid and requires no handling of blood products. Zhuang and coworkers [18] evaluated FDG-PET in 74 joint prostheses, 21 of which were infected. Studies were considered positive for infection when an area of increased uptake was identified at the bone prosthesis interface. They reported a sensitivity, specificity, and accuracy of 90%, 89.3%, and 89.5%, respectively, for prosthetic hip infection, and sensitivity, specificity, and accuracy of 90.9%, 72%, and 77.8%, respectively, for prosthetic knee infection. Though, the FDG PET/CT patterns for infected elbow prostheses have not been reported, pattern of aseptic loosening has been described [19].

5.6 Labeled antibiotics

Ciprofloxacin, a broad spectrum antibiotic was labeled with 99m- Technetium. It was hypothesized that this tracer will be concentrated only in the sites of infection and thus may be useful in differentiating sterile inflammation and infection (Fig.4). However, further studies have shown that localization is primarily due to tracer extravasation and stasis at the sites of increased vascular permeability. The tracer is rapidly cleared from circulation by the kidneys and shows no uptake in the bone marrow. Minimal localization is noted in the liver. Several studies have shown the ease of usage and good sensitivity of labeled ciprofloxacin in detection of osteomyelitis [20-23] . Recently, radiolabeled –third generation cephalosporin (Ceftriaxone) has been shown (Fig.5) to have improved sensitivity and specificity for the accurate diagnosis of active bacterial bony infections [24]. Labeled antibiotics can be used both in acute as well as chronic infections and it has also been tried in diabetic foot infections (Fig.6).

6. Imaging acute osteomyelitis

6.1 Imaging diabetic foot infections

Diabetic foot infections are one of the major causes of morbidity in diabetics. Imaging of diabetic foot infection poses several challenges. Infectious and non-infectious conditions affecting the foot of a diabetic often present clinically in a similar way. The conventional imaging techniques often are unable to ascertain the cause of the problem. Nuclear medicine techniques are of immense utility in differentiating and monitoring the different pathologies affecting the foot of a diabetic.

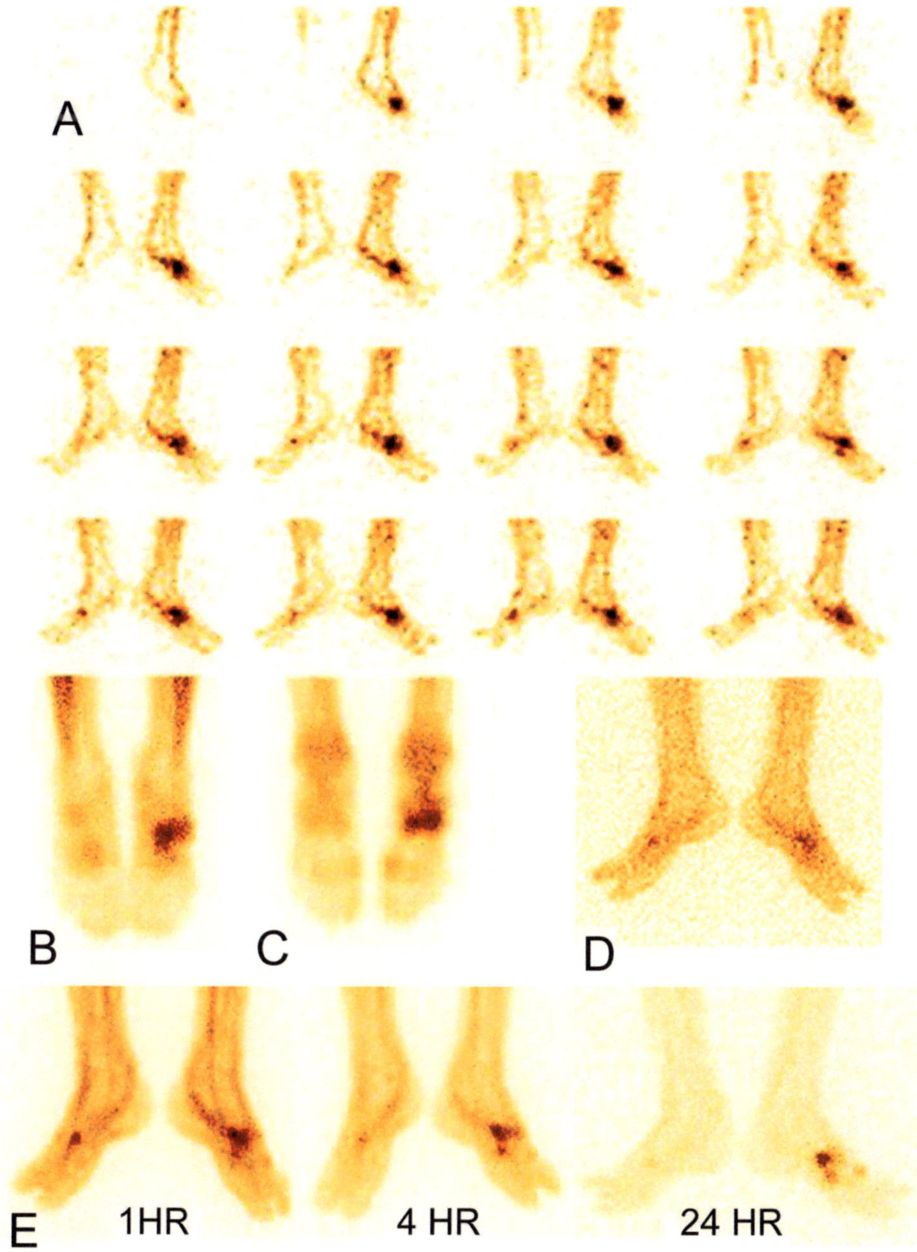

Fig. 3. Three phase bone scintigraphy of the feet with 99mTc-MDP showing increased flow (A) and soft tissue concentration (B) of tracer in the mid part of the left foot. The delayed images (C) at 3h shows focally increased bony uptake of tracer in the mid-tarsal region, indicating active bony infection. 99mTc-HMPAO labeled leukocyte images (E) at 1, 4, 24-h show focal tracer concentration in the mid-tarsal region of the left foot indicative of active infection. Bone marrow scan (D) performed 1-h after injection of 4.0 mCi of filtered 99mTc-Sulfo-colloid shows mild uptake in the mid-tarsal region less than 99mTc-MDP and labeled leukocyte uptake.

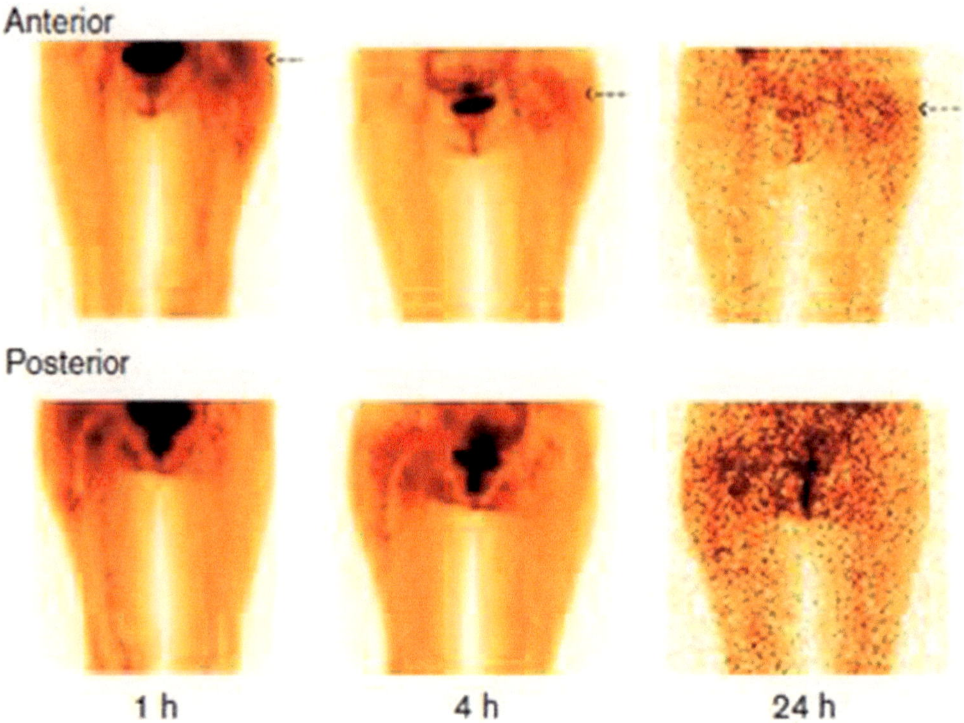

Fig. 4. 99mTc-Ciprofloxacin (Diagnobact™) scan (static anterior and posterior images) acquired at 1, 4 & 24h indicating increased radiotracer concentration in the region of left hip joint prosthetic (arrows)

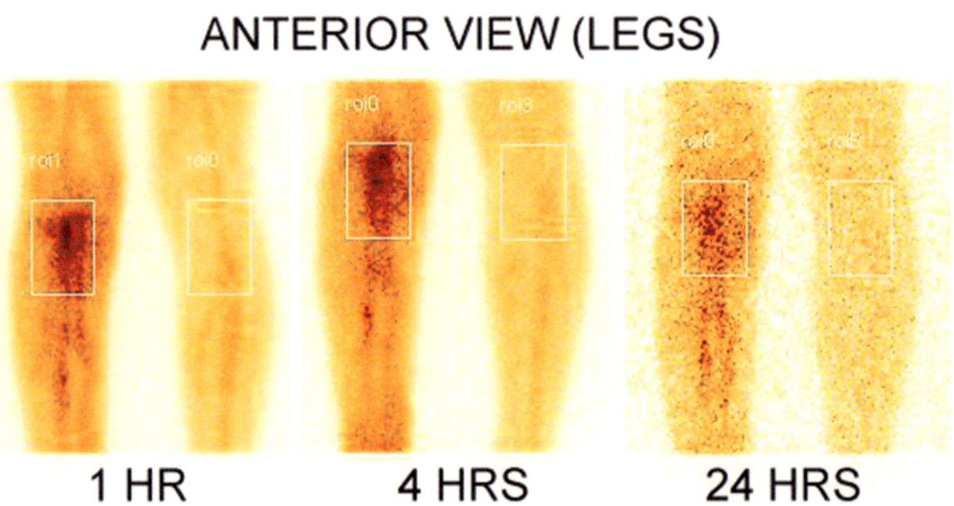

Fig. 5. 99mTc-Ceftriaxone (Scintibact) images of the legs showing focally increased concentration of the radiotracer in the proximal part of the right tibia. The radiotracer concentration remained consistent till 24-h of imaging time indicating active tibial infection

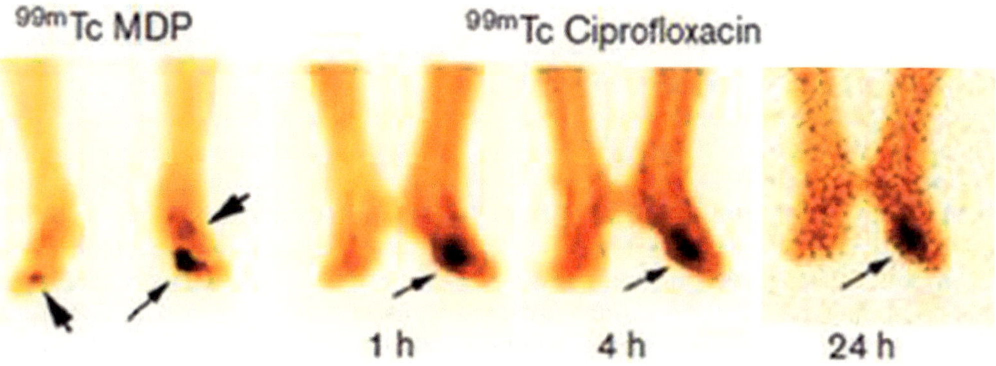

Fig. 6. 99mTc-MDP bone scan in the diabetic foot showing two foci of abnormal tracer uptake in the left foot and one focus in the right foot with 99mTc-ciprofloxacin scan indicating only one focus of increased tracer concentration in the left foot (arrow) at 1, 4 & 24h.

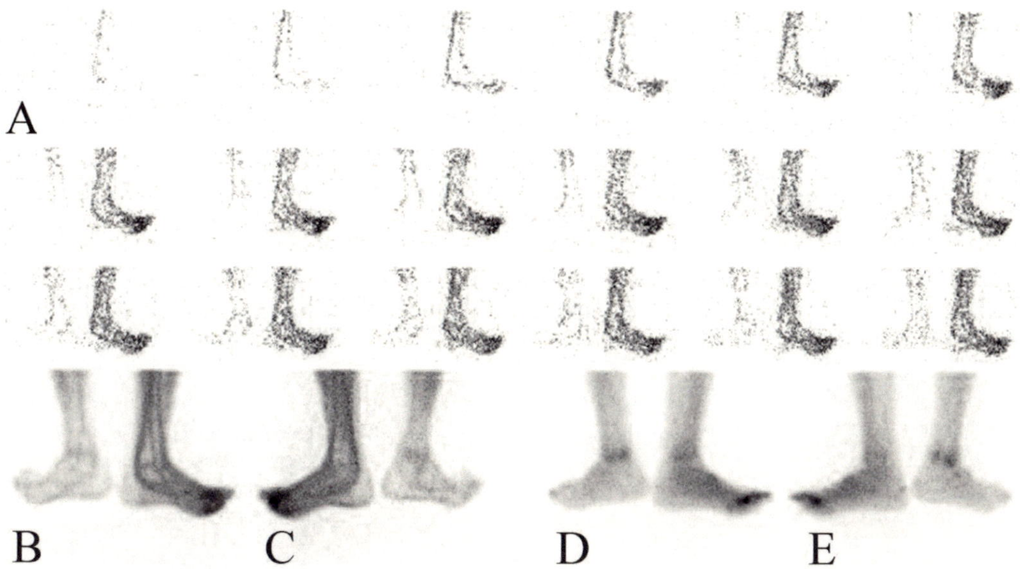

Fig. 7. Three phase bone scintigraphy in a diabetic patient with an ulcer in the left foot showing increased flow of tracer in the perfusion phase (A) images. Blood pool images in the medial (B) and lateral (C) and bone phase images in the medial (D) and lateral (E) views also show increased soft tissue pooling and increased tracer uptake in the fore foot region indicating active infection. SPECT CT (not shown here) localized the tracer uptake in the head of 2nd metatarsal.

Up to 25% of diabetic patients are at risk of developing pedal ulcers. Diagnosis of osteomyelitis is often overlooked in diabetic patients because of the lack of pain and systemic inflammatory response. Bone scintigraphy has low specificity in diabetic patients. The sensitivity may reach up to 100%. Low specificity is due to conditions that mimic osteomyelitis i.e. trauma, fracture and neuropathic joints (Fig.7). An attempt to increase the specificity of bone scintigraphy is the fourth phase bone scan. This is based on the fact that tracer accumulation in woven or immature bone continues for several hours leading to an increase in the lesion to background ratio in the fourth phase than the third phase bone scan. However, woven bone is also present in fractures and degenerative changes apart from osteomyelitis. Labeled leukocyte imaging is one of the most sensitive and specific investigation for diabetic foot infections [25-27]. The results are read in conjunction with the findings of the bone scintigraphy findings. One of the main disadvantages of labeled leukocytes imaging in diabetic patients is the co-existence of neuropathic joints. Labeled leukocytes accumulate both in infected and uninfected neuropathic joints. This is due to the presence of hematopoietically active bone marrow in neuropathic joints. Combining with bone marrow imaging helps in distinguishing infected from non-infected neuropathic joints. Addition of SPECT/CT helps in differentiating soft tissue from bone infection, though the lower resolution of SPECT images makes this difficult in the foot. FDG PET/CT is also being tried in diabetic foot. Some studies have shown the ability of PET to differentiate between infected and neuropathic joints using SUV values.

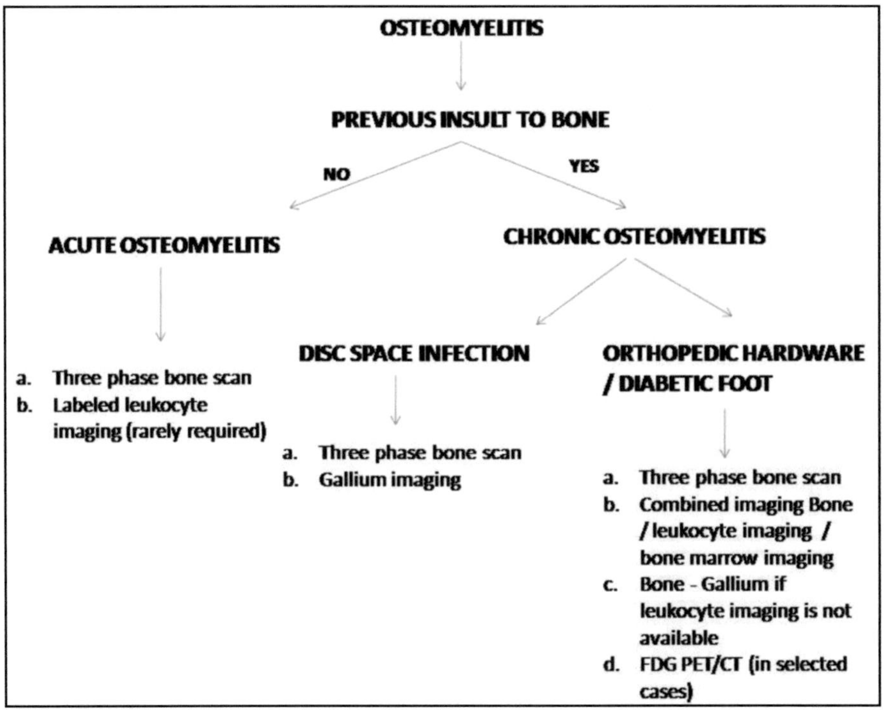

Table 4.

7. Conclusion

Diagnosis of osteomyelitis can be made clinical in a majority of patients without previous insult to the bone. However, with history of previous insult like fracture, surgery or previous infection, the diagnosis becomes more and more difficult. Conventional imaging modalities often fail in these patients. Nuclear medicine techniques owing to the functional information provided, is ideally suited for these patients. A variety of nuclear medicine and PET techniques are available for evaluation of these patients. Each of the nuclear medicine modalities has their own strengths and weaknesses. The decision to subject the patient to a particular nuclear medicine technique is to be taken on a case by case basis and is illustrated as a Flow chart (table 4).

Nuclear medicine techniques add a new dimension to the diagnosis of osteomyelitis. They are also extremely effective monitoring tools. With the advent of fusion imaging such as SPECT/CT and PET/CT, the combined morphologic and functional information available has made significant impact in the effectiveness of nuclear medicine investigations.

8. References

[1] Ranklin JA: Biologic mediators of acute inflammation. Clin Issues 2004; 15: 3-17.
[2] Stumpe KD, Strobel K. Osteomyelitis and arthritis. Semin Nucl Med. 2009;39:27-35.
[3] Goldsmith SJ, Vallabhajosula S. Clinically proven radiopharmaceuticals for infection imaging: mechanisms and applications. Semin Nucl Med. 2009;39:2-10.
[4] Gemmel F, Dumarey N, Welling M. Future diagnostic agents. Semin Nucl Med. 2009;39:11-26.
[5] Aigner RM, Fueger GF, Ritter G. Results of three-phase bone scintigraphy and radiography in 20 cases of neonatal osteomyelitis. Nucl Med Commun. 1996;17:20-8.
[6] Termaat MF, Raijmakers PG, Scholten HJ, Bakker FC, Patka P, Haarman HJ. The accuracy of diagnostic imaging for the assessment of chronic osteomyelitis: a systematic review and meta-analysis. J Bone Joint Surg Am. 2005;87:2464-71.
[7] Stumpe KD, Zanetti M, Weishaupt D, Hodler J, Boos N, Von Schulthess GK. FDG positron emission tomography for differentiation of degenerative and infectious endplate abnormalities in the lumbar spine detected on MR imaging. AJR Am J Roentgenol. 2002;179:1151-7.
[8] Kurtz S, Ong K, Lau E, Mowat F, Halpern M. Projections of primary and revision hip and knee arthroplasty in the United States from 2005 to 2030. J Bone Joint Surg Am. 2007;89:780-5.
[9] Ostlere S, Soin S. Imaging of prosthetic joints. Imaging 2003:15:270-85
[10] Love C, Tomas MB, Marwin SE, Pugliese PV, Palestro CJ. Role of nuclear medicine in diagnosis of the infected joint replacement. Radiographics. 2001;21:1229-38.
[11] Pandey R, Drakoulakis E, Athanasou NA. An assessment of the histological criteria used to diagnose infection in hip revision arthroplasty tissues. J Clin Pathol. 1999;52:118-23.
[12] Hanssen AD, Rand JA. Evaluation and treatment of infection at the site of a total hip or knee arthroplasty. Instr Course Lect. 1999;48:111-22.
[13] Palestro CJ, Love C, Miller TT. Infection and musculoskeletal conditions: Imaging of musculoskeletal infections. Best Pract Res Clin Rheumatol. 2006;20:1197-218.
[14] Magnuson JE, Brown ML, Hauser MF, Berquist TH, Fitzgerald RH Jr, Klee GG. In-111-labeled leukocyte scintigraphy in suspected orthopedic prosthesis infection: comparison with other imaging modalities. Radiology. 1988;168:235-9.
[15] Weiss PE, Mall JC, Hoffer PB, Murray WR, Rodrigo JJ, Genant HK. 99mTc-methylene diphosphonate bone imaging in the evaluation of total hip prostheses. Radiology. 1979;133:727-9.

[16] Williamson BR, McLaughlin RE, Wang GW, Miller CW, Teates CD, Bray ST. Radionuclide bone imaging as a means of differentiating loosening and infection in patients with a painful total hip prosthesis. Radiology. 1979;133:723-5.

[17] Reing CM, Richin PF, Kenmore PI. Differential bone-scanning in the evaluation of a painful total joint replacement. J Bone Joint Surg Am. 1979;61:933-6.

[18] Zhuang H, Duarte PS, Pourdehnad M, Maes A, Van Acker F, Shnier D et al. The promising role of 18F-FDG PET in detecting infected lower limb prosthesis implants. J Nucl Med. 2001;42:44-8.

[19] Balasubramanian Harisankar Natrajan C, Mittal BR, Bhattacharya A, Parmar M, Singh B. Interesting image. Aseptic loosening of elbow prostheses diagnosed on F-18 FDG PET/CT. Clin Nucl Med. 2010;35:886-7.

[20] Singh B, Sunil HV, Sharma S, Prasad V, Kashyap R, Bhattacharya A et al. Efficacy of indigenously developed single vial kit preparation of 99mTc-ciprofloxacin in the detection of bacterial infection: an Indian experience. Nucl Med Commun. 2008;29:1123-9

[21] Singh B, Prasad V, Bhattacharya A, Singh AK, Bhatnagar A, Mittal BR et al. Diagnosis of mandibular osteomyelitis in probable coexisting tumor recurrence: role of Tc-99m ciprofloxacin imaging. Clin Nucl Med. 2008;33:525-7.

[22] Dutta P, Bhansali A, Mittal BR, Singh B, Masoodi SR. Instant 99mTc-ciprofloxacin scintigraphy for the diagnosis of osteomyelitis in the diabetic foot. Foot Ankle Int. 2006;27:716-22.

[23] Singh B, Mittal BR, Bhattacharya A, Aggarwal A, Nagi ON, Singh AK. Technetium-99m ciprofloxacin imaging in the diagnosis of postsurgical bony infection and evaluation of the response to antibiotic therapy: A case report. J Orthop Surg (Hong Kong). 2005;13:190-4.

[24] Singh B, Babbar A, Sharma Sarika, Kaur A, Bhattacharya, A, Mittal BR, Mishra A, Tripathi RP. To evaluate the clinical efficacy of a single vial kit preparation of 99mTc-ceftriaxone (Scintibact) for the diagnosis of orthopedic infections –First results. J Nucl Med , 2010 ; 51 (S 2): 373.

[25] Devillers A, Moisan A, Hennion F, Garin E, Poirier JY, Bourguet P.: Contribution of technetium- 99m hexamethylpropylene amine oxime labeled leucocyte scintigraphy to the diagnosis of diabetic foot infection. Eur J Nucl Med: 1998; 25:132-138

[26] Harvey J, Cohen MM: Technetium-99-labeled leukocytes in diagnosing diabetic osteomyelitis in the foot. J Foot Ankle Surg: 1997;36:209-14.

[27] Poirier JY, Garin E, Derrien C, Devillers A, Moisan A, Bourguet P et al: Diagnosis of osteomyelitis in the diabetic foot with 99mTc-HMPAO leukocyte scintigraphy combined with a 99mTc-MDP bone scintigraphy. Diabetes Metab: 2002; 28:485-90

3

Skull Osteomyelitis

Myoung Soo Kim
Department of Neurosurgery, Seoul Paik Hospital,
Inje University College of Medicine
Republic of Korea

1. Introduction

Osteomyelitis is an inflammatory process accompanied by bone destruction and caused by an infecting microorganism. The decline of fulminant osteomyelitis of the skull from a routine event to a rare occurrence has largely paralleled the emergence of potent antibiotics. Today, osteomyelitis of the skull usually presents as a chronic process that occasionally complicates craniotomies and scalp injuries. Despite the relative infrequency of this entity, it is essential that the well-trained neurosurgeon be skilled in the recognition and treatment of this potentially dangerous condition.

In this review we describe the history of skull osteomyelitis and development of preventive methods against skull osteomyelitis after trephination. We also review postoperative skull osteomyelitis and its prevention. We discuss skull osteomyelitis associated with special conditions (skull base, fungal, pediatric, syphilitic, tuberculous osteomyelitis, and skull osteomyelitis associated with immunodeficiency virus infection (HIV)).

2. Skull osteomyelitis

2.1 History of skull osteomyelitis

2.1.1 Skull osteomyelitis in the prehistoric period

Trephination was performed in many parts of the ancient world and remains in use today in some traditional communities. Authors of comparative osteologic studies (Liu & Apuzzo, 2003) have demonstrated that using primitive stone or metal instruments, prehistoric surgeons achieved an average survival rate of 50%–90% in patients undergoing skull trephination. Interestingly, some of these primitive surgeons covered the trephined opening with discs cut from shells or sometimes with thin gold plates (Froeschner, 1992). Although the exact incidence of infection after trephination is not known, some skulls showed infection and various stages of healing (Froeschner, 1992). The rate of infection for trephination, as represented by skeletal inflammatory reactions, was only 15%. As an example, severe periostitis after the trephination resulted in the death of individuals (Gerstzen et al., 1998).

Trauma related to conflict is evident in many prehistoric cultures. In human skulls recovered from archaeological excavations, several cases of traumatic skull injury were found. One report described a man having survived an arrow injury to his forehead.

However, he subsequently developed severe osteomyelitis, probably resulting in a generalized fatal infection (Gerstzen et al., 1998). Some skulls also showed evidence of osteomyelitis.

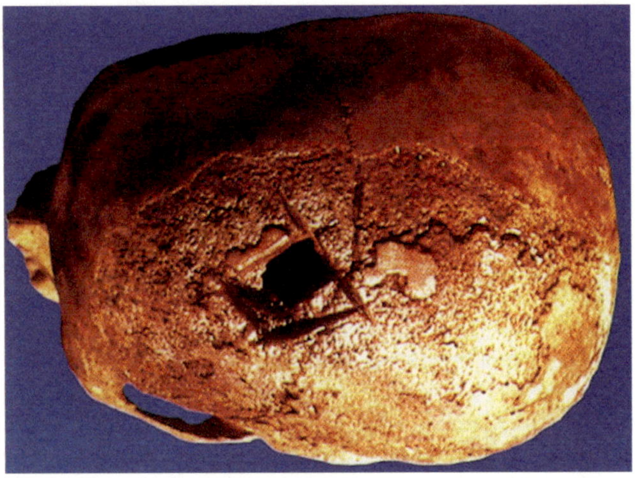

Fig. 1. A crosscut opening was made in the parietal bone of this trephined skull after a fracture. A subsequent infection resulted in severe periostitis. (Reproduced with permission from Gerszten, PC., Gerszten, E., & Allison, MJ. (1998). Diseases of the skull in pre-Columbian South American mummies. *Neurosurgery,* Vol.42, No.5, (May 1998), pp. 1145-1152, ISSN 0148-396X) (Gerszten et al., 1998)

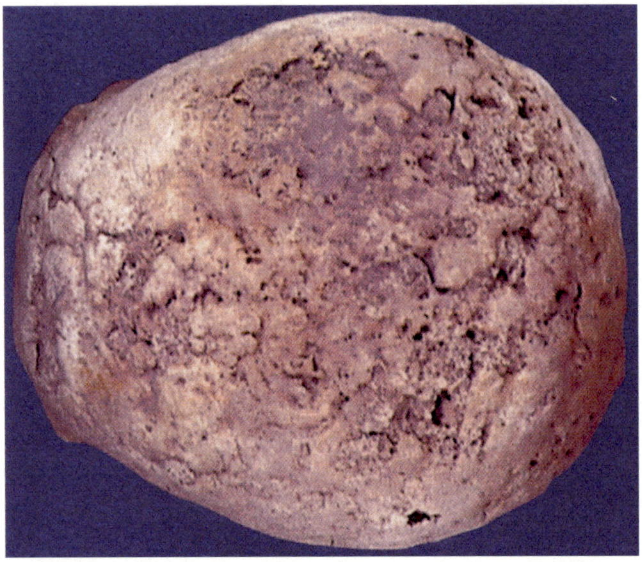

Fig. 2. *Treponema peritonitis* and osteitis of the calvaria in a man of the Atacameña (AD 300). He was also found to have "saber shins". (Reproduced with permission from Gerszten, PC., Gerszten, E., & Allison, MJ. (1998). Diseases of the skull in pre-Columbian South American mummies. *Neurosurgery,* Vol.42, No.5, (May 1998), pp. 1145-1152, ISSN 0148-396X) (Gerszten et al., 1998).

Bone lesions resembling tertiary syphilis caused by *Treponema pallidum* or another of the *treponematoses* have been observed in nearly every Andean culture from Peru and Chile, dating back nearly 8000 years (Gerstzen et al., 1998).

The lesions are similar in each case, with periostitis, osteitis, and osteomyelitis attacking the skull and the long bone, particularly the tibia. This tibial involvement results in the classic "saber shin". Several of the skulls observed with such lesions had been "treated" during life by repeated trephination using a scraping technique.

2.1.2 Greek and early Byzantine period

The intellectual evolution of neurological surgery originated in the golden age of Greece with the founding of the Alexandrian school in 300 BC. Because of both sporting injuries, in particular gladiator injuries, and wars, head injuries appear to have been plentiful, and provided opportunities to develop neurosurgical skills (Goodrich & Flamm, 2011). In this early era of medicine, the risk of infection, lack of antiseptic technique, and minimal anesthesia prevented generations of surgeons from performing any serious or aggressive surgical intervention for head injury (Goodrich & Flamm, 2011).

Galen of Pergamon (AD 129–200) detailed a safer and more reliable use of the trephine, and in particular argued for continuous irrigation during trephination to avoid delivering excessive heat and injury to the underlying brain (Goodrich, 2005).

Paul of Aegina (AD 625–690), trained in the Alexandrian school, was the last great Byzantine physician. His wound management was quite sophisticated for prevention of infection. He used wine (helpful in antisepsis, although this concept was then unknown) (Goodrich, 2005).

2.1.3 Medieval Europe

Inventive medieval surgeon Theodoric Borgognoni of Cervia (1205–1298) is remembered as a pioneer in the use of the aseptic technique—not the "clean" aseptic technique of today, but rather a method based on avoidance of "laudable pus". He attempted to discover the ideal conditions for good wound healing, and concluded that they comprised control of bleeding, removal of contaminated or necrotic material, avoidance of dead space, and careful application of a wound dressing bathed in wine (Goodrich & Flamm, 2011). Control of bleeding, removal of contaminated or necrotic material, and avoidance of dead space are principles that can also apply in today's neurosurgical operations. He also argued for primary closure of all wounds when possible and avoiding "laudable pus" (Goodrich & Flamm, 2011).

Lanfranchi of Milan (1250–1306) noted that the head should be shaved prior to surgery to prevent hair from getting into the wound and interfering with primary healing. Today, most neurosurgeons also shave hair before an operation. However, the time of shaving is currently controversial. When dealing with depressed skull fractures, Lanfranchi advocated putting wine into the depression to assist healing (Goodrich & Flamm, 2011).

Guy de Chauliac (1300–1368) was clearly the most influential European surgeon of the 14th and 15th centuries. Chauliac also provided an interesting discussion of techniques that he devised for the treatment of head injuries. Before beginning surgery, he advocated shaving the head, stating that shaving of the hair would prevent it from getting into the wound and interfering with primary healing. For depressed skull fractures, Chauliac preferred to put wine-soaked cloth into the injured site to assist healing (Goodrich & Flamm, 2011).

Leonard of Bertapalia (1380?–1460) was a prominent figure in 15th century surgery. He recommended always avoiding materials that might cause pus (Goodrich, 2005).

However, in the medieval period, the combination of a lack of anatomic knowledge and poor surgical outcomes naturally led physicians to recommend against operating on the brain, except in simple cases (Goodrich, 2005).

2.1.4 Sixteenth century

Ambroise Paré (1510–1590) is considered to be the father of modern surgery. Although not original to Paré, he advanced an interesting technique of elevating a depressed skull fracture using the Valsalva maneuver. This maneuver enabled the expulsion of blood and pus. He advocated debridement of wounds for good healing, emphasizing that all foreign bodies must be removed. He was skilled at removing osteomyelitis bone, incising dura, and evacuating blood clots and pus (Goodrich & Flamm, 2011). Paré's most useful advance in surgery was the discovery that boiling oil should not be used in gunshot wounds (Goodrich, 2005).

2.1.5 Eighteenth century

Percival Pott (1714–1788) was the greatest English surgeon of the 18th century. He described an osteomyelitic condition of the skull with a collection of pus under the pericranium, now called Pott's puffy tumor. In 1760, Pott described the almost constant relationship between the acute forehead swelling of frontal osteomyelitis and an underlying extradural abscess (Paramore, 1996). He felt strongly that these lesions should be trephined to remove the pus and decompress the brain. Although the frequency of Pott's puffy tumor has decreased since the introduction of antibiotics, it should be treated using the same principles.

Until early in the 19th century, surgery for pyogenic infections of the brain had an extremely high mortality rate, and was often performed by pure chance after cases of trauma. The first documented case of a successful operation was performed by François-Sauveur Morand (1697–1773) in 1752 (Guyot et al., 2006). Morand had a patient who developed otitis and subsequently mastoiditis with a temporal abscess. He trephined over the carious bone and discovered pus. Drainage of pus after two operations resulted in healing of the abscess and survival of the patient.

Benjamin Bell (1749–1806) stressed the importance of relieving compression of the brain, whether it be caused by a depressed skull fracture or pressure caused by pus or blood—a remarkably aggressive approach for this period (Goodrich, 2005). However, Lorenz Heister (1683–1758) felt that trephination in wounds involving only concussion and contusion might be too dangerous (Goodrich, 2005).

2.1.6 Nineteenth and twentieth centuries

Even with the best surgical technique, the patient might well die postoperatively of suppuration and infection. Fever, purulent material, brain abscess, and draining wounds all defeated the best surgeons. Surgery was revolutionized when, using concepts developed by

Louis Pasteur, Joseph Lister introduced antisepsis into the operating room. For the first time, a surgeon, using aseptic techniques and a clean operating theater, could operate on the brain with a reasonably small likelihood of infection (Goodrich, 2005). Certainly, the development of the technique of antiseptic surgery by Lister, which stressed the treatment of the surgeon's hands with 1:20 carbolic acid, was a major advance (Leedom & Holtom, 1993).

William Macewen (1848–1924) had operated on 21 neurosurgical cases with only three deaths and 18 successful recoveries, and considered his success to be the result of excellent cerebral localization and good aseptic technique (Goodrich, 2005).

Fedor Krause (1857–1937), like William Macewen, was a major advocate of aseptic techniques in neurosurgery (Goodrich, 2005).

William W. Keen (1837–1932), professor of surgery at Jefferson Medical College in Philadelphia, was one of the strongest American advocates for the use of Listerian techniques in surgery, advancing the concepts of surgical bacteriology, asepsis, and antisepsis. A description of Keen's surgical setup provides a contemporary view of this innovative surgeon's approach to antisepsis (Goodrich, 2005).

In 1929, Alexander Fleming (1881–1955) published a report on the first observation of a substance that appeared to block the growth of a bacterium. This substance, identified as penicillin, heralded a new era of medicine and surgery. During World War II, the use of antibiotics in the treatment of bacterial infection was perfected, reducing even further the risk of infection during craniotomy (Goodrich, 2005).

2.2 Postoperative skull osteomyelitis

2.2.1 Risk factors for postoperative skull osteomyelitis

The frequency of surgical site infections (SSIs) in a clean neurosurgical operation in randomized controlled trials is from 4.0% to 12.0% without prophylactic antibiotics and from 0.3% to 3.0% with prophylactic antibiotics (Erman, 2005).

Specific risk factors associated with postoperative skull osteomyelitis have not been reported. A variety of risk factors for SSIs in neurosurgery have been reported. SSIs may involve any or all surgical layers from the surface to deeper tissues causing superficial cellulitis, bone-flap osteomyelitis, meningitis, encephalitis, and brain abscesses (Vogelsang et al., 1998). Mollman and Haines (Mollman & Haines, 1986) reported that the presence of a cerebrospinal fluid (CSF) leak and a concurrent non-central nervous system infection increased the estimated relative risk of infection to 13:1 and to 6:1, and use of perioperative antibiotics decreased the risk of infection to approximately 20% of control levels. Korinek (Korinek, 1997) reported the presence of a CSF leak, emergency surgery, clean-contaminated and dirty surgery, an operative time longer than 4 hours, and recent neurosurgery as independent predictive risk factors for SSIs. Other retrospective studies reported that obesity, surgical reexploration, steroid administration, and increased hospital stay for patients with infection have no relation to SSIs.

2.2.2 Clinical manifestations and diagnosis of postoperative skull osteomyelitis

Early diagnosis of skull osteomyelitis is very important in its treatment. However, early diagnosis is difficult. Postoperative osteomyelitis presents with findings referable to the site of the wound. A bone infection may cause high fever and marked local reaction and suppuration, or it may appear as a stubborn fistula.

Since progression of the disease is relatively slow and the presenting symptoms are initially subtle, the diagnosis is often made after considerable advance of the disease, which occasionally makes treatment difficult. The diagnosis of skull osteomyelitis is based primarily on the clinical findings, with data from the initial history, physical examination, and laboratory tests.

Despite the immense improvements that have taken place in medicine, we still use the same basic methods to identify infections. Blood leukocyte count and erythrocyte sedimentation rate (ESR) are methods still in use. An elevated ESR provides a useful marker to monitor the efficacy of therapy using serial determinations. C-reactive protein (CRP) is a useful indication of infection. Like ESR, it is nonspecific; its advantage is that CRP levels rise and fall rapidly after surgery, thus making it a good indicator of acute infections, recovery, and relapse (Blomstedt, 1992). Operations cause a detectable rise in CRP levels within 6 hours. The level peaks after 2 days and then falls rapidly. Daily CRP tests for all patients with an elevated temperature are recommended; a secondary increase indicates infection (van Lente, 1982). Blood cultures are obtained before initiating therapy. Bacterial culturing remains the most important method. Aspiration of the incision and bone biopsy provide the definitive diagnostic tests. Histopathological and microbiological examination of bone is the criterion standard for diagnosing osteomyelitis.

Radiographic diagnosis of osteomyelitis can be particularly difficult when there is concurrent bone destruction or repair because of a noninfectious process. Plain radiographs lack both the sensitivity and the specificity to establish a diagnosis of osteomyelitis (Tumeh et al., 1987).

Computed tomography (CT) is the best imaging modality for demonstrating bony erosion and destruction in osteomyelitis. It depicts detailed pathological changes, including focal osteopenia, subtle erosion of inner and outer tables, and gross lytic destruction. However, if bone has been altered by trauma, surgery, or infection, CT abnormalities are no longer diagnostic of active osteomyelitis. Furthermore, neither skull X-ray nor CT scan are useful for monitoring the response of osteomyelitis to therapy, because it takes several months to years for skull X-ray nor CT scan to appear normal after successful treatment (Rubin et al., 1990; Mendelson et al., 1983)

Bone scintigraphy using technetium technetium 99 and gallium citrate scans, and positron emission tomography have also been used for diagnosis, with great accuracy. These modalities can also be used to evaluate a patient's therapeutic response (Koorbusch et al., 1992). In a three-phase bone scan, initial hyperemia represents increased blood flow because of inflammation, while delayed bone images demonstrate increased radiotracer concentration. Photopenic or cold patterns may also be seen in acute hematogenous osteomyelitis. The specificity of bone scintigraphy is not sufficiently high to confirm a diagnosis of osteomyelitis in many clinical situations. On a bone scan, osteomyelitis is often not distinguished from soft tissue infections and postsurgical changes. Compared with bone scintigraphy, magnetic resonance imaging (MRI) has equivalent or greater sensitivity, specificity, and accuracy for the detection of osteomyelitis. However, MRI is usually not useful in monitoring the response to therapy in patients with osteomyelitis, because marrow changes caused by inflammation take 2–6 months to return to normal (Gherini et al., 1986). Gallium-67-labeled and ^{111}In-labeled white blood cell scans are fairly sensitive, albeit nonspecific, tests whose use appears to be helpful during the follow-up period. Single photon emission CT improves the monitoring of therapy.

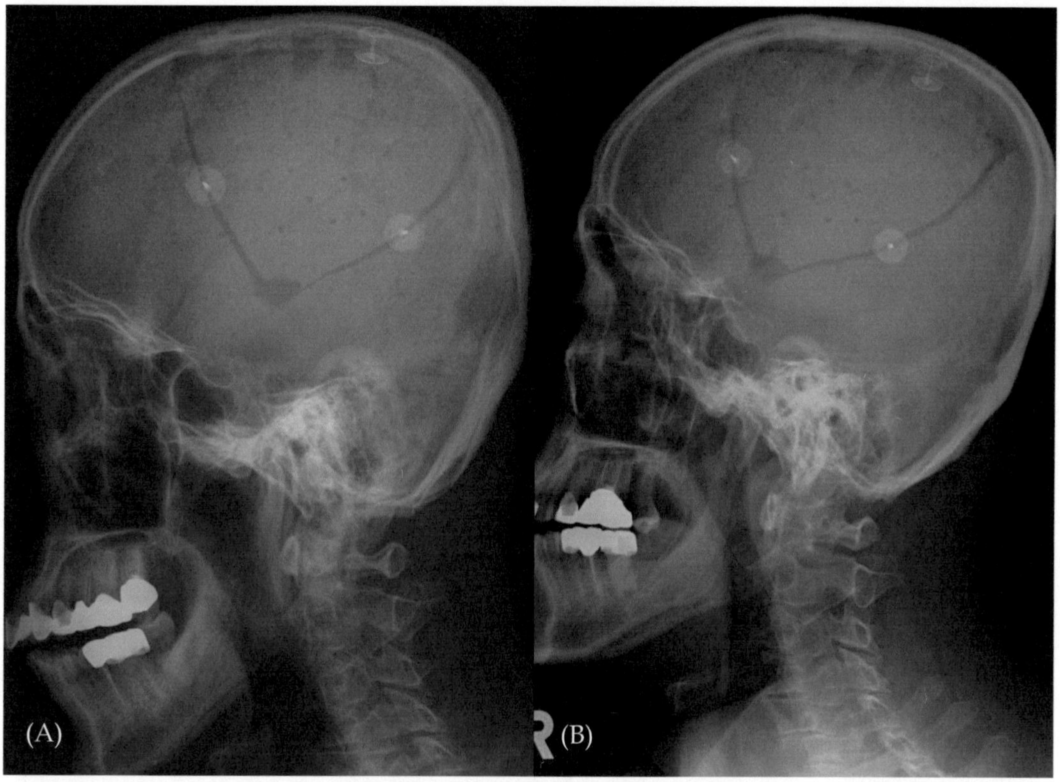

Fig. 3. Simple skull X-ray images taken 20 days (A) and 66 days (B) after a craniotomy showing the progression of an osteolytic lesion in the upper portion of the bone flap and in the adjacent surrounding bone. *Staphylococcus epidermidis* was cultured from blood. (Reproduced with permission from Nam, JR., Kim, MS., Lee, CH., & Whang, DH. (2008). Linezolid Treatment for Osteomyelitis due to Staphylococcus Epidermidis with Reduced Vancomycin Susceptibility. *J Korean Neurosurg Soc*, Vol.43, No.6, (June 2008), pp. 307-310, ISSN 2005-3711) (Nam et al., 2008)

2.2.3 Treatment

The treatment of cranial osteomyelitis is often surgical debridement, removal of infected bone flaps, and 4–6 weeks of parenteral antibiotics. In addition, in cases arising from the sinuses or an auditory canal, surgical debridement needs to be conducted by an otologist.

Empirical therapy should be started with antibiotics broadly effective for *Escherichia coli* and *Staphylococcus aureus (S. aureus)*. The antibiotics should be changed appropriately once the culture sensitivity reports are available. In advanced cases where the underlying bone is grossly eroded, a partial craniectomy may be required.

Chou and Erickson (Chou & Erickson, 1976) introduced a treatment with closed suction irrigation with topical antibiotics; this treatment, they claimed, may save 50% of infected bone flaps.

2.2.4 New treatments for postoperative skull osteomyelitis with a high risk factor

2.2.4.1 Hyperbaric oxygen (HBO) therapy

HBO therapy is used to treat a variety of infected, hypoperfused, and hypoxic wounds. Oxygen tension plays an important role in the outcome of infection (Park et al., 1992). Leukocyte bactericidal capacity is substantially impaired at low oxygen tensions often observed in wounds (Allen et al., 1997). HBO therapy increases the oxygen tension in infected tissues, including bone (Mader et al., 1980), resulting in a direct bactericidal effect of HBO treatment on aerobic organisms such as *S. aureus* (Korinek, 1997). HBO therapy improves host defenses and has been proven as a useful adjunct to antibiotics and surgery for the treatment of infectious wound complications after surgery in the irradiated head and neck (Neovius et al., 1997). In radiation-injured tissues, HBO therapy facilitates the formation of new capillaries, thus improving tissue oxygen tensions and host defenses, and improving osseointegration and reducing implant failure rates (Larsson et al., 2002).

The use of HBO therapy for the treatment of uncomplicated wound infections (osteomyelitis of a free cranial bone flap after craniotomy, without additional risk factors) with osteomyelitis of a bone flap is controversial. However, in complicated cranial wound infections (osteomyelitis, with or without remaining bone/acrylic flap, after craniotomy with additional risk factors, such as repeated surgery, foreign material, malignant disease, or previous radiotherapy), HBO therapy is particularly useful (Larsson et al., 2002). Infection control and establishment of the healing process can be quite rapid, and many patients continue to exhibit improvement after cessation of HBO therapy (Larsson et al., 2002).

2.2.4.2 One-stage reconstruction of cranial defects using a titanium mesh plate enclosed in an omental flap

Treatment of chronic cranial osteomyelitis is difficult. Asai et al. (Asai et al., 2004) developed a reconstructive technique for osteomyelitis-related cranial defects that fills the dead space with an omental flap and uses a titanium mesh plate as a structural element.

Cranial defects have been reconstructed with split rib, split calvarial bone, biocompatible osteoconductive polymers, and by many other methods. However, if there is an infection at the site, autogenous bone should be selected as a reconstructive material, even though autogenous bone itself may become infected. The advantages of using an omental flap are that there is sufficient tissue volume to cover a large wound, it can be cut to any space, and it shapes relatively large blood vessels, making vascular anastomoses easier to perform. Titanium mesh plates make an excellent prosthesis in many ways, but carry the risk of exposure associated with thinning of overlying skin (Asai et al., 2004). Asai et al. (Asai et al., 2004) described the first case of an omental flap–mesh–omental flap "sandwich". To reduce the risk of prosthesis exposure and infection, Asai et al.'s technique places the omental flap both superficial and deep to the titanium mesh plates, thus vascularizing the graft. The use of an omental flap has several advantages in cranial reconstruction, and its flexible consistency facilitates the obliteration of dead space because it adapts to the size and shape of the defect (Asai et al., 2004).

2.2.4.3 Vacuum-Assisted Closure (VAC)

VAC therapy was introduced by Argenta and Morykwas in 1997 (Argenta & Morykwas, 1997) and has been in routine clinical use for the treatment of difficult wounds. The mechanism of treatment is exposure of the wound bed to negative pressure, resulting in removal of edema fluid, improvement in the blood supply, and stimulation of cellular proliferation of reparative granulation tissue (Subotic et al., 2011). Reconstruction of scalp and calvarial defects can be challenging because of the poor vascularity of the cortical bone. The aims of VAC therapy are the formation of new granulation tissue, wound cleansing, and bacterial clearance.

Subotic et al. (Subotic et al., 2011) reported successful treatment of chronic scalp wounds with exposed dura using VAC. The VAC device is feasible for use in the treatment of scalp wounds with exposed dura and chronic infection to create a setting for wound closure, e.g., secondary healing and skin transplantation (Subotic et al., 2011).

2.2.4.4 Preservation of bone flap in patients with post-craniotomy infections

The standard care for the management of post-craniotomy wound infections consists of operative debridement and removal of the devitalized bone flap followed by delayed cranioplasty performed several months later. This strategy, although successful in treating most patients, adversely affects patient satisfaction by necessitating an additional surgical procedure for cranioplasty, as well as leaving a cosmetic deformity and lack of brain protection before cranioplasty can be performed.

Standard operative debridement for preservation of the bone flap consists of reopening of the wound and re-elevation of the bone flap. All visible suture material and hemostatic agents are removed. The purulent material is cultured and analyzed for anaerobic and aerobic organisms, and for antibiotic sensitivities. Necrotic and purulent debris is removed by mechanical debridement and copious irrigation with bacitracin solution followed by saline. The bone flap is vigorously scrubbed and soaked in Betadine solution. In no instance is the bone flap autoclaved, and the bone edges are not routinely drilled. Hemostasis is achieved with the aid of bipolar cautery and a hemostatic agent such as Avitene (Avicon, Fort Worth, TX, USA) or FloSeal (Fusion Medical Technologies, Fremont, CA, USA) (J.N. Bruce & S.S. Bruce 2003).

Simple operative debridement is sufficient in patients with uncomplicated post-craniotomy infections, making it unnecessary to discard bone flaps and perform later cranioplasties. Even patients with risk factors such as prior surgery, skull base procedures, chemotherapy, or radiotherapy can be successfully treated using this strategy in most cases. However, patients with craniofacial surgery involving the nasal sinuses are at higher risk and might be best treated with bone flap removal and delayed cranioplasty (J.N. Bruce & S.S. Bruce 2003). J.N. Bruce and S.S. Bruce (J.N. Bruce & S.S. Bruce 2003) reported the highly favorable results of a prospective study in which aggressive surgical debridement was performed to preserve bone flaps without cranioplasty in patients who had post-craniotomy wound infections.

2.2.4.5 Prevention of neurosurgical infection

Specific methods for prevention of postoperative skull osteomyelitis have not been reported. A variety of methods for prevention of SSIs in neurosurgery have been reported.

Leaper (Leaper, 1995) reviewed the principles given for prevention such as an emphasis on surgical skill to minimize tissue damage and residual hematoma formation that could also apply to neurosurgery. In compound depressed skull fractures, the most effective way of avoiding subsequent meningitis, abscess, or empyema is rapid and thorough debridement and elevation of the fracture.

For antimicrobial prophylaxis, Baker (Baker, 1994) performed a meta-analysis to determine with more confidence whether antimicrobial prophylaxis for craniotomy is effective. He concluded that there was a significant advantage of antimicrobial prophylaxis over placebo, but no significant differences between regimens that did or did not cover Gram-negative organisms or between single- and multiple-dose regimens. The impact of prophylaxis noted in clean procedures may be diminished in contaminated procedures because of the larger biomass of contaminating bacteria and hence the need for additional measures such as debridement with the latter.

The general surgical literature contains significant evidence for decreased wound infection rates with careful skin preparation, but without shaving (Alexander et al., 1983). That shaving the day before operation causes higher rates of infection is well known, but even same-day shaving or clipping have been implicated. Surgery without shaving the scalp is technically feasible, and does appear to reduce the infection rate (Hosein et al., 1999).

2.3 Skull Base Osteomyelitis (SBO)

SBO has been described most often as a complication of malignant otitis externa (MOE) secondary to *Pseudomonas aeruginosa (P. aeruginosa)* infection (Chandler, 1989). Increasing age, diabetes mellitus, and microvascular disease are common risk factors (Rothholtz et al., 2008). SBO, however, may also occur in the absence of MOE and with pathogens other than *P. aeruginosa,* including fungi. Fungal SBO has been reported to be mostly caused by *Aspergillus* species, and less commonly by *Scedosporium* spp. (Lee et al., 2008; Stodulski et al., 2006).

Early diagnosis, identification of the causative pathogens, prompt initiation of appropriate antimicrobial or surgical therapies, and continuation of therapy for an adequate period are essential when managing SBO. Identification of the pathogen often requires surgical biopsy. Because this may be delayed for medical or technical reasons, clinical features or risk factors that discriminate between SBO caused by bacterial and fungal infections could guide selection of empiric antimicrobial therapy pending a definitive diagnosis (Blyth et al., 2011).

2.3.1 Typical type (SBO secondary to MOE)

In 1959, Meltzer and Keleman (Meltzer & Keleman, 1959) reported a case of external otitis caused by *P. aeruginosa* in a patient with poorly controlled diabetes mellitus who later died despite progressive medical and surgical treatment. The term "MOE" was introduced by Chandler (Chandler, 1968) in 1968 when he published a review of his personal experience with 13 patients. He detailed what are now considered the classical physical examination and histology findings and deduced the currently accepted pathophysiology. However, in contrast with today's therapies, he believed that radical surgical debridement offered the only chance of cure. Advances in imaging and antibiotic therapy have changed this belief; these advances and greater awareness of the disease have brought a dramatic improvement in the prognosis of MOE (Sreepada & Kwartler, 2003).

The most common predisposing factor in the development of temporal bone osteomyelitis secondary to MOE is diabetes mellitus (Chandler, 1989). Driscoll et al. (Driscoll et al., 1993) found that cerumen from the ears of patients with diabetics had a higher average pH compared with that from the ears of nondiabetics, and they postulated that such alkaline pH could provide a beneficial environment for bacterial overgrowth. Diabetic patients' increased predisposition to temporal bone osteomyelitis is also because of their increased susceptibility to microangiopathic changes and an altered immune response (Alva et al., 2009).

SBO is a serious, life-threatening condition seen most commonly in elderly diabetic or immunocompromised patients. Usually, it is a complication of otitis externa when repeated episodes fail to resolve with topical medication and aural cleansing. Pain may become worse, granulation tissue is seen within the auditory canal, the bone of the external auditory canal becomes involved, and cranial neuropathies may arise. These patients usually have only minimal constitutional symptoms. The typical patient has headaches and ear pain as the primary complaints. Cranial nerve palsies occur less frequently and indicate advanced disease. This MOE can be difficult to treat, but it is a reasonably well-recognized clinical entity that should be straightforward to diagnose in an ears, nose, and throat setting. This condition has been described most often as complication of MOE secondary to *P. aeruginosa* infection. *P. aeruginosa* is by far the commonest pathogen implicated in MOE, being responsible for 50%–98% of all cases. Fungal SBO is increasingly reported in the literature (Marr et al., 2002; Roden et al., 2005).

The warning signs of temporal bone osteomyelitis followed as: deep pain (temporal, parietal, postauricular, or retro-orbital); intermittent, foul otorrhea and spiking fever; preauricular cellulitis; woody induration of the pinna; chronic mastoid cutaneous fistula; fibrotic mastoid granulation tissue; intermittent facial twitching suggestive of facial canal dehiscence; and persistent leukocytosis and an elevated ESR. It is widely accepted that clinical suspicion of MOE should be heightened when otalgia persists in adequately treated patients with otitis externa. The diagnosis is based on a combination of clinical findings, history, imaging, microbiology, and histology (Cohen & Friedman, 1987). Identification of skull base osteitis in imaging studies seems to be an indispensable indicator. However, imaging studies are particularly useful in determining the extent of the inflammatory process. In such cases, deep surgical biopsies are mandatory, and are now the main indication for surgery in patients with suspected MOE (Rubin et al., 2004). The imaging studies lack specificity in differentiating MOE from diseases with similar symptoms, such as nasopharyngeal and skull base tumors. A bacterial or a fungal species should always be isolated. The role of histology is mainly to differentiate this entity from malignant tumor. CT defines the location and extent of the disease at initial evaluation (Alva et al., 2009). MRI has the advantage of better soft tissue discrimination than CT, and is particularly useful for assessing soft tissue planes around the skull base and abnormalities of the medullary cavity of bone. MRI features that are highly sensitive but nonspecific for osteomyelitis include marrow T1 hypointensity and T2 hyperintensity (Chang et al., 2003).

Treatment for osteomyelitis consists of broad-spectrum antibiotics for not less than 3 months, along with surgical debridement and wide meatoplasty (Alva et al., 2009). Antimicrobial therapy in SBO is targeted to eradication of the causative pathogen. The role of surgical resection is also likely to be influenced by a pathogen. Aggressive surgical debridement is recommended in fungal SBO, but is probably unnecessary in patients with bacterial SBO.

Early diagnosis is very important, because MOE may not always be slow and gradual, but sometimes rapid and fulminant. Some patients present with a venous sinus thrombosis, cerebral infarct, or cerebral abscess (Vourexakis et al., 2010). Other central nervous system complications, such as meningitis, have also been reported (Sreepada & Kwartler, 2003).

2.3.2 Atypical type (central SBO)

Atypical SBO is an uncommon condition that is potentially life threatening if not promptly recognized and properly treated (Chandler et al., 1986). Atypical SBO occurs much less frequently and does not begin with otitis externa (Chang et al., 2003). These patients may have headaches as the initial symptom and only later develop cranial abnormalities (Grobman et al., 1989). Whereas MOE primarily affects the temporal bone, central or atypical SBO can be seen affecting the sphenoid and occipital bone, often centered on the clivus, and can be considered a variant of MOE (Chang et al., 2003).

It can present with headache and a variety of cranial neuropathies, often a combination of abducens and lower cranial nerve neuropathies. The imaging findings are of particular concern because they frequently mimic malignancy, which makes accurate histological diagnosis all the more important. However, once diagnosed and treated with appropriate antibiotics, it is one of the few times when cranial nerve palsies can be seen to resolve. Several potentially serious complications can arise as a result of SBO, including cranial neuropathy, soft tissue involvement of the cavernous sinus with or without cavernous sinus thrombosis, and meningeal and brain parenchymal extension. Cranial nerve involvement is commonly seen because of the proximity of the clivus to the brain stem, basal cisterns, cavernous sinuses, and skull base foramina (Chang et al., 2003). Other complications of SBO reported in the literature have included epidural abscess of the cervical spine as a result of the spread of infection through the prevertebral space (Azizi et al., 1995) and petroclival abscess (Hoistad & Duvall, 1999).

The imaging findings are of particular interest. The bone erosion and marrow infiltrate of the basiocciput or petrous apex, as well as mass-like soft tissue swelling below the skull base, often raises concerns that there is an underlying malignant process, such as a nasopharyngeal carcinoma or skull base metastases. Imaging of the skull base in the setting of cranial neuropathy and probable infection is best accomplished with MRI. MRI has the advantage of superior soft tissue discrimination without the beam-hardening artifacts of CT. Clival enhancement can be seen with both infectious and neoplastic processes, but it should not be observed under normal circumstances. The use of fat suppression on postgadolinium study is of course necessary to assess skull base enhancement accurately (Chang et al., 2003). Other imaging techniques can help support the diagnosis of SBO. Technetium scans may be helpful for initial diagnosis, although they may remain "hot" for months following resolution of infection (Seabold et al., 1995). Gallium scan abnormalities have been shown to be useful to monitor response to treatment and evaluate recurrence (Grobman et al., 1989).

A tissue-sampling procedure is often required for definitive diagnosis of this condition, because the imaging appearance alone is highly suggestive but nonspecific for SBO. Diagnosis is made by endoscopic sphenoidotomy or open craniotomy. Potentially complicating the diagnosis is the fact that a low burden of infectious organisms within the clival bone or preclival soft tissue can lead to a false-negative biopsy (Chang et al., 2003). New modalities such as MRI-guided biopsy of soft tissue surrounding the skull base may prove to be useful under these circumstances (Kacl et al., 1999). An important point is to always send biopsy material for microbiological analysis as well as histology; ultimately, this may lead to the correct diagnosis. In this lesion, biopsy is inevitably required both to ensure the absence of malignancy and to aid subsequent microbiological advice.

2.3.3 Fungal SBO

Fungal SBO involves an immunocompromised host, prior antibiotic therapy, and steroid therapy. In contrast with bacterial SBO, fungal SBO has not been definitively associated with diabetes mellitus. Invasive fungal disease is usually caused by *A. fumigatus* and less commonly by *A. flavus* (Bickley et al., 1988). Given the rarity of fungal SBO, it is not surprising that almost all prior cases involving a several-week delay in diagnosis are secondary to misdiagnosis of necrotizing external otitis (Hanna et al., 1993).

Fungal SBO is increasingly reported in the literature. This apparent rise may reflect the increasing use of immunosuppressive therapies in parallel with the rise of other forms of invasive fungal disease (Roden et al., 2005). Importantly, however, fungal SBO may also occur in immunocompetent individuals (Shelton et al., 2002) and should be considered in all patients presenting with symptoms or signs of SBO, especially given evidence from other forms of invasive fungal disease that a delay in antifungal therapy results in increased mortality (Chamilos et al., 2008). Fungal SBO is often only considered following failure of antibacterial therapy (Kountakis et al., 1997). In a study by Blyth et al. (Blyth et al., 2011), 55% of patients with fungal SBO were treated with antibacterial drugs for a median of 5 weeks prior to diagnosis.

Most cases of fungal SBO result from *Aspergillus* or *Scedosporium* spp., reportedly arising from the contiguous spread of ear infection (Shelton et al., 2002). Patients with fungal SBO were more likely to have underlying chronic sinus disease, symptoms attributable to invasive sinus infection (sinofacial pain, periorbital swelling, nasal stuffiness/discharge), but with a relative paucity of features attributable to ear infection (Blyth et al., 2011).

Definitive diagnosis of fungal SBO usually requires pathological demonstration of tissue invasion. Technetium bone scan is very sensitive for osteomyelitis, and this is strongly positive. Gallium scan is also positive, further supporting the diagnosis of osteomyelitis. CT reveals definite evidence of bone destruction (Shelton et al., 2002) (Figs. 4 and 5) (Lee et al., 2005).

Calcium oxalate production has been frequently noted with *A. niger* infection. The presence of calcium oxalate crystals may assist in early diagnosis before the return of culture results in this rare clinical entity (Shelton et al., 2002). Early diagnosis, identification of the causative pathogen, prompt initiation of appropriate antimicrobial or surgical therapies, and continuation of therapy for an adequate period are essential when managing SBO.

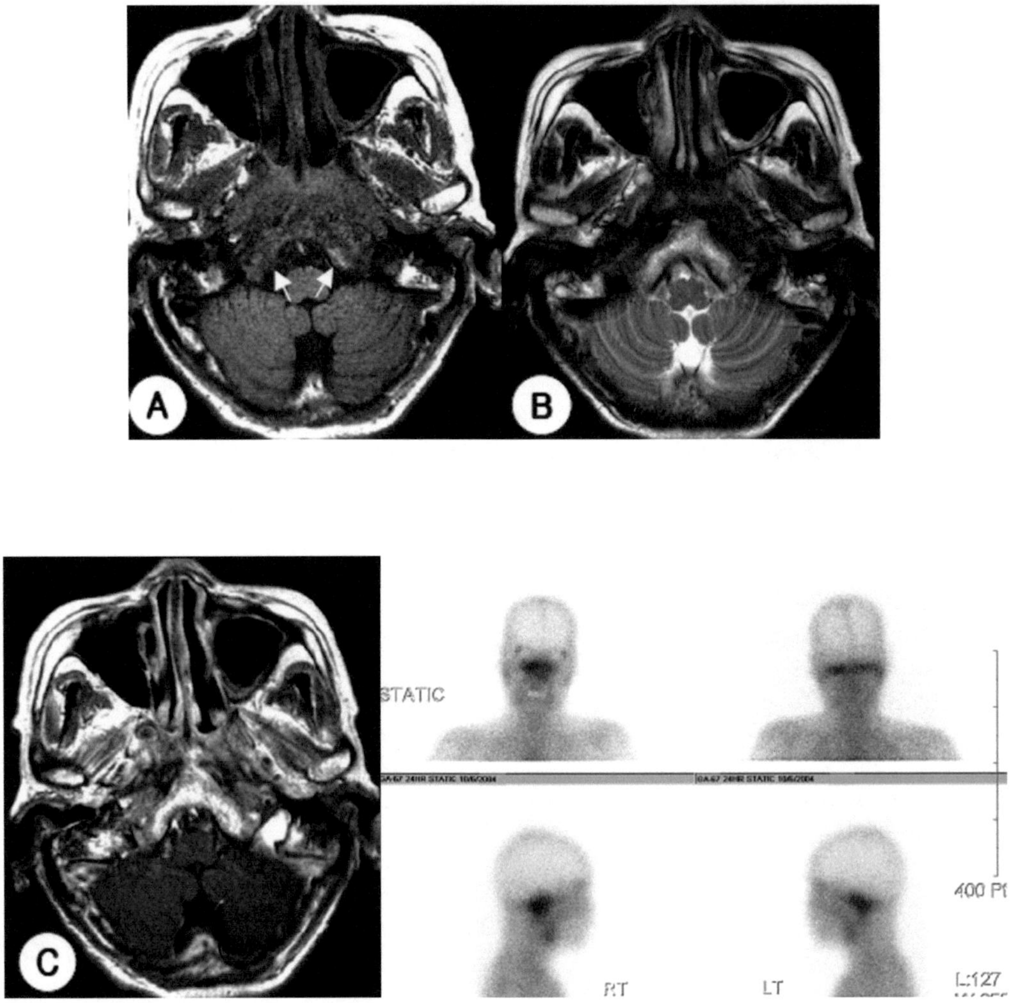

Fig. 4. (A) On axial T1-weighted MR imaging, a high signal intensity of normal fatty marrow within clivus (arrows) is replaced by inhomogeneous low signal intensity. Abnormal soft tissue intensity signals infiltrate the nasopharynx submucosally and adjacent parapharyngeal space. (B) On axial T2-weighted MR imaging, nasopharyngeal soft tissues show low signal intensity compared with normal muscle. In addition, there is fluid in the mastoid air cells. (C) With Gd-enhancement, nasopharyngeal soft tissues and prevertebral muscles show diffuse enhancement. (D) A gallium scan shows intense uptake in the right petrous temporal bone. (Reproduced with permission from Lee, SS., Son, JY., Lee, JH., & Kim, OK. (2005). A Case of Invasive Fungal Sinusitis Accompanied with Inflammatory Pseudotumor in Skull Base. *Korean J Otolaryngol-Head Neck Surg*, Vol.48, No.9, (September 2005), pp. 1173-1176, ISSN 1225-035X) (Lee et al., 2005).

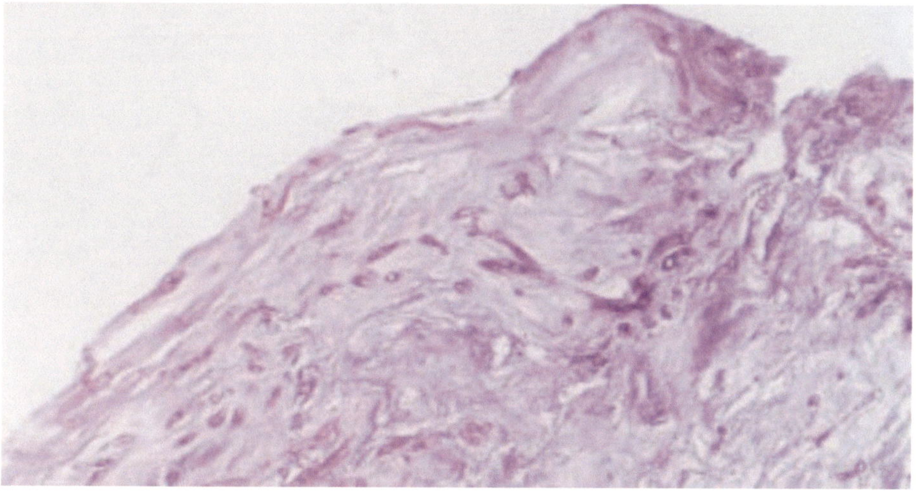

Fig. 5. (A)

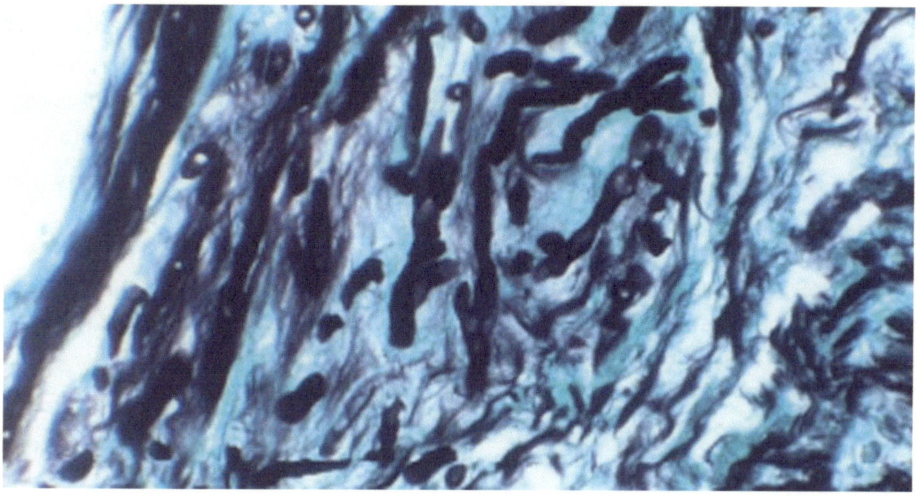

Fig. 5. (B)

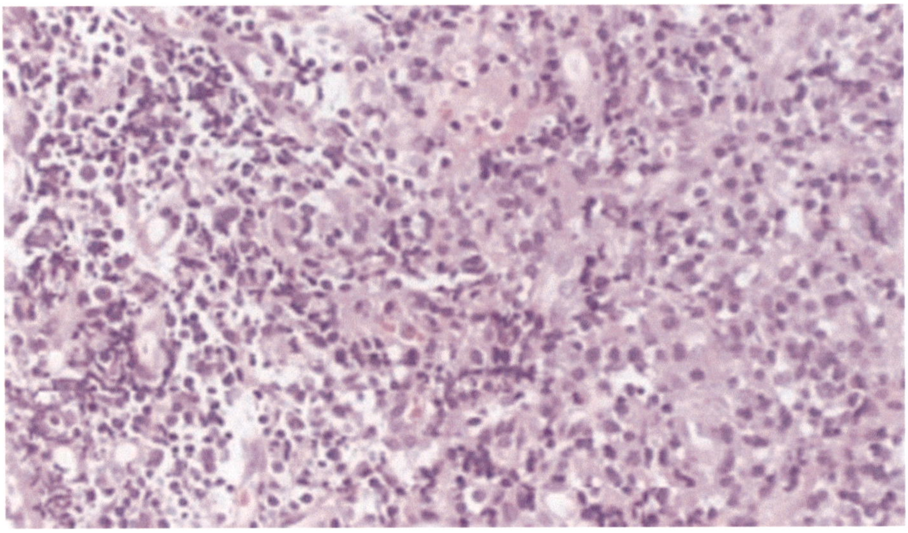

Fig. 5. (C)

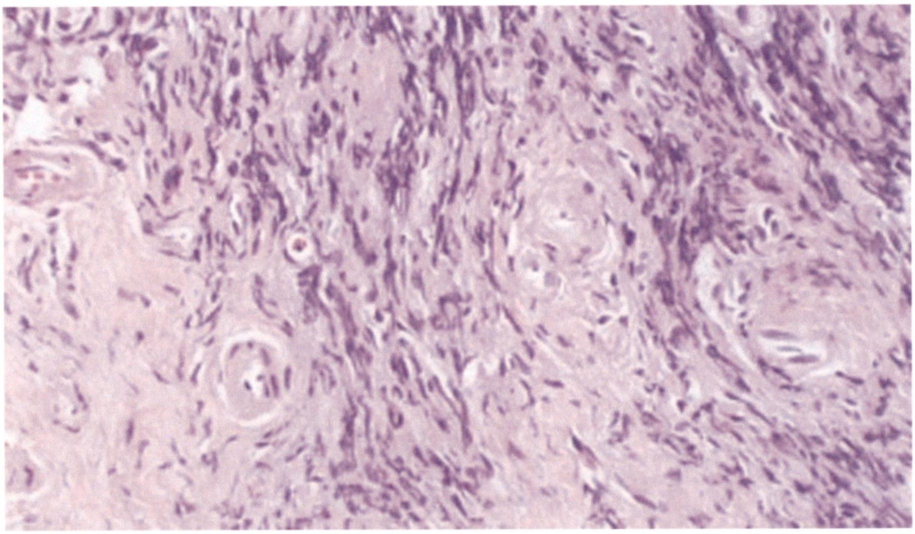

Fig. 5. (D)

Fig. 5. Histological findings show fungal hyphae compatible with *Aspergillus* within the mucosa of the sphenoid sinus (A, B). (A: hematoxylin and eosin, ×200, B : Gomori's methenamine silver, ×400). Histological findings of a nasopharyngeal biopsy (C, D). C: There is diffuse infiltration of inflammatory cells, especially lymphocytes and plasma cells (hematoxylin and eosin, original magnification ×200). D: Increased fibroblastic activity and collagen deposition are noted in submucosa adjacent to infiltrated inflammatory cells (hematoxylin and eosin, ×200). (Reproduced with permission from Lee, SS., Son, JY., Lee, JH., & Kim, OK. (2005). A Case of Invasive Fungal Sinusitis Accompanied with Inflammatory Pseudotumor in Skull Base. *Korean J Otolaryngol-Head Neck Surg*, Vol.48, No.9, (September 2005), pp. 1173-1176, ISSN 1225-035X) (Lee et al.., 2005)

Antimicrobial therapy in SBO is targeted to eradication of the causative pathogen. Because *P. aeruginosa* infection predominates in most case series of bacterial SBO, initiation of antibiotics with activity against *P. aeruginosa* is appropriate pending microbiological diagnosis (Blyth et al., 2011). Blyth et al. (Blyth et al., 2011) recommended the use of regimens including high-dose amphotericin B formulations pending definitive diagnosis. Aggressive surgical debridement is recommended in fungal SBO (Stodulski et al., 2006) but is probably unnecessary in patients with bacterial SBO (Blyth et al., 2011).

The diagnosis of invasive fungal SBO requires a high index of suspicion as it is often misdiagnosed as bacterial otitis externa.

2.4 Pediatric skull infection

Osteomyelitis of the skull in pediatric patients is most common complication of a compound skull wound following either surgery or trauma. It may also occur in the frontal bone secondary to sinus infection or in the parietal and temporal bones from ear infection. Osteomyelitis may develop in the skull of a newborn as a complication of an infected scalpwound from the use of forceps or secondary to intrauterine monitoring. Rarely, it occurs opportunistically in a child with a suppressed immune mechanism, and may be the result of a fungal infection. In this section, we discuss unique types of skull osteomyelitis seen in the pediatric patient.

2.4.1 Skull osteomyelitis complicating infected cephalohematoma

Osteomyelitis of the skull in the neonatal period is very rare. All reported cases are secondary to an infected cephalohematoma (Miedema et al., 1999), and complications of infected cephalohematoma, such as osteomyelitis or epidural abscess, may develop. Placement of a scalp electrode, scalp-vein line insertion, or trauma to the scalp by instruments are thought to be common routes for the introduction of infection (Miedema et al., 1999).

However, no source of infection can be identified in 50% of cases, so cephalohematoma should be considered as a potential site of infection, even without a history of scalp trauma (Miedema et al., 1999). Prasad et al. (Prasad et al., 2011) described one case of skull osteomyelitis without a history of scalp trauma. They reported that delayed swelling was first noted on the tenth day after birth, which is very unusual for a cephalohematoma. Their explanation is as follows; a small cephalohematoma that remained unnoticed may have been present at birth, until it was infected and started to progressively increase in size, or osteomyelitis resulted from hematogenous spread (Prasad et al., 2011).

The most common pathogens in infected cephalohematomas are *E. coli* and *S. aureus* (Chang et al., 2005; Goodwin et al., 2000). CT is the best imaging modality to demonstrate bony erosion and destruction in osteomyelitis complicating infected cephalohematoma (Chan et al., 2002). It depicts detailed pathological changes, including focal osteopenia, subtle erosion of inner and outer tables, and gross lytic destruction.

Management consists of surgical drainage, together with a prolonged course of intravenous antibiotics. Empirical therapy should be started with antibiotics covering for *E. coli* and *S. aureus*. The antibiotics should be changed appropriately once the culture sensitivity reports are available. Typically, osteomyelitis caused by infected cephalohematoma requires 4–6 weeks of intravenous antibiotics (Chang et al., 2005). In advanced cases, where the underlying bone is grossly eroded, a partial craniectomy may be required (Chan et al., 2002).

2.4.2 Pott's puffy tumor in children

Pott's puffy tumor was first described in 1760 by Percival Pott, a surgeon at St. Bartholomew's Hospital in London, as "a puffy, circumscribed, indolent tumor of the scalp and a spontaneous separation of the pericranium from the skull under such tumor" in observation of the natural course of head trauma. Currently, it is defined as a forehead-localized swelling with overlying subperiosteal abscess and osteomyelitis of the frontal bone (Bambakidis & Cohen, 2001; Tattersall, 2002). It was considered a rare entity in the postantibiotics era, and the majority of reported cases were adolescents and young adults. The incidence of Pott's puffy tumor showed a trend of increasing incidence in the review of articles (Rao et al., 2003; Tattersall, 2002). This may be attributed to partial antibiotics treatment for chronic sinusitis, and delayed diagnosis of potentially serious complications of frontal sinusitis (Rao et al., 2003).

Pott's puffy tumor is often associated with antecedent frontal sinusitis, and less commonly with trauma (Rao et al., 2003; Karaman et al., 2008). Other rarer risk factors for Pott's puffy tumor include osteocartilaginous necrosis secondary to chronic intranasal cocaine abuse, dental sepsis, or delayed complications of neurosurgery (Rao et al., 2003; Karaman et al., 2008).

Gradually tendered tumefaction of the scalp at the forehead is a typical sign. Osteomyelitis arising from paranasal sinusitis presents with the findings of the underlying process (nasal discharge, localized pain, and tenderness over the affected sinus, headache, localized edema, and inconsistently, fever). The initial symptoms and signs of Pott's puffy tumor often exhibit inconspicuously, which represents frontal sinusitis. Nasal obstruction and fever are less common. Acute worsening of symptoms, particularly headache and fever, or presenting with signs of increased intracranial pressure (nausea, vomiting, lethargy), periorbital complaints, or failure of resolution of symptoms with antibiotics treatment warrant image evaluation to look for silent intracranial involvement, even in the absence of neurological symptoms (Bambakidis & Cohen, 2001; Rao et al., 2003; Karaman et al., 2008). Intracranial involvement including meningitis, subdural empyema, cerebral abscess, epidural abscess, and rarely cavernous or superior sagittal sinus thrombosis and epidural frontocutaneous fistulas has been reported (Forgie & Marrie, 2008; Gupta et al., 2004; Yucel & Ogretmenoglu, 1998).

CT scan is the diagnostic modality for Pott's puffy tumor, but MRI is the criterion standard for the diagnosis of intracranial complications (Durur-Subasi et al., 2008).

Because of the high incidence of intracranial complications, both imaging studies should be performed when Pott's puffy tumor is suspected, especially for those having neurological symptoms or periorbital involvement.

The use of antibiotics should be prolonged for at least 6–8 weeks postoperatively (Bambakidis & Cohen, 2001; Brook, 2009). In consideration of rapid intracranial expansion, aggressive debridement should be prompt, and reoperation is often needed to evacuate the abscess of sinusitis, the subperiosteal abscess, the infected bone, and the epidural or subdural abscess, because the septic material may continuously disperse, which will lead to recurrence or disease progression.

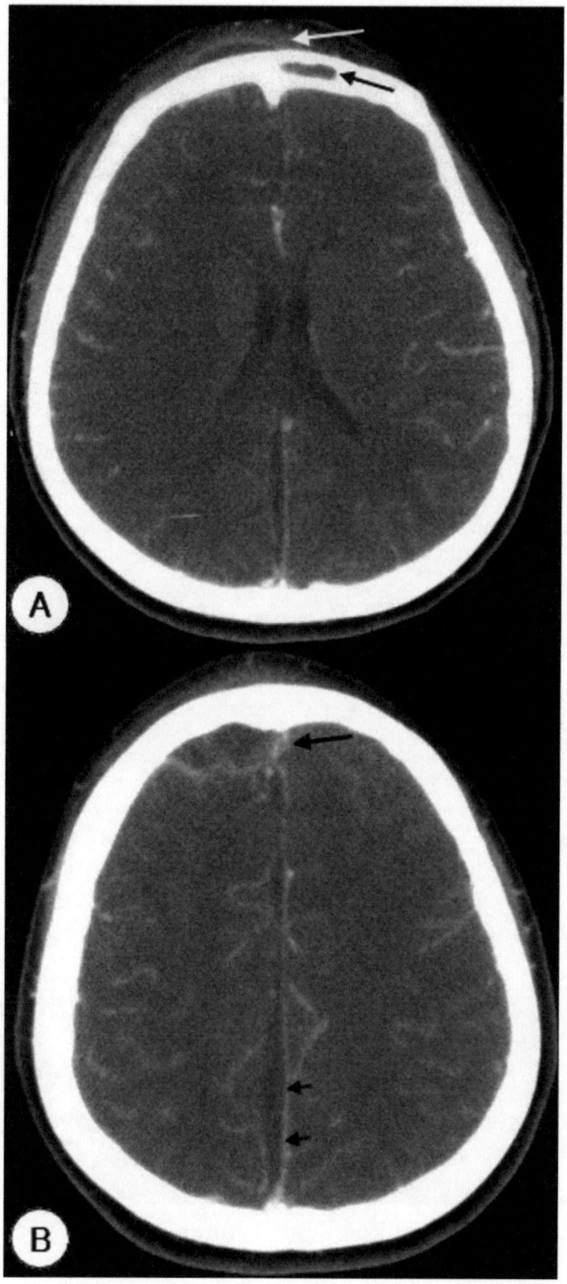

Fig. 6. Enhanced axial CT images of Pott's puffy tumor in a 12-year-old girl. A: Left frontal sinusitis (black arrow) and right subperiosteal abscess (white arrow). B: Right epidural abscess (black arrow) and subdural empyema along the falx cerebri (arrowheads). (Reproduced with permission from Lim, HW., Jang, YJ., Lee, BJ., & Chung, YS. (2006). A Case of Pott's Puffy Tumor as a Complication of Contralateral Frontal Sinusitis. *Korean J Otolaryngol-Head Neck Surg,* Vol.49, No.1, (January 2006), pp. 109-112, ISSN 1225-035X) (Lim et al., 2006)

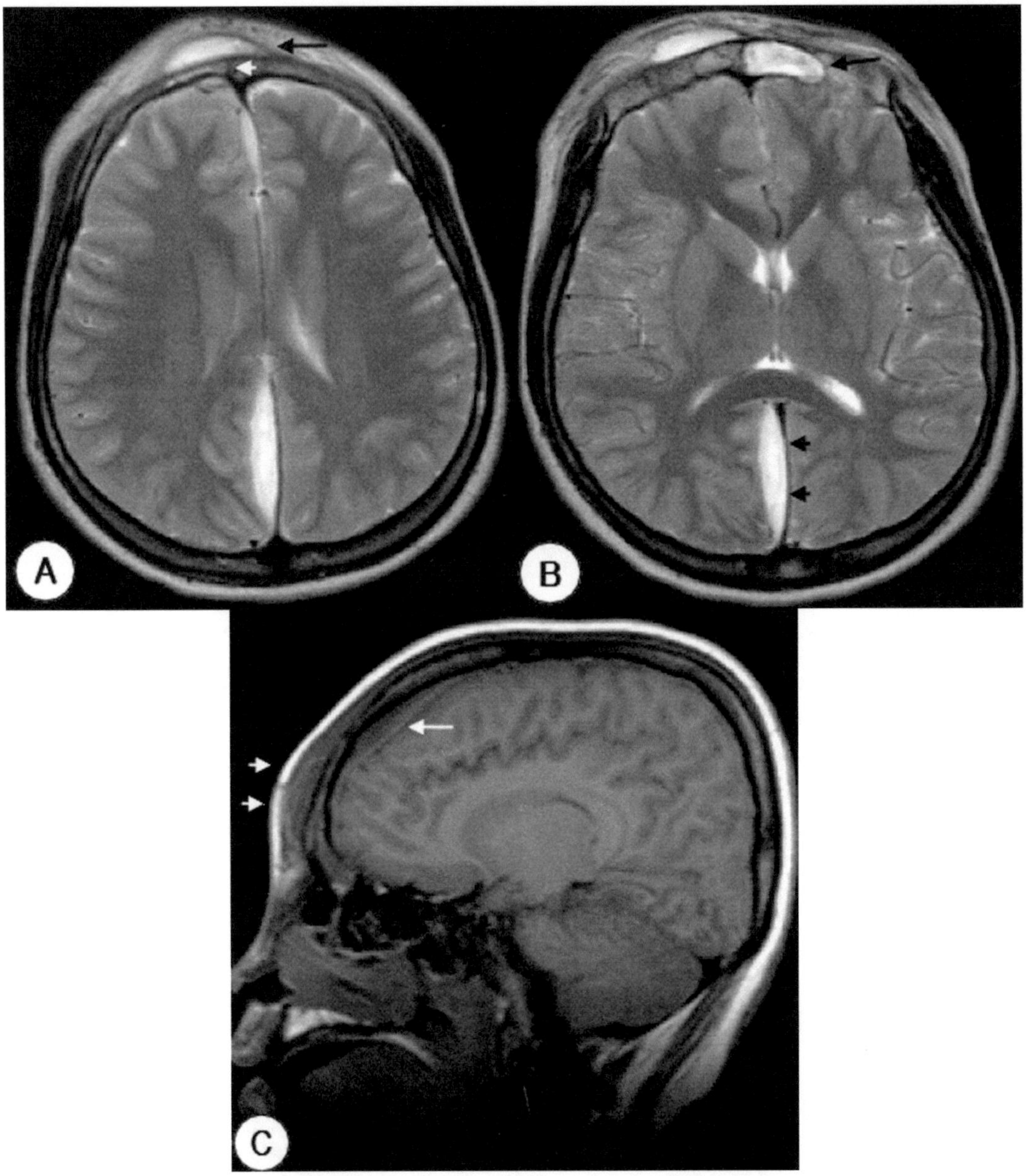

Fig. 7. Magnetic resonance images of Pott's puffy tumor in a 12-year-old girl. A: T2-weighted axial MR finding of osteomyelitis. Note the high signal lesion of the right frontal bone marrow (arrowhead) under the right subperiosteal abscess (black arrow). B: T2-weighted axial MR. Left frontal sinusitis (black arrow) accompanied with right subperiosteal abscess and subdural empyema along the falx cerebri (arrowheads). C: T1-weighted sagittal MR. Note the swelling of the forehead, and subperiosteal abscess (arrowheads) and epidural abscess formation (white arrow). (Reproduced with permission from Lim, HW., Jang, YJ., Lee, BJ., & Chung, YS. (2006). A Case of Pott's Puffy Tumor as a Complication of Contralateral Frontal Sinusitis. *Korean J Otolaryngol-Head Neck Surg,* Vol.49, No.1, (January 2006), pp. 109-112, ISSN 1225-035X) (Lim et al., 2006)

2.4.3 Clival osteomyelitis

Osteomyelitis of the clivus is an uncommon condition in the pediatric population. Previous authors have suggested various other causes of clivus osteomyelitis, which include direct spread of an infectious process involving the paranasal sinuses or adjacent bones of the skull base (Rusconi et al., 2005). Prabhu et al. (Prabhu et al., 2009) proposed that the fossa navicularis magna can be a potential source of transmission of infection through the skull base from the lymphatic tissue in the pharynx. The presence of an emissary vein in addition to lymphatics in the fossa navicularis magna may be a potentiating factor for the unusual route of spread of infection through this skull base foramen (Prabhu et al., 2009). Anecdotal cases have been reported in adult patients, but there are few published pediatric cases (Rusconi et al., 2005). Rusconi et al. (Rusconi et al., 2005) reported that clivus osteomyelitis with an effusive abscess in the retropharyngeal space had been treated by abscess drainage via the posterior wall of the pharyngeal tract and antibiotics therapy. In this case, Rusconi et al. (Rusconi et al., 2005) suggested that this patient may have lacerated the retropharyngeal space with a stick or toy picked up from soil contaminated by Enterococcus (thus allowing the entry of the bacteria and subsequent clivus osteomyelitis).

2.4.4 Garré's osteomyelitis (chronic sclerosing osteomyelitis)

Garré's osteomyelitis, first described in 1893, is synonymously used for chronic sclerosing osteomyelitis, periostitis ossificans, and similar forms of osteomyelitis (Braun & Kreipe, 1979; Wood et al., 1988). Imaging findings in the long bones and jaw have previously been reported, but to our knowledge imaging findings in the skull have been reported in only one case (Klisch et al., 2002).

The calvarium is an uncommon location of sclerosing osteomyelitis, which is still not completely understood. It is assumed that the chronic process is maintained by a slow active infection. The bone responds to stimulation with new bone formation, resorption, or a combination of both. Sclerosis may be the result of either decreased resorption or excessive bone formation. Because sclerosis of the bone and calvarial thickening are the predominant imaging findings, the differential diagnosis includes more sclerotic than lytic lesions in the skull (Klisch et al., 2002). Bacterial infection is thought to reach the calvarium by hematogenous spread, or rarely by direct penetration, but in most cases no bacterial growth is obtained in culture, and radionuclide scans for osteomyelitis may be falsely negative (Tumeh et al., 1986).

The imaging findings are not specific, and a wide range of differential diagnoses have to be considered in calvarial lesions in children (Arana et al., 1996): intraosseous hemangioma, or metabolic diseases, e.g., hyperparathyroidism, Langerhans cell histiocytosis, and anemias. The differential diagnosis furthermore includes neoplasms such as osteoid osteoma, Ewing's sarcoma, intraosseous hyperostotic meningioma, osteoblastic metastasis, or fibrous dysplasia.

Treatment of Garré's osteomyelitis is based on individual decision. A conservative approach with antibiotics therapy may lead to a temporary improvement; however, complete resection of the diseased bone is necessary in order to achieve a permanent cure. Klisch et al. (Klisch et al., 2002) performed an extended frontal and parietal trephination and construction with a titanium implant.

Sclerosing osteomyelitis of the calvarium has to be included in the differential diagnosis of osteolytic and sclerosing lesions of the skull coinciding with persistent swelling of the head (Klisch et al., 2002).

2.4.5 Spontaneous cranial osteomyelitis in an otherwise healthy child

In children, three origins for cranial osteomyelitis appear to dominate: Pott's puffy tumor, skull base osteomyelitis secondary to ear infection, or postsurgical complications. However, on extremely rare occasions, risk factors or etiology may not be ascertained (Arnold et al., 2009). Arnold et al. (Arnold et al., 2009) reported a case of spontaneous cranial osteomyelitis in an otherwise healthy child.

Researchers have proposed several theories regarding the etiology of frontal bone osteomyelitis. In Arnold et al.'s reported case, cultures from the wound grew *Streptococcus intermedius*, a microaerophilic streptococcus in the *milleri* group that resides in the mouth, upper respiratory tract, and the gastrointestinal and genitourinary tracts. This patient also had poor dental hygiene. Arnold et al. (Arnold et al., 2009) proposed that an infected tooth could have caused bacteremia either before or after the appearance of the scalp hematoma. The bacteremia then possibly seeded the hematoma, resulting in a subperiosteal abscess, which led to osteomyelitis and then to the epidural abscess.

2.4.6 Skull osteomyelitis after varicella infection

Superficial bacterial infection is a well-known complication of varicella infection, but serious superinfection requiring hospitalization and intravenous antibiotic therapy is uncommon (Fleisher et al., 1981). Rarely do these lead to deep-seated, suppurative complications such as osteomyelitis. A 5.5-month-old girl presented with a pox lesion of the scalp associated with a 1-cm-diameter lytic lesion of the right parietal bone (Gallagher, 1990). This lesion was treated by debridement and intravenous antibiotics therapy. Patients with varicella-related superficial bacterial infections should receive close follow-up and, when indicated, antibiotic therapy should be started.

2.5 Fungal skull osteomyelitis

Most invasive fungal infections occur in patients with prolonged neutropenia, critically ill patients in intensive care, patients undergoing chemotherapy for solid tumors, patients with acquired immunodeficiency syndrome (AIDS), and patients who have received an organ transplant. A secondary infection by an opportunistic fungus in an already immunocompromised patient is not easy to diagnose or treat, and the prognosis for patients with this life-threatening complication is poor (Safaya et al., 2006).

2.5.1 Cryptococcal osteomyelitis of the skull

Cryptococcosis is an opportunistic mycosis caused by members of the *Cryptococcus neoformans (C. neoformans)* complex. Although it has been known since the beginning of the 20th century when it occasionally affected immunocompetent humans, it has recently become more important because of its association with the human immunodeficiency virus (HIV) epidemic. *C. neoformans* infections typically involve the lungs and the central nervous system, but can also affect other organs, e.g., the skin, eye, prostate, and, rarely, the skeletal system (Chayakulkeeree & Perfect, 2006).

Cryptococcal osteomyelitis is often preceded by dissemination of the etiologic agent from the portal of entry. Bone involvement is found in 10% of patients with disseminated disease. Osteomyelitis without fungemia is uncommon, appearing in a little more than 50 reported cases. In addition to systemic infection, cryptococcal osteomyelitis has been typically associated with sarcoidosis, tuberculosis, steroid therapy, and diabetes (Liu, 1998). When bone infections do occur, *Cryptococcus* is most commonly associated with the vertebrae, pelvis, ribs, femur, and tibia, with one-quarter of patients having involvement of more than one bone (Liu, 1998; Witte et al., 2000). The skull is a less frequent target, with only 18 previously reported cases (Corral et al., 2011).

Cryptococcal osteomyelitis in the skull shares many characteristics with cutaneous cryptococcosis. Direct inoculation after trauma is a common cause, although hematogenous dissemination from adjacent areas of infection is also responsible for many cases of osteomyelitis. Predisposing risk factors are very similar for both entities, i.e., corticosteroid use, solid organ transplantation, diabetes mellitus, and T-cell deficiency (Corral et al., 2011).

Diagnosis was accomplished in all cases through excision biopsy. Smears should be prepared with india ink and Wright's stain. Mucicarmine stains can help distinguish *Cryptococcus* from other fungal infections (Armonda et al., 1993). The identification of the fungi recovered from patients is accomplished by conventional methods and culture of the isolate on 3,4-dihydroxyphenylalanine (DOPA) agar and canavanine glycine bromothymol blue (CGB) media.

Treatment for cryptococcal skull osteomyelitis includes a combination of surgical debridement and systemic antifungals (Christianson et al., 2003; Corral et al., 2011). If cerebrospinal fluid was sterile, surgical curettage and oral fluconazole without amphotericin B could be a good regimen for treating these cases (Corral et al., 2011). However, amphotericin B should be included in the regimen if meningitis is coincident.

Cryptococcal osteomyelitis of the skull probably has a worse outcome, with a mortality of 16% (2/12) compared with 5% (2/40) for nonskull osteomyelitis as reported by Liu in 1998 (Liu, 1998).

2.5.2 *Aspergillus* infection

Although human exposure to *Aspergillus* is common, infections are infrequent. *Aspergillus* osteomyelitis is often seen in patients who are immunodeficient, taking cytotoxic medications, of advanced age, receiving antimicrobial therapy, or taking chronic systemic steroids (Rinaldi, 1983). Invasive fungal disease is usually caused by *A. fumigatus* and less commonly by *A. flavus* (Bickley et al., 1988). In some cases, *A. niger* was isolated (Shelton et al., 2002). Invasive skull base mastoiditis, also known as malignant or necrotizing otitis externa, typically affects immunocompromised patients and is usually caused by *P. aeruginosa*. Patients with invasive aspergillosis can have similar clinical presentation and physical findings as those with an infection caused by *P. aeruginosa*. Failure to identify *Aspergillus* as the causative pathogen of invasive temporal bone infection is the principal reason for delay in initiating potentially life-saving therapy.

Definitive diagnosis of fungal SBO usually requires pathological demonstration of tissue invasion. However, a technetium bone scan is very sensitive for osteomyelitis, and is a strongly positive indicator. Gallium scans are also positive indicators, further supporting the diagnosis of osteomyelitis (Shelton et al., 2002).

Although the ideal treatment for cases of post-traumatic cranial osteomyelitis caused by *Aspergillus* spp. has not yet been described, the authors of some previously reported cases of MOE affecting the temporal bone used a treatment consisting of surgical debridement of the wound and intravenous long-term treatment with amphotericin B (Gordon & Giddings, 1994). Therefore, treatment of *Aspergillus* mastoiditis is threefold. Aggressive surgical debridement and resection is required, and antifungal therapy should be instituted once the diagnosis is made. HBO therapy should be considered postoperatively, although clear evidence to demonstrate its effectiveness is still lacking. Treatment failure could also be the result of suboptimal therapeutic management as a consequence of antifungal agent toxicity. In particular, the side effects of amphotericin B, especially renal failure, may require interruption of antifungal agents or a decrease in dosage (Parize et al., 2009). Parize et al. (Parize et al., 2009) recommended that based on its favorable bone penetration, its tolerance, and its efficacy, voriconazole may be considered an attractive first-line therapeutic option for *Aspergillus* SBO.

2.5.3 Blastomycotic skull osteomyelitis

Blastomycotic cranial osteomyelitis is a rare disease that warrants consideration in persistent otologic infections despite adequate antimicrobial therapy. Temporal bone blastomycotic osteomyelitis is extremely rare and difficult to diagnose, because it appears to present as common serous otitis media. In one case, it was approximately 1 year between the initial presentation and the final diagnosis of blastomycosis (Farr et al., 1992). In another case, it was 5 years between the initial presentation with serous otitis media and the final diagnosis of blastomycosis, despite numerous attempts at fungal stains and cultures (Louis & Lockey, 1974). Progression of the disease despite antimicrobial therapy should cause consideration of alternative diagnosis such as *Mycobacterium tuberculosis*, *Pseudomonas* sp., other fungi, and tumors.

Hematoxylin and eosin staining commonly reveals pseudoepitheliomatous hyperplasia, dense granulomatous infiltration, microabscesses, or giant cells. A relatively unusual pattern of inflammation that is characteristic of this infection is granuloma with central suppuration. A definitive diagnosis requires culture on Sabouraud's agar, or one of the enriched agars such as Sabhi or brain heart infusion, at 30°C, and reveals a characteristic white mold (Farr et al., 1992).

The mainstay of treatment of blastomycosis is amphotericin B, which has significantly reduced the 60% mortality rate of the infection since its introduction in the 1950s (Farr et al., 1992).

2.5.4 Cerebral mycetoma with cranial osteomyelitis

Mycetoma is a chronic granulomatous infection caused by true fungi (eumycetoma) or bacterial actinomycetes (actinomycetoma). Mycetoma is characterized by the presence of a subcutaneous mass and multiple sinuses draining pus, blood, and fungal grains. Traumatic injury to the local tissue is considered to be its route into the subcutaneous tissue, where these saprophytic fungi cause chronic granulomatous inflammation. The infection then spreads through the fascial planes and destroys connective tissue and bone. In the bone, the cortex is invaded and masses of grains gradually replace osseous tissue and marrow. The appearance of various granules on pathological examination is characteristic and allows a specific diagnosis of the causative organism (Beeram et al., 2008).

Mycetoma is clinically manifested by the appearance of painless papules or nodules that swell up and rupture, leading to sinus tract formation. As the infection spreads, similar lesions appear in adjacent skin and soft tissue. The tissue undergoes a recurring cycle of swelling, suppuration, and scarring. Ultimately, the infected site becomes a swollen, deformed mass of destroyed tissue with many fistulas through which grains are discharged (Beeram et al., 2008).

Currently, itraconazole and ketoconazole are the best treatment options. The duration of treatment varies with the severity of the infection and the general health status of individual adults (Welsh et al., 1995). It may be necessary to continue treatment for years, and the liver function of such patients requires regular monitoring. After treatment with itraconazole, these lesions remain well-encapsulated, localized, and easily excisable. Early diagnosis followed by antifungal treatment in combination with surgical excision appears to be a reasonable treatment (Beeram et al., 2008).

2.5.5 Mucormycosis SBO

A few reports of chronic invasive mucormycotic sinusitis causing SBO have appeared in the literature (Bahna et al., 1980; Finn & Farmer, 1982). Mucormycosis is the third most common opportunistic fungal infection in immunocompromised and diabetic patients (Safaya et al., 2006). However, skull base involvement is generally a late and uncommon finding in this situation. More frequently, mucormycosis results in sinonasal, orbital, and deep facial soft-tissue infiltration and intracranial involvement, cerebral abscesses, and infarcts. The late occurrence of bony involvement is explained by the angioinvasive nature of the fungus and characteristically deep extension of the infection through perivascular channels that precedes frank bony destruction (Gamba et al., 1986). Mucormycotic SBO is rare, but has been described as a late finding.

In the appropriate clinical context, the imaging findings of rhinocerebral mucormycosis on CT and MR imaging are diagnostic (Gamba et al., 1986). These include soft-tissue opacification of sinuses with hyperdense material, nodular mucosal thickening, and an absence of fluid levels (Gamba et al., 1986).

Management of chronic rhinocerebral mucormycosis is not well established. Wide surgical debridement where feasible, prolonged high-dose systemic amphotericin B, control of underlying comorbid factors, and HBO are used. Survival rates range from 21% to 70% (Blitzer et al., 1980).

2.6 Skull infection in human immunodeficiency virus (HIV)-infected patients

2.6.1 MOE in HIV and AIDS

MOE is a necrotizing infection of the external ear canal that may spread to include the mastoid and petrous parts of the temporal bone, leading to SBO. It is almost exclusively caused by infection with *P. aeruginosa,* and usually occurs in elderly non-insulin-dependent diabetic patients. Patients with HIV infection and AIDS are at risk because many take multiple chemotherapeutic medications, including cotrimoxazole, and have defects in both cell-mediated and humoral immunity. Factors contributing to the neutropenia include the effect of the HIV infection itself, administration of zidovudine, toxic effects of other drugs, and bone marrow suppression secondary to opportunistic infections and neoplasia (Kielhofner et al., 1992). Another factor in the susceptibility of HIV and AIDS patients to *Pseudomonas* infection is the effect of concurrent infection with cytomegalovirus. Cytomegalovirus itself may have immunosuppressive effects and enhance the ability of *P. aeruginosa* to cause disease (Hamilton & Overall, 1978).

Since the advent of AIDS, several cases of MOE have been reported in afflicted patients. The first published case of MOE was documented in 1990 in an HIV-seropositive Hispanic male (Rivas & Pumarola, 1990). Sporadic cases of this invasive infection have been reported in HIV and AIDS patients (Chandler, 1989; Kielhofner et al., 1992; Reiss et al., 1991; Scott et al., 1984). None of the patients had underlying diabetes, and all were severely immunocompromised with either markedly decreased CD4 cell counts or neutropenia.

Factors implicated in MOE include preexisting dermatitis of the external ear canal, concurrent medication with antibiotics, recent ear syringing, and immunosuppressive defects.

Treatment should include combination anti-*Pseudomonas* antibiotic therapy such as ciprofloxacin and ceftazidime. Mendelson et al. (Mendelson et al., 1994), in a study of 27 episodes of *Pseudomonas* bacteremia in AIDS patients, found that in an analysis of the effect of the number of agents used in the total intravenous course of treatment, mortality was 44.4% for one agent and 26.7% for two agents (p=0.036). Thus, the combination of two antimicrobial agents was found to be significantly more beneficial in treating *Pseudomonas* infection (Hern et al., 1996).

If a patient with HIV and AIDS presents with a history of intense otalgia and purulent otorrhea, a diagnosis of MOE should be considered and appropriate investigations undertaken.

2.6.2 Salmonella osteomyelitis

Nontyphoidal salmonella infections are recognized with increasing frequency in HIV-infected individuals. Recurrent bacteremia is the most common manifestation, while localized infections have rarely been described in patients with HIV infection (Sperber & Schleupner, 1987). It is known that *Salmonella* organisms can produce local pyogenic infections in any anatomic site (Cohen et al, 1987). Before the AIDS epidemic, suppurative complications were described in about 7% of salmonellosis cases (Sperber & Schleupner, 1987). There have been few reports of extraintestinal foci of infection with abscess formation in AIDS patients. However, a location in the bone is rare. Cohen et al. (Cohen et al, 1987) reported 150 cases of osteomyelitis, of which only three were localized in flat bones. Curiously, lesions were localized in flat cranial bones (parietal) in two of them (Mastroianni et al., 1992; Gato et al., 1989). The number of CD4-positive lymphocytes reflects a severe stage of immunocompromisation (Belzunegui et al., 1997).

One case with cranial *Salmonella* abscess with parietal bone osteomyelitis in an HIV-infected patient showed good recovery (Mastroianni et al., 1992). The use of an appropriate antibiotic, ciprofloxacin, with a high bactericidal activity against *Salmonella* and good intracellular penetration, allowed a favorable clinical outcome from the infection without surgical drainage or further complications. The antimicrobial susceptibility of these pathogens in patients with HIV infection does not appear to differ from that in other patients. They should be treated with ampicillin, amoxicillin, a third-generation cephalosporin or ciprofloxacin for 6 weeks or longer, and long-term therapy with an oral antimicrobial may be required in localized forms such as endocarditis or osteomyelitis in an effort to prevent relapse (Belzunegui et al., 1997).

Because bacteremia resulting from *Salmonella* organisms is common in HIV-infected individuals, it seems likely that more cases of *Salmonella* arthritis and osteomyelitis will be encountered in the future.

2.6.3 Mycobacterium osteomyelitis

Nontuberculous mycobacterial disease is common in patients with AIDS. Disseminated nontuberculous mycobacterium disease is a common problem for patients with advanced AIDS. *Mycobacterium avium complex* (MAC) accounts for 96% of reported cases, while *Mycobacterium kansasii (M. kansasii)* accounts for only 2.9% (Horsburgh & Selik, 1989). *M. kansasii* can cause tenosynovitis and soft-tissue infections. A few cases of skull osteomyelitis caused by *M. kansasii* have been reported (Weinroth et al., 1994).

Reports have described *M. kansasii* infections in patients with HIV infections (Valainis et al., 1991); disseminated disease is a common manifestation in these patients. It is also common to have mixed mycobacterial infections, usually including MAC.

Treatment of *M. kansasii* infections in non-HIV-infected patients usually involves administration of isoniazid, rifampin, and ethambutol for a period of 18–24 months. HIV-positive patients have been treated with the same regimen. However, most patients die prior to completion of therapy. Disseminated disease is universally fatal; the mean survival time is ~6 months from initial diagnosis (Weinroth et al., 1994).

2.7 Syphilitic osteomyelitis

Although there was no evidence by serologic test or pathological evaluations, *Treponema pallidum (T. pallidum)* infection is reported to have existed prior to AD 300 (Gerszten et al., 1998). Syphilis is a chronic systemic infectious disease caused by the spirochete *T. pallidum*. In acquired syphilitic infection, the organism has an incubation period lasting about 3 weeks, after which the disease exhibits four classically described clinical stages. In the primary stage, infection is characterized by a non-painful skin lesion (chancre) that is usually associated with regional lymphadenopathy and initial bacteremia. A secondary bacteremic or disseminated stage is associated with generalized mucocutaneous lesions, lymphadenopathy, and variable array of clinical findings. Latent syphilis, having no clinical manifestations, is detected only by reactive serologic tests. A late or tertiary stage occurs in up to one-third of untreated patients 10–30 years later, with typical involvement of the ascending aorta and central nervous and skeletal systems (Fenton et al., 2008).

Syphilitic osteomyelitis of the skull is a destructive bone disease that occurs as a complication of syphilis. Bone and joint involvement is well described in cases of congenital syphilis, but bone involvement is an unusual manifestation of acquired syphilis (Gurland et al., 2001). The incidence of symptomatic syphilitic osteomyelitis among patients with primary and secondary syphilis is quite rare. In a retrospective review of 854 patients who were diagnosed with secondary syphilis, osteomyelitis was found in only two patients (0.2%) (Mindel et al., 1989). Destructive bone lesions are rare complications of early-stage syphilis. However, because the clinical presentation is often nonspecific, the diagnosis can be overlooked in the absence of other syphilitic symptoms. Acquired syphilitic osteomyelitis has been described in only a few case reports in the literature (Chung et al., 1994; Gurland et al., 2001; Huang et al., 2007; Kang et al., 2010). Symptomatic bone involvement in association with syphilis is very unusual.

Presentations have varied, but bone pain is routinely found. Lymphadenopathy is also frequently reported. In early-acquired syphilis, the secondary spirochetemia that resulted after primary infection can lead to infection and involvement of the deeper vascular areas of the periosteum with production of perivascular inflammatory infiltrates and highly cellular granulation tissue. The inflammatory process extends into the Haversian canals, with resultant osteitis and osteomyelitis (Ehrlich & Kricun, 1976). The medullary canals enlarge with increasing osteolysis. With continued inflammation and bone lysis, an irregular macerated appearance of the bone results. New bone formation can occur, sometimes in a prominent manner, typically along the periphery of the lesion (Turk, 1995).

Radiography of affected bones can demonstrate an osteolytic lesion. Pathological examination can demonstrate a plasma cell and lymphocytic perivascular infiltration of the bone and the surrounding tissue (Gurland et al., 2001). Radiologically, it is difficult to distinguish syphilitic osteomyelitis from other radiolucent lesions of the skull, such as eosinophilic granuloma, multiple myeloma, or cystic fibrous dysplasia. MRI can demonstrate marrow space involvement, the periosteal process, and the degree of intracranial extension more completely than CT. MRI findings in acquired syphilitic osteitis of the calvaria showed a focal enhancing calvarial lesion and adjacent soft tissue abnormality in the scalp (Gurland et al., 2001) (Fig. 8).

The differential diagnosis for lytic bone lesions is very extensive. We suggest that a diagnosis of syphilis be considered for at-risk patients with lytic bone lesions. In addition, since osteomyelitis is a manifestation of secondary syphilis, a serum rapid plasma reagin test, or venereal disease research laboratory (VDRL) test, or *T. pallidum* haemagglutination assay (TPHA) should be sufficient to exclude syphilis as a possibility. The presence of organisms on biopsy material is variably seen and is less common in late-stage disease. One report notes that spirochete visualization by dark field microscopy is present in only 50% of biopsied cases of bone involvement in early-stage syphilis (Halm, 1979).

Syphilitic osteomyelitis can be treated with antibiotic therapy, benzathine penicillin, or ceftriaxone (Dismukes et al., 1976; Fenton et al., 2008). Although symptomatic relief after therapy is typically rapid, the osseous lesions in early-phase syphilis resolve more slowly and can persist for up to 7-11 months. With proper therapy, there can be complete conventional radiographic and imaging resolution of lesions, with little residual abnormality (Gurland et al., 2001). Early recognition will result in prompt therapy of this treatable condition.

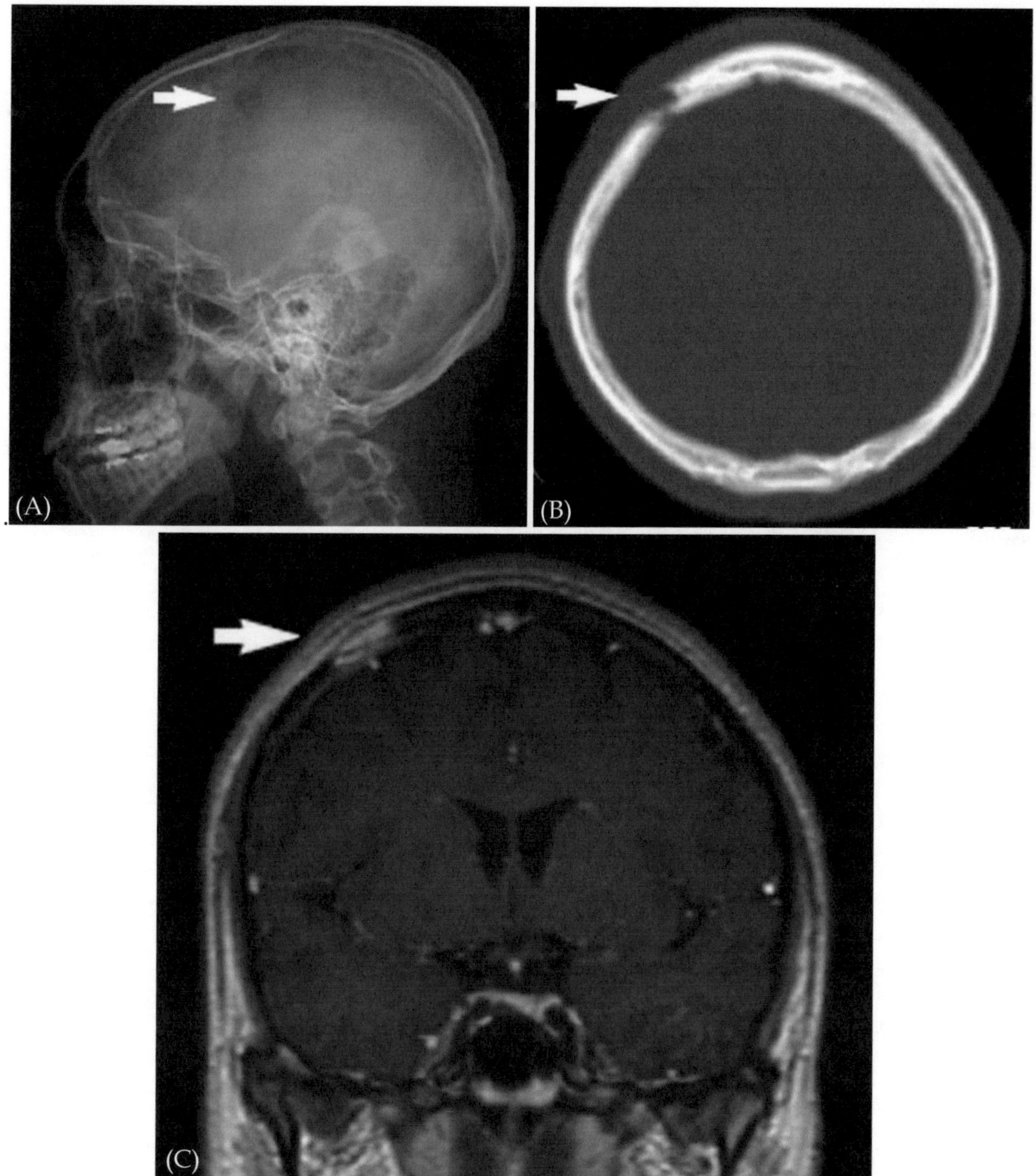

Fig. 8. The imaging study of syphilitic osteomyelitis in a 20-year-old man. A: Skull lateral X-ray image shows a 17-mm radiolucent skull lesion (arrow) of the parietal bone. B: Computed tomography shows a 17-mm osteolytic skull lesion (arrow) involving the whole thickness of the right parietal bone. C: A coronal magnetic resonance imaging section shows a well-enhanced mass lesion involving the whole thickness of the skull (arrow) at the right parietal area and surrounding soft tissue swelling. (Reproduced with permission from. Kang, SH., Park, SW., Kwon, KY., & Hong, WJ. (2010). A solitary skull lesion of syphilitic osteomyelitis. *J Korean Neurosurg Soc,* Vol.48, No.1, (July 2010), pp. 85-87, ISSN 2005-3711) (Kang et al., 2010)

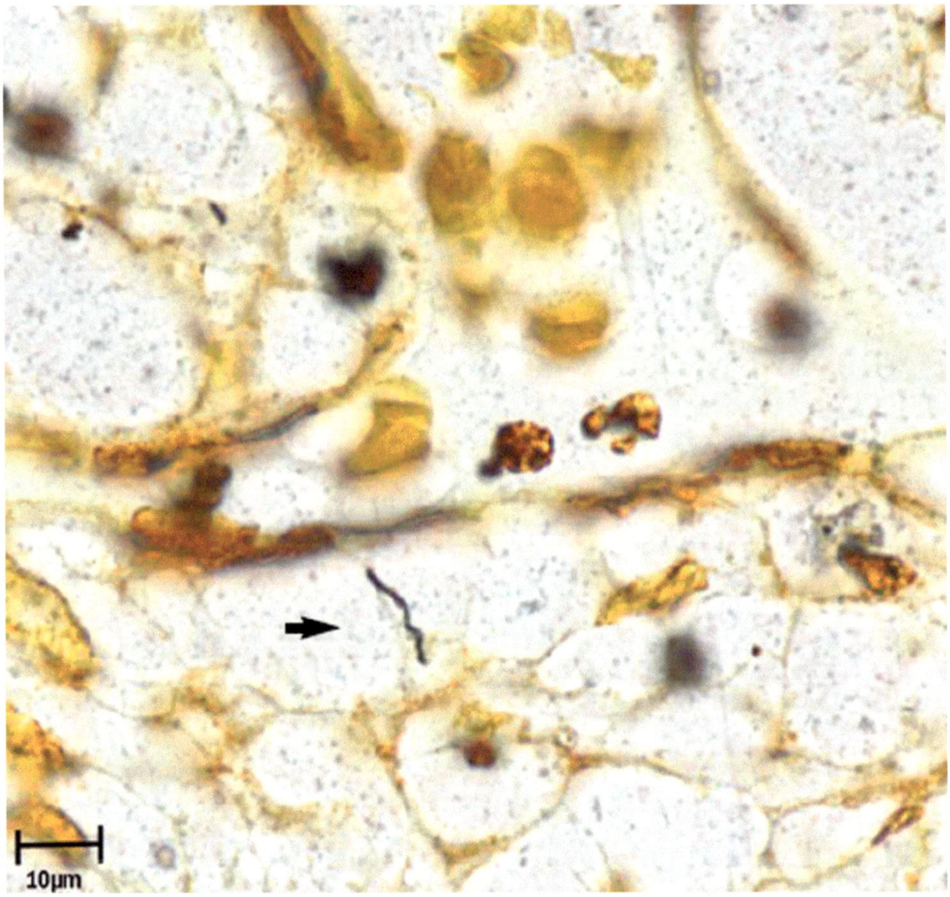

Fig. 9. Identification of spirochetes by Warthin-Starry staining in a skull bone specimen (×1000). Arrow indicates the *Treponema pallidum*. (Reproduced with permission from. Kang, SH., Park, SW., Kwon, KY., & Hong, WJ. (2010). A solitary skull lesion of syphilitic osteomyelitis. *J Korean Neurosurg Soc,* Vol.48, No.1, (July 2010), pp. 85-87, ISSN 2005-3711) (Kang et al., 2010)

2.8 Tubercular osteomyelitis

Skull osteomyelitis may also result from infection of the bone by tubercular bacilli (Bhatia et al., 1980). Calvarial tuberculosis is an uncommon form of tuberculosis and is usually seen in younger patients. Most cases reported in the literature are from countries with a high incidence of tuberculosis. The incidence of bone tuberculosis appears to be falling (LeRoux et al., 1990). The overall incidence of skull tuberculosis is approximately 1/10,000 cases of tuberculosis (Davidson & Horowitz, 1970; Prinsloo & Kirsten, 1977). Tubercular osteomyelitis is caused by haematogenous or by lymphatic dissemination of bacilli from an active focus, usually in the lungs (Bhatia et al., 1980; Joseph et al., 1989). Many authors have stressed the importance of lymphatics in the spread of tuberculosis. The relative paucity of lymphatics in the cranium has been considered to account for the infrequent tuberculosis infections of the skull bones (Scoggin et al., 1976).

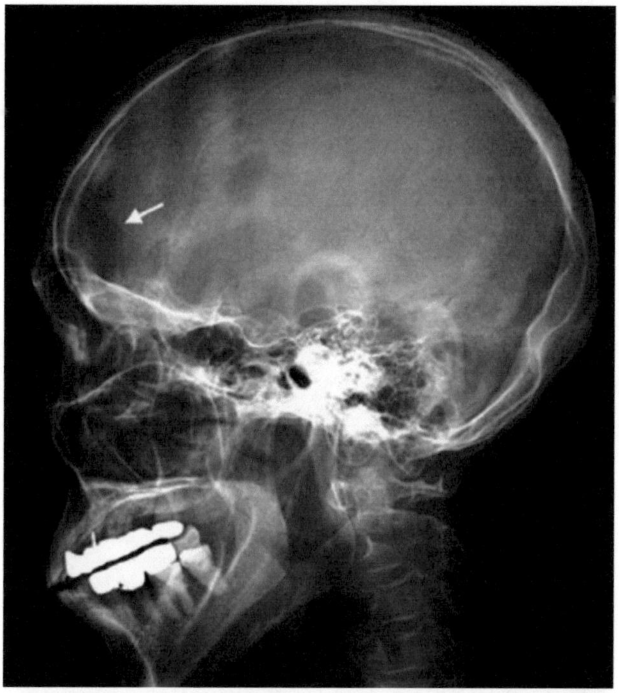

Fig. 10. (A)

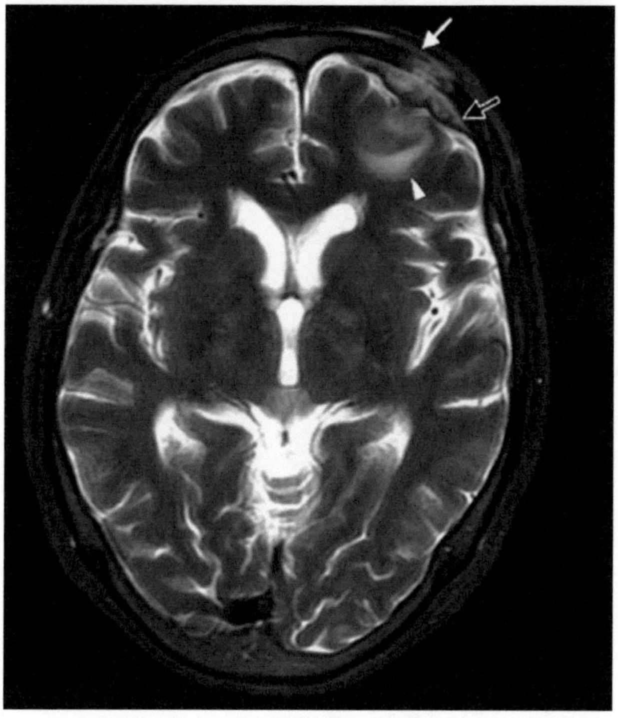

Fig. 10. (B)

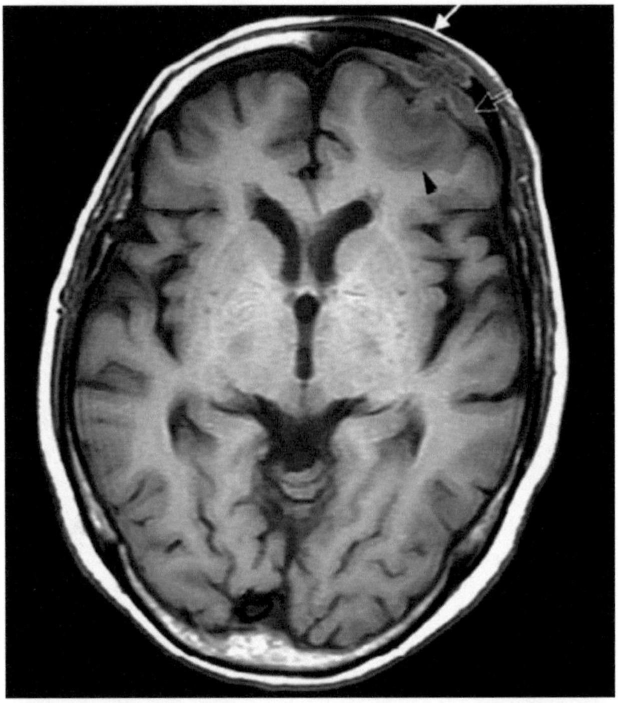

Fig. 10. (C)

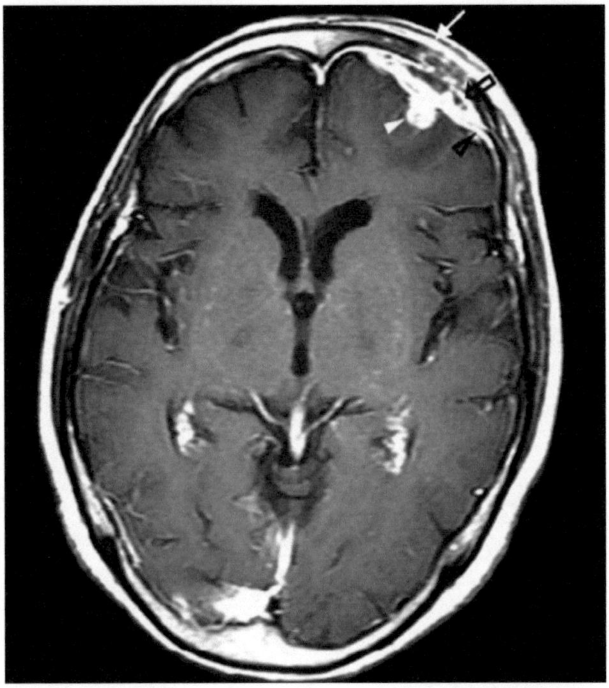

Fig. 10. (D)

Fig. 10. Simple radiography (A) and magnetic resonance imaging (B–D). A: Skull lateral radiography shows the ovoid osteolytic lesion (arrow) without sclerosis in the left frontal bone. B. T2-weighted image shows high signal intensity lesions on the left frontal bone diploe, subgaleal space (white arrow), and extradural space (open arrow). High signal intensity is also noted on the left frontal lobe (arrowhead). C. T1-weighted image shows low signal intensity lesions in the left frontal bone and the adjacent frontal lobe. D. Contrast-enhanced T1-weighted image shows homogeneous enhancement on the subgaleal space (arrow), peripheral rim enhancement on the extradural space (open arrow), and small nodular enhancement on the right frontal lobe cortex (arrowhead). Thick enhancement along dura (open arrowhead) is also noted. (Reproduced with permission from Kang, M., Cho, JH., Choi, S., Yoon, SK., Kim, KN., & Lee, JH. (2008). The MRI Findings of Skull Tuberculosis: A Case Report. *J Korean Radiol Soc*, Vol.58, No.1, (January 2008), pp. 17-20, ISSN 1738-2637) (Kang et al., 2008).

Tuberculosis of the skull is commonly associated with tuberculosis elsewhere in the body. The setting of the bacillus in the diploe marks the onset of acute inflammation surrounded by fibroblasts. Granulation tissue takes place in the bone trabeculae, and Langhans giant cells and epithelioid histiocytes appear (LeRoux et al., 1990). Because the dura is extremely resistant to calvarial tuberculosis, tuberculosis meningitis is rare (LeRoux et al., 1990). With further development, cold abscess formation appears. Tuberculosis of the skull usually appears as a painless mass or ulcer. Systemic manifestations are unusual; headache may occur, but fever is rarely present. Intracranial extension is uncommon, although complications such as tuberculous meningitis or encephalitis have been reported (Scoggin et al., 1976). Clinically, the disease is characterized by lack of early symptoms, and the appearance of fluctuant swelling is usually the first symptom (it is one of the causes of Pott's puffy tumor). The swelling has a soft, fluctuant center with a surrounding firmly attached base, and can thus be differentiated from cephalohematoma. Skin attachment, discoloration, and sinus formation are late features. Headache can occur, but pain localized to the site of the lesion is more common (Malhotra et al., 1993).

Radiologically, tubercular osteomyelitis showed lytic lesions with or without areas of sclerosis. A similar radiological picture may be seen in congenital syphilis, eosinophilic granuloma, or secondary malignant deposits (Bhandari et al., 1981; Bhatia et al., 1980). Radiological findings are nonspecific. The commonest radiological lesion of tubercular osteitis is a single calvarial defect in the frontal or parietal region (Shahat et al., 2004). Both osteolytic and osteoblastic features are seen. Lesions that are usually lytic at first can normally be seen on plain X-ray images of the skull, and are helpful for diagnosis (Schuster et al., 1984). A technetium scan can be helpful to delineate the expansion of the lesion and to rule out meningeal or cerebral involvement.

Cases of tubercular osteomyelitis have been diagnosed on the basis of pathological evaluation of fine needle aspirates and tissue biopsies from the infected bones (Sethi et al., 2008). In all cases, histopathological evaluation has showed epithelioid, caseating granulomas. The presence of caseating granulomas is strongly suggestive of tuberculosis (Bhatia et al., 1980; Joseph et al., 1989). Diagnosis is further supported by positive acid-fast bacilli (AFB) staining, indicating enzyme-linked immunosorbent assay seropositivity for *M. tuberculosis.* Another test that can be used in the diagnosis of tuberculosis is the polymerase chain reaction, which is considered to have a high sensitivity and specificity. The identification of tuberculous bacillus at the site of the lesion confirms the diagnosis (Gupta et al., 1989; LeRoux et al., 1990). The differential diagnosis of tuberculosis includes pyogenic osteomyelitis, calvarial metastasis, hemangiomas, aneurismal bone cysts, meningiomas, and histiocytosis (Gupta et al., 1989).

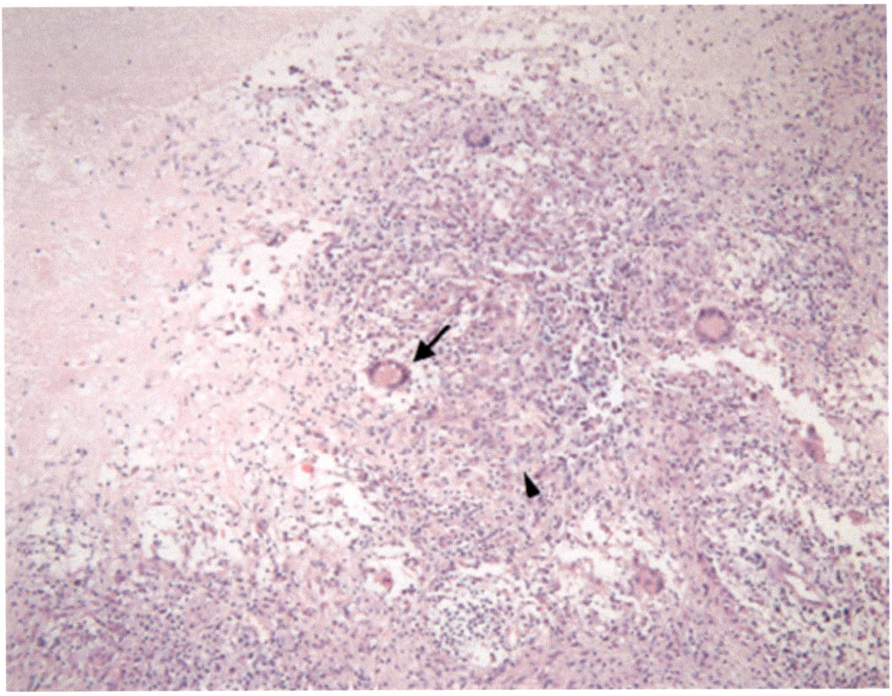

Fig. 11. Microscopic findings (hematoxylin and eosin, ×100). Characteristic granuloma composed of central caseous necrosis surrounding epithelioid histiocytes (arrowhead), multinucleated giant cells (arrow), and lymphocytes. The finding is compatible with tuberculosis. (Reproduced with permission from Kang, M., Cho, JH., Choi, S., Yoon, SK., Kim, KN., & Lee, JH. (2008). The MRI Findings of Skull Tuberculosis: A Case Report. *J Korean Radiol Soc*, Vol.58, No.1, (January 2008), pp. 17-20, ISSN 1738-2637) (Kang et al., 2008)

The available treatment options are antituberculous chemotherapy and surgery. The role of surgery in the treatment of tuberculous osteomyelitis has declined markedly with the advent of effective antituberculous chemotherapy. Current indications for surgery include the treatment of a subperiosteal abscess and the removal of a sequestrum. Surgical treatment is also considered when the lesion creates a mass effect, when there is an increase in intracranial pressure, or when the patient has a large collection of caseous material (Gupta et al., 1989). However, the treatment of tubercular osteomyelitis is primarily medical, in the form of antituberculous chemotherapy (Sethi et al., 2008).

Tuberculosis of the skull should be suspected in any case of secreting lesions of the scalp that are apparently sterile or fail to respond to conventional antibiotic therapy. It is also important to consider tuberculosis as a cause of postoperative osteomyelitis, as its treatment is quite distinct from pyogenic osteomyelitis, which is the commonest cause of postoperative osteomyelitis. Hence, all bone flaps that are removed for suspected osteomyelitis should be sent for histopathological examination and for AFB and fungal cultures, in addition to routine cultures (Biniwale & Rajshekhar, 2000). Especially in developing countries, tuberculosis should be borne in mind in the differential diagnosis of skull osteomyelitis. Prognosis depends on the gravity of the local disease, but currently, with chemotherapy, it is usually good (Malhotra et al., 1993).

Tuberculosis focused in the calvarium can extend subperiosteally as a swelling under the scalp, and the same lesion could extend into the epidural space as a granuloma. However, an efficient antituberculous regimen and supportive therapy have virtually eliminated such lesions.

3. Conclusion

Greater awareness, new diagnostic methods, and better treatment for people with ready access to modern health care have led to a decrease in the rate of treatment failure in acute skull osteomyelitis. Infection control strategies and prophylactic antibiotics have further lowered the rate of postoperative infection. However, skull osteomyelitis has recently become more important because of its association with HIV infection, prolonged neutropenia, critically ill patients in intensive care, chemotherapy for solid tumors, and organ transplant. Early diagnosis, identification of the causative pathogens, prompt initiation of appropriate antimicrobial or surgical therapies, and continuation of therapy for an adequate period are essential when managing skull osteomyelitis. The most important thing in diagnosing skull osteomyelitis is suspicion. Early recognition will result in prompt therapy of this treatable condition.

4. Acknowledgement

This work was supported by research grant from an Inje University College of Medicine.

5. References

Alexander, JW., Fischer, JE., Boyajian, M., Palmquist, J., & Morris, MJ. (1983). The influence of hair-removal methods on wound infections. *Arch Surg,* Vol.118, No.3, (March 1983), pp. 347-352, ISSN 0004-0010

Alva, B., Prasad, KC., Prasad, SC., & Pallavi, S. (2009). Temporal bone osteomyelitis and temporoparietal abscess secondary to malignant otitis externa. *J Laryngol Otol,* Vol.123, No.11, (November 2009), pp. 1288-1291, ISSN 0022-2151

Allen, DB., Maguire, JJ., Mahdavian, M., Wicke, C., Marcocci, L., Scheuenstuhl, H., Chang, M., Le, AX., Hopf, HW., & Hunt, TK. (1997). Wound hypoxia and acidosis limit neutrophil bacterial killing mechanisms. *Arch Surg,* Vol.132, No.9, (September 1997), pp. 991-996, ISSN 0004-0010

Arana, E., Diaz, C., Latorre, FF., Menor, F., Revert, A., Beltrán, A., & Navarro, M. (1996). Primary intraosseous meningiomas. *Acta Radiol,* Vol.37, No.6, (November 1996), pp. 937-942, ISSN 0284-1851

Argenta, LC., & Morykwas, MJ. (1997). Vacuum-assisted closure: a new method for wound control and treatment: clinical experience. *Ann Plast Surg,* Vol.38, No.6, (Junuary 1997), pp. 563-577, ISSN 0148-7043

Armonda, RA., Fleckenstein, JM., Brandvold, B., & Ondra, SL. (1993). Cryptococcal skull infection: a case report with review of the literature. *Neurosurgery,* Vol.32, No.6, (June 1993), pp. 1034-1036, ISSN 0148-396X

Arnold, PM., Govindan, S., & Anderson, KK. (2009). Spontaneous cranial osteomyelitis in an otherwise healthy ten-year-old male. *Pediatr Neurosurg, Vol.*45, No.6, (2009). pp. 407-409, ISSN 1016-2291

Asai, S., Kamei, Y., & Torii, S. (2004). One-stage reconstruction of infected cranial defects using a titanium mesh plate enclosed in an omental flap. *Ann Plast Surg,* Vol.52, No.2, (February 2004), pp. 144-147, ISSN 0148-7043

Azizi, SA., Fayad, PB., Fulbright, R., Giroux, ML., & Waxman, SG. (1995). Clivus and cervical spinal osteomyelitis with epidural abscess presenting with multiple cranial neuropathies. *Clin Neurol Neurosurg,* Vol.97, No.3, (August 1995), pp. 239-244, ISSN 0303-8467

Bahna, MS., Ward, PH., & Konrad, HR. (1980). Nasopharyngeal mucormycotic osteitis: a new syndrome characterized by initial presentation of multiple cranial nerve palsies. *Otolaryngol Head Neck Surg,* Vol.88, No.2, (March-April 1980), pp. 146-153, ISSN 0194-5998

Bambakidis, NC., & Cohen, AR. (2001). Intracranial complications of frontal sinusitis in children: Pott's puffy tumor revisited. *Pediatr Neurosurg,* Vol.35, No.2, (August 2001), pp. 82-89, ISSN 1016-2291

Barker, FG, 2nd. (1994). Efficacy of prophylactic antibiotics for craniotomy: a meta-analysis. *Neurosurgery,* Vol.35, No.3, (September 1994), pp. 484-492, ISSN 0148-396X

Beeram, V., Challa, S., & Vannemreddy, P. (2008). Cerebral mycetoma with cranial osteomyelitis. *J Neurosurg Pediatr,* Vol.1, No.6, (June 2008), pp. 493-495, ISSN 1933-0707

Belzunegui, J., Lopez, L., Arrizabalaga, J., Gonzalez, C., & Figueroa, M. (1997). Salmonella osteomyelitis in a patient with human immunodeficiency virus infection. *Clin Rheumatol,* Vol.16, No.3, (May 1997), pp. 319-320, ISSN 0770-3198

Bhandari, B., Mandowara, SL., & Joshi, H. (1981). Tubercular osteomyelitis of skull. *Indian J Pediatr,* Vol.48, No.390, (January-February 1981), pp. 113-115, ISSN 0019-5456

Bhatia, PL., Agarwal, MK., Gupta, OP., & Khanna, S. (1980). Tubercular osteomyelitis of facial bones. *Ear Nose Throat J,* Vol.59, No.8, (August 1980), pp. 310-317, ISSN 0145-5613

Bickley, LS., Betts, RF., & Parkins, CW. (1988). Atypical invasive external otitis from Aspergillus. *Arch Otolaryngol Head Neck Surg,* Vol.114, No.9, (September 1988), pp. 1024-1028, ISSN 0886-4470

Biniwale, SN., & Rajshekhar, V. (2000). Tuberculous osteomyelitis of the bone flap following craniotomy for a glioma. *Neurol India,* Vol.48, No.1, (March 2000), pp. 91-92, ISSN 0028-3886

Blitzer, A., Lawson, W., Meyers, BR., & Biller, HF. (1980). Patient survival factors in paranasal sinus mucormycosis. *Laryngoscope,* Vol.90, No.4, (April 1980), pp. 635-648, ISSN 0023-852X

Blomstedt, GC. (1992). Craniotomy infections. *Neurosurg Clin N Am,* Vol.3, No.2, (April 1992), pp. 375-385, ISSN 1042-3680

Blyth, CC., Gomes, L., Sorrell, TC., da Cruz, M., Sud, A., & Chen, SC. (2011). Skull-base osteomyelitis: fungal vs. bacterial infection. *Clin Microbiol Infect,* Vol.17, No.2, (February 2011), pp. 306-311, ISSN 1198-743X

Braun, OH., & Kreipe, U. (1979). Rare forms of chronic osteomyelitis in children (author's transl). *Klin Padiatr,* Vol.191, No.5, (September 1979), pp. 511-521, ISSN 0300-8630

Brook, I. (2009). Microbiology and antimicrobial treatment of orbital and intracranial complications of sinusitis in children and their management. *Int J Pediatr Otorhinolaryngol,* Vol.73, No.9, (September 2009), pp. 1183-1186, ISSN 0165-5876

Bruce, JN., & Bruce, SS. (2003). Preservation of bone flaps in patients with postcraniotomy infections. *J Neurosurg,* Vol.98, No.6, (June 2003), pp. 1203-1207, ISSN 0022-3085

Chamilos, G., Lewis, RE., & Kontoyiannis, DP. (2008). Delaying amphotericin B-based frontline therapy significantly increases mortality among patients with hematologic malignancy who have zygomycosis. *Clin Infect Dis,* Vol.47, No.4, (August 2008), pp. 503-509, ISSN 1058-4838

Chan, MS., Wong, YC., Lau, SP., Lau, KY., & Ou, Y. (2002). MRI and CT findings of infected cephalhaematoma complicated by skull vault osteomyelitis, transverse venous sinus thrombosis and cerebellar haemorrhage. *Pediatr Radiol,* Vol.32, No.5, (May 2002), pp. 376-379, ISSN 0301-0449

Chandler, JR. (1968). Malignant external otitis. *Laryngoscope,* Vol.78, No.8, (August 1968), pp. 1257-1294, ISSN 0023-852X

Chandler, JR. (1989). Malignant external otitis and osteomyelitis of the base of the skull. *Am J Otol,* Vol.10, No.2, (March 1989), pp. 108-110, ISSN 0192-9763

Chandler, JR., Grobman, L., Quencer, R., & Serafini, A. (1986). Osteomyelitis of the base of the skull. *Laryngoscope,* Vol.96, No.3, (March 1986), pp. 245-251, ISSN 0023-852X

Chang, HY., Chiu, NC., Huang, FY., Kao, HA., Hsu, CH., & Hung, HY. (2005). Infected cephalohematoma of newborns: experience in a medical center in Taiwan. *Pediatr Int,* Vol.47, No.3, (June 2005), pp. 274-277, ISSN 1328-8067

Chang, PC., Fischbein, NJ., & Holliday, RA. (2003). Central skull base osteomyelitis in patients without otitis externa: imaging findings. *AJNR Am J Neuroradiol,* Vol.24, No.7, (August 2003), pp. 1310-1316, ISSN 0195-6108

Chayakulkeeree, M., & Perfect, JR. (2006). Cryptococcosis. *Infect Dis Clin North Am,* Vol.20, No.3, (September 2006), pp. 507-544, ISSN 0891-5520

Chou, SN., & Erickson, DL. (1976). Craniotomy infections. *Clin Neurosurg,* Vol.23, pp. 357-362, ISSN 0069-4827

Christianson, JC., Engber, W., & Andes, D. (2003). Primary cutaneous cryptococcosis in immunocompetent and immunocompromised hosts. *Med Mycol,* Vol.41, No.3, (June 2003), pp. 177-188, ISSN 1369-3786

Chung, KY., Yoon, J., Heo, JH., Lee, MG., Jang, JW., & Lee, JB. (1994). Osteitis of the skull in secondary syphilis. *J Am Acad Dermatol,* Vol.30, No.5 Pt 1, (May 1994), pp. 793-794, ISSN 0190-9622

Cohen, D., & Friedman, P. (1987). The diagnostic criteria of malignant external otitis. *J Laryngol Otol,* Vol.101, No.3, (March 1987), pp. 216-221, ISSN 0022-2151

Cohen, JI., Bartlett, JA., & Corey, GR. (1987). Extra-intestinal manifestations of salmonella infections. *Medicine (Baltimore),* Vol.66, No.5, (September 1987), pp. 349-388, ISSN 0025-7974

Corral, JE., Lima, S., Quezada, J., Samayoa, B., & Arathoon, E. (2011). Cryptococcal osteomyelitis of the skull. *Med Mycol,* Vol.49, No.6, (August 2011), pp. 667-671, ISSN 1369-3786

Davidson, PT., & Horowitz, I. (1970). Skeletal tuberculosis. A review with patient presentations and discussion. *Am J Med,* Vol.48, No.1, (January 1970), pp. 77-84, ISSN 0002-9343

Dismukes, WE., Delgado, DG., Mallernee, SV., & Myers, TC. (1976). Destructive bone disease in early syphilis. *JAMA,* Vol.236, No.23, (December 1976), pp. 2646-2648, ISSN 0098-7484

Driscoll, PV., Ramachandrula, A., Drezner, DA., Hicks, TA., & Schaffer, SR. (1993). Characteristics of cerumen in diabetic patients: a key to understanding malignant external otitis? *Otolaryngol Head Neck Surg,* Vol.109, No.4, (October 1993), pp. 676-679, ISSN 0194-5998

Durur-Subasi, I., Kantarci, M., Karakaya, A., Orbak, Z., Ogul, H., & Alp, H. (2008). Pott's puffy tumor: multidetector computed tomography findings. *J Craniofac Surg,* Vol.19, No.6, (November 2008), pp. 1697-1699, ISSN 1049-2275

Ehrlich, R., & Kricun, ME. (1976). Radiographic findings in early acquired syphilis: case report and cirtical review. *AJR Am J Roentgenol,* Vol.127, No.5, (November 1976), pp. 789-792, ISSN 0361-803X

Erman, T., Demirhindi, H., Gocer, AI., Tuna, M., Ildan, F., & Boyar, B. (2005). Risk factors for surgical site infections in neurosurgery patients with antibiotic prophylaxis. *Surg Neurol,* Vol.63, No.2, (February 2005), pp. 107-113, ISSN 0090-3019

Farr, RC., Gardner, G., Acker, JD., Brint, JM., Haglund, LF., Land, M., Schweitzer, JB., & West, BC. (1992). Blastomycotic cranial osteomyelitis. *Am J Otol,* Vol.13, No.6, (November 1992), pp. 582-586, ISSN 0192-9763

Fenton, KA., Breban, R., Vardavas, R., Okano, JT., Martin, T., Aral, S., & Blower, S. (2008). Infectious syphilis in high-income settings in the 21st century. *Lancet Infect Dis,* Vol.8, No.4, (April 2008), pp. 244-253, ISSN 1473-3099

Finn, DG., & Farmer, JC, Jr. (1982). Chronic mucormycosis. *Laryngoscope,* Vol.92, No.7Pt 1, (July 1982), pp. 761-766, ISSN 0023-852X

Fleisher, G., Henry, W., McSorley, M., Arbeter, A., & Plotkin, S. (1981). Life-threatening complications of varicella. *Am J Dis Child,* Vol.135, No.10, (October 1981), pp. 896-899, ISSN 0002-922X

Forgie, SE., & Marrie, TJ. (2008). Pott's puffy tumor. *Am J Med,* Vol.121, No.12, (December 2008), pp. 1041-1042, ISSN 0002-9343

Froeschner, EH. (1992). Two examples of ancient skull surgery. *J Neurosurg,* Vol.76, No.3, (March 1992), pp. 550-552, ISSN 0022-3085

Gallagher, PG. (1990). Osteomyelitis of the skull after varicella infection. *Clin Pediatr (Phila),* Vol.29, No.1, (January 1990), pp. 29, ISSN 0009-9228

Gamba, JL., Woodruff, WW., Djang, WT., & Yeates, AE. (1986). Craniofacial mucormycosis: assessment with CT. *Radiology,* Vol.160, No.1, (July 1986), pp. 207-212, ISSN 0033-8419

Gato, DA., Perez, GV., Ballesteros, MP., & Gaspar, AVG. (1989). Salmonella osteomyelitis in an AIDS patient. *An Med Interna,* Vol.6, No.11, (November 1989), pp. 603, ISSN 0212-7199

Gerszten, PC., Gerszten, E., & Allison, MJ. (1998). Diseases of the skull in pre-Columbian South American mummies. *Neurosurgery,* Vol.42, No.5, (May 1998), pp. 1145-1152, ISSN 0148-396X

Gherini, SG., Brackmann, DE., & Bradley, WG. (1986). Magnetic resonance imaging and computerized tomography in malignant external otitis. *Laryngoscope,* Vol.96, No.5, (May 1986), pp. 542-548, ISSN 0023-852X

Goodrich, JT. (2005). Landmarks in the history of neurosurgery, In: *Principles of neurosurgery 2nd ed,* S.S. Rengachary & R.G. Ellenbogen, (Eds.), pp. 1-37, Elsevier Mosby, ISBN 978-0-7234-3222-7, Philadelphia, PA, U.S.A.

Goodrich, JT., & Flamm, ES. (2011). Historical overview of neurosurgery, In: *Youmans Neurological Surgery 6th ed,* H.R. Winn, (Ed.), pp. 3-37, Elsevier Sanuders, ISBN 978-1-4160-5316-3, Philadelphia, PA, U.S.A.

Goodwin, MD., Persing, JA., Duncan, CC., & Shin, JH. (2000). Spontaneously infected cephalohematoma: case report and review of the literature. *J Craniofac Surg,* Vol.11, No.4, (July 2000), pp. 371-375, ISSN 1049-2275

Gordon, G., & Giddings, NA. (1994). Invasive otitis externa due to Aspergillus species: case report and review. *Clin Infect Dis,* Vol.19, No.5. (November 1994), pp. 866-870, ISSN 1058-4838

Grobman, LR., Ganz, W., Casiano, R., & Goldberg, S. (1989). Atypical osteomyelitis of the skull base. *Laryngoscope,* Jul;Vol.99, No.7 Pt 1, (July 1989), pp. 671-676, ISSN 0023-852X

Gupta, M., El-Hakim, H., Bhargava, R., & Mehta, V. (2004). Pott's puffy tumour in a pre-adolescent child: the youngest reported in the post-antibiotic era. *Int J Pediatr Otorhinolaryngol,* Vol.68, No.3, (March 2004), pp. 373-378, ISSN 0165-5876

Gupta, PK., Kolluri, VR., Chandramouli, BA., Venkataramana, NK., & Das, BS. (1989). Calvarial tuberculosis: a report of two cases. *Neurosurgery,* Vol.25, No.5, (November 1989), pp. 830-833, ISSN 0148-396X

Gurland, IA., Korn, L., Edelman, L., & Wallach, F. (2001). An unusual manifestation of acquired syphilis. *Clin Infect Dis,* Vol.32, No.4, (February 2001), pp. 667-669, ISSN 1058-4838

Guyot, LL., Duffy, CB., Guthikonda, M., & Natarajan, SK. (2006). Epidural abscess, subdural empyema, and brain abscess, In: *Atlas of neurosurgical techniques. Brain,* L.N. Sekhar & R.G. Fessler, (Eds.), pp. 975-980, Thieme Medical Publishers, Inc., ISBN 0-86577-920-1, New York, NY, U.S.A.

Halm, DE. (1979). Bone lesions in early syphilis, case report. *Nebr Med J,* Vol.64, No.10, (October 1979), pp. 310-312, ISSN 0091-6730

Hamilton, JR., & Overall, JC, Jr. (1978). Synergistic infection with murine cytomegalovirus and Pseudomonas aeruginosa in mice. *J Infect Dis,* Vol.137, No.6, (June 1978), pp. 775-782, ISSN 0022-1899

Hanna, E., Hughes, G., Eliachar, I., Wanamaker, J., & Tomford, W. (1993). Fungal osteomyelitis of the temporal bone: a review of reported cases. *Ear Nose Throat J,* Vol.72, No.8, (August 1993), pp. 532, 537-41, ISSN 0145-5613

Hern, JD., Almeyda, J., Thomas, DM., Main, J., & Patel, KS. (1996). Malignant otitis externa in HIV and AIDS. *J Laryngol Otol,* Vol.110, No.8, (August 1996), pp. 770-775, ISSN 0022-2151

Hoistad, DL., & Duvall AJ, 3rd. (1999). Sinusitis with contiguous abscess involvement of the clivus and petrous apices. Case report. *Ann Otol Rhinol Laryngol,* Vol.108, No.5, (May 1999), pp. 463-466, ISSN 0003-4894

Horsburgh CR, Jr., & Selik, RM. (1989). The epidemiology of disseminated nontuberculous mycobacterial infection in the acquired immunodeficiency syndrome (AIDS). *Am Rev Respir Dis,* Vol.139, No.1, (January 1989), pp. 4-7, ISSN 0003-0805

Hosein, IK., Hill, DW., & Hatfield, RH. (1999). Controversies in the prevention of neurosurgical infection. *J Hosp Infect,* Vol.43, No.1, (September 1999), pp. 5-11, ISSN 0195-6701

Huang, I., Leach, JL., Fichtenbaum, CJ., & Narayan, RK. (2007). Osteomyelitis of the skull in early-acquired syphilis: evaluation by MR imaging and CT. *AJNR Am J Neuroradiol,* Vol.28, No.2, (February 2007). pp. 307-308, ISSN 0195-6108

Joseph, T., Mishra, HB., & Singh, JP. (1989). Primary tuberculous osteomyelitis of skull: report of two cases. *Br J Neurosurg,* Vol.3, No.6, pp. 705-707, ISSN 0268-8697

Kacl, GM., Carls, FR., Moll, C., & Debatin, JF. (1999). Interactive MR-guided biopsies of maxillary and skull-base lesions in an open-MR system: first clinical results. *Eur Radiol,* ;Vol.9, No.3, pp. 487-492, ISSN 0938-7994

Kang, M., Cho, JH., Choi, S., Yoon, SK., Kim, KN., & Lee, JH. (2008). The MRI Findings of Skull Tuberculosis: A Case Report. *J Korean Radiol Soc,* Vol.58, No.1, (January 2008), pp. 17-20, ISSN 1738-2637

Kang, SH., Park, SW., Kwon, KY., & Hong, WJ. (2010). A solitary skull lesion of syphilitic osteomyelitis. *J Korean Neurosurg Soc,* Vol.48, No.1, (July 2010), pp. 85-87, ISSN 2005-3711

Karaman, E., Hacizade, Y., Isildak, H., & Kaytaz, A. (2008). Pott's puffy tumor. *J Craniofac Surg,* Vol.19, No.6, (November 2008), pp. 1694-1697, ISSN 1049-2275

Kielhofner, M., Atmar, RL., Hamill, RJ., & Musher, DM. (1992). Life-threatening Pseudomonas aeruginosa infections in patients with human immunodeficiency virus infection. *Clin Infect Dis,* Vol.14, No.2, (February 1992), pp. 403-411, ISSN 1058-4838

Klisch, J., Spreer, J., Bötefür, I., Gellrich, NC., Adler, CP., Zentner, J., & Schumacher, M. (2002). Calvarial sclerosing osteomyelitis. *Pediatr Neurosurg,* Vol.36, No.3, (March 2002), pp. 128-132, ISSN 1016-2291

Koorbusch, GF., Fotos, P., & Goll, KT. (1992). Retrospective assessment of osteomyelitis. Etiology, demographics, risk factors, and management in 35 cases. *Oral Surg Oral Med Oral Pathol,* Vol.74, No.2, (August 1992), pp. 149-154, ISSN 0030-4220

Korinek, AM. (1997). Risk factors for neurosurgical site infections after craniotomy: a prospective multicenter study of 2944 patients. The French Study Group of Neurosurgical Infections, the SEHP, and the C-CLIN Paris-Nord. Service Epidemiologie Hygiene et Prevention. *Neurosurgery,* Vol.41, No.5, (November 1997), pp. 1073-1081, ISSN 0148-396X

Kountakis, SE., Kemper, JV, Jr., Chang, CY., DiMaio, DJ., & Stiernberg, CM. (1997). Osteomyelitis of the base of the skull secondary to Aspergillus. *Am J Otolaryngol,* Vol.18, No.1, (January-February 1997), pp. 19-22, ISSN 0196-0709

Larsson, A., Engstrom, M., Uusijarvi, J., Kihlstrom, L., Lind, F., & Mathiesen, T. (2002). Hyperbaric oxygen treatment of postoperative neurosurgical infections. *Neurosurgery,* Vol.50, No.2, (February 2002), pp. 287-296, ISSN 0148-396X

Leaper, DJ. (1995). Risk factors for surgical infection. *J Hosp Infect,* Vol.30, (June 1995), pp. Suppl 127-139, ISSN 0195-6701

Lee, S., Hooper, R., Fuller, A., Turlakow, A., Cousins, V., & Nouraei, R. (2008). Otogenic cranial base osteomyelitis: a proposed prognosis-based system for disease classification. *Otol Neurotol,* Vol.29, No.5, (August 2008), pp. 666-672, ISSN 1531-7129

Lee, SS., Son, JY., Lee, JH., & Kim, OK. (2005). A Case of Invasive Fungal Sinusitis Accompanied with Inflammatory Pseudotumor in Skull Base. *Korean J Otolaryngol-Head Neck Surg,* Vol.48, No.9, (September 2005), pp. 1173-1176, ISSN 1225-035X

Leedom, JM. & Holtom, PD. (1993). Infectious complications, In: *Brain surgery complication avoidance and management,* M.L.J. Apuzzo, (Ed.), pp. 127-144, Churchill Livingstone Inc., ISBN 0-443-08709-1, New York, NY, U.S.A.

LeRoux, PD., Griffin, GE., Marsh, HT., & Winn, HR. (1990). Tuberculosis of the skull--a rare condition: case report and review of the literature. *Neurosurgery,* Vol.26, No.5, (May 1990), pp. 851-856, ISSN 0148-396X

Lim, HW., Jang, YJ., Lee, BJ., & Chung, YS. (2006). A Case of Pott's Puffy Tumor as a Complication of Contralateral Frontal Sinusitis. *Korean J Otolaryngol-Head Neck Surg,* Vol.49, No.1, (January 2006), pp. 109-112, ISSN 1225-035X

Liu, CY., & Apuzzo, ML. (2003). The genesis of neurosurgery and the evolution of the neurosurgical operative environment: part I-prehistory to 2003. *Neurosurgery,* Vol.52, No.1, (January 2003), pp. 3-19, ISSN 0148-396X

Liu, PY. (1998). Cryptococcal osteomyelitis: case report and review. *Diagn Microbiol Infect Dis,* Vol.30, No.1, (January 1998), pp. 33-35, ISSN 0732-8893

Louis T, 3rd., & Lockey, MW. (1974). Blastomycosis of the middle ear cleft. *South Med J,* Vol.67, No.12, (December 1974), pp. 1489-1491, ISSN 0038-4348

Mader, JT., Brown, GL., Guckian, JC., Wells, CH., & Reinarz, JA. (1980). A mechanism for the amelioration by hyperbaric oxygen of experimental staphylococcal osteomyelitis in rabbits. *J Infect Dis,* Vol.142, No.6, (December 1980), pp. 915-922, ISSN 0022-1899

Malhotra, R., Dinda, AK., & Bhan, S. (1993). Tubercular osteitis of skull. *Indian Pediatr,* Vol.30, No.9, (September 1993), pp. 1119-1123, ISSN 0019-6061

Marr, KA., Carter, RA., Crippa, F., Wald, A., & Corey, L. (2002). Epidemiology and outcome of mould infections in hematopoietic stem cell transplant recipients. *Clin Infect Dis,* Vol.34, No.7, (April 2002), pp. 909-917, ISSN 1058-4838

Mastroianni, CM., Vullo, V., & Delia, S. (1992). Cranial Salmonella abscess with parietal bone osteomyelitis in an HIV-infected patient. *AIDS,* Vol.6, No.7, (July 1992), pp. 749-750, ISSN 0269-9370

Meltzer, PE., & Keleman, G. (1959). Pyocutaneous osteomyelitis of the temporal bone, mandible, and zygoma. *Laryngoscope,* Vol.69, pp. 1300-1316, ISSN 0023-852X

Mendelson, DS., Som, PM., Mendelson, MH., & Parisier, SC. (1983). Malignant external otitis: the role of computed tomography and radionuclides in evaluation. *Radiology,* Vol.149, No.3, (December 1983), pp. 745-749, ISSN 0033-8419

Mendelson, MH., Gurtman, A., Szabo, S., Neibart, E,, Meyers, BR., Policar, M., Cheung, TW., Lillienfeld, D., Hammer, G., Reddy, S., Choi, K., Hirschman, SZ. (1994). Pseudomonas aeruginosa bacteremia in patients with AIDS. *Clin Infect Dis,* Vol.18, No.6, (June 1994), pp. 886-895, ISSN 1058-4838

Miedema, CJ., Ruige, M., & Kimpen, JL. (1999). Primarily infected cephalhematoma and osteomyelitis in a newborn. *Eur J Med Res,* Vol.26, No.4(1), (January 1999), pp. 8-10, ISSN 0949-2321

Mindel, A., Tovey, SJ., Timmins, DJ., & Williams, P. (1989). Primary and secondary syphilis, 20 years' experience. 2. Clinical features. *Genitourin Med,* Vol.65, No.1, (January 1989), pp. 1-3, ISSN 0266-4348

Mollman, HD., & Haines, SJ. (1986). Risk factors for postoperative neurosurgical wound infection. A case-control study. *J Neurosurg,* Vol.64, No.6, (June 1986), pp. 902-906, ISSN 0022-3085

Nam, JR., Kim, MS., Lee, CH., & Whang, DH. (2008). Linezolid Treatment for Osteomyelitis due to Staphylococcus Epidermidis with Reduced Vancomycin Susceptibility. *J Korean Neurosurg Soc,* Vol.43, No.6, (June 2008), pp. 307-310, ISSN 2005-3711

Neovius, EB., Lind, MG., & Lind, FG. (1997). Hyperbaric oxygen therapy for wound complications after surgery in the irradiated head and neck: a review of the literature and a report of 15 consecutive patients. *Head Neck,* Vol.19, No.4, (July 1997), pp. 315-322, ISSN 1043-3074

Paramore, CG. (1996). Infections of the scalp and osteomyelitis of the skull, In: *Neurosurgery 2nd ed,* R.H. Wilkins & S.S. Rengachary, (Eds.), pp. 3317-3331, McGraw-Hill Companies, ISBN 0-07-113545-6, New York, NY, U.S.A.

Parize, P., Chandesris, MO., Lanternier, F., Poirée, S., Viard, JP., Bienvenu, B., Mimoun, M., Méchai, F., Mamzer, MF., Herman, P., Bougnoux, ME., Lecuit, M., & Lortholary, O. (2009). Antifungal therapy of Aspergillus invasive otitis externa: efficacy of voriconazole and review. *Antimicrob Agents Chemother,* Vol.53, No.3, (March 2009), pp. 1048-1053, ISSN 0066-4804

Park, MK., Myers, RA., & Marzella, L. (1992). Oxygen tensions and infections: modulation of microbial growth, activity of antimicrobial agents, and immunologic responses. *Clin Infect Dis,* Vol.14, No.3, (March 1992), pp. 720-740, ISSN 1058-4838

Prabhu, SP., Zinkus, T., Cheng, AG., & Rahbar, R. (2009). Clival osteomyelitis resulting from spread of infection through the fossa navicularis magna in a child. *Pediatr Radiol,* Vol.39, No.9, (September 2009), pp. 995-998, ISSN 0301-0449

Prasad, R., Verma, N., Mishra, OP., & Srivastava, A. (2011). Osteomyelitis of skull with underlying brain abscess. *Indian J Pediatr,* Vol.78, No.8, (August 2011), pp. 1005-1007, ISSN 0019-5456

Prinsloo, JG., & Kirsten, GF. (1977). Tuberculosis of the skull vault: a case report. *S Afr Med J, Vol.*19, No.51(8), (February 1977), pp. 248-250, ISSN 0256-9574

Rao, M., Steele, RW., & Ward, KJ. (2003). A "hickey". Epidural brain abscess, osteomyelitis of the frontal bone, and subcutaneous abscess (pott puffy tumor). *Clin Pediatr (Phila),* Vol.42, No.7, (September 2003), pp. 657-660, ISSN 0009-9228

Reiss, P., Hadderingh, R., Schot, LJ., & Danner, SA. (1991). Invasive external otitis caused by Aspergillus fumigatus in two patients with AIDS. *AIDS,* Vol.5, No.5, (May 1991), pp. 605-606, ISSN 0269-9370

Rinaldi, MG. (1983). Invasive aspergillosis. *Rev Infect Dis,* Vol.5, No.6, (November-December 1983), pp. 1061-1077, ISSN 0162-0886

Rivas, Lacarte MP, & Pumarola, SF. (1990). Malignant otitis externa and HIV antibodies. A case report. *An Otorrinolaringol Ibero Am,* Vol.17, No.5, pp. 505-512, ISSN 0303-8874

Roden, MM., Zaoutis. TE., Buchanan, WL., Knudsen, TA., Sarkisova, TA., Schaufele, RL., Sein, M., Sein, T., Chiou, CC., Chu, JH., Kontoyiannis, DP., & Walsh, TJ. (2005). Epidemiology and outcome of zygomycosis: a review of 929 reported cases. *Clin Infect Dis,* Vol.1, No.41(5), (September 2005), pp. 634-653, ISSN 1058-4838

Rothholtz, VS., Lee, AD., Shamloo, B., Bazargan, M., Pan, D., & Djalilian, HR. (2008). Skull base osteomyelitis: the effect of comorbid disease on hospitalization. *Laryngoscope,* Vol.118, No.11, (November 2008), pp. 1917-1924, ISSN 0023-852X

Rubin, GJ., Branstetter, BFt., & Yu, VL. (2004). The changing face of malignant (necrotising) external otitis: clinical, radiological, and anatomic correlations. *Lancet Infect Dis,* Vol.4, No.1, (January 2004), pp. 34-39, ISSN 1473-3099

Rubin, J., Curtin, HD., Yu, VL., & Kamerer, DB. (1990). Malignant external otitis: utility of CT in diagnosis and follow-up. *Radiology,* Vol.174, No.2, (February 1990), pp. 391-394, ISSN 0033-8419

Rusconi, R., Bergamaschi, S., Cazzavillan, A., & Carnelli, V. (2005). Clivus osteomyelitis secondary to Enterococcus faecium infection in a 6-year-old girl. *Int J Pediatr Otorhinolaryngol,* Vol.69, No.9, (September 2005), pp. 1265-1268, ISSN 0165-5876

Safaya, A., Batra, K., & Capoor, M. (2006). A case of skull base mucormycosis with osteomyelitis secondary to temporal bone squamous cell carcinoma. *Ear Nose Throat J,* Vol.85, No.12, (December 2006), pp. 822-824, ISSN 0145-5613

Schuster, JD., Rakusan, TA., Chonmaitree, T., & Box, QT. (1984). Tuberculous osteitis of the skull mimicking histiocytosis X. *J Pediatr,* Vol.105, No.2, (August 1984), pp. 269-271, ISSN 0022-3476

Scoggin, CH., Schwarz, MI., Dixon, BW., & Durrance, JR. (1976). Tuberculosis of the skull. *Arch Intern Med,* Vol.136, No.10, (October 1976), pp. 1154-1156, ISSN 0003-9926

Scott, GB., Buck, BE., Leterman, JG., Bloom, FL., & Parks, WP. (1984). Acquired immunodeficiency syndrome in infants. *N Engl J Med,* Vol.12, No.310(2), (January 1984), pp. 76-81, ISSN 0028-4793

Seabold, JE., Simonson, TM., Weber, PC., Thompson, BH., Harris, KG., Rezai, K., Madsen, MT., & Hoffman, HT. (1995). Cranial osteomyelitis: diagnosis and follow-up with In-111 white blood cell and Tc-99m methylene diphosphonate bone SPECT, CT, and MR imaging. *Radiology,* Vol.196, No.3, (September 1995), pp. 779-788, ISSN 0033-8419

Sethi, A., Sethi, D., Agarwal, AK., Nigam, S., & Gupta, A. (2008). Tubercular and chronic pyogenic osteomyelitis of cranio-facial bones: a retrospective analysis. *J Laryngol Otol,* Vol.122, No.8, (August 2008), pp. 799-804, ISSN 0022-2151

Shahat, AH., Rahman, NU., Obaideen, AM., Ahmed, I., & Zahman, AA. (2004). Cranial-epidural tuberculosis presenting as a scalp swelling. *Surg Neurol,* Vol.61, No.5, (May 2004), pp. 464-467, ISSN 0090-3019

Shelton, JC., Antonelli, PJ., & Hackett, R. (2002). Skull base fungal osteomyelitis in an immunocompetent host. *Otolaryngol Head Neck Surg,* Vol.126, No.1, (January 2002), pp. 76-78, ISSN 0194-5998

Sperber, SJ., & Schleupner, CJ. (1987). Salmonellosis during infection with human immunodeficiency virus. *Rev Infect Dis,* Vol.9, No.5, (September-October 1987), pp. 925-934, ISSN 0162-0886

Sreepada, GS., & Kwartler, JA. (2003). Skull base osteomyelitis secondary to malignant otitis externa. *Curr Opin Otolaryngol Head Neck Surg,* Vol.11, No.5, (October 2003), pp. 316-323, ISSN 1068-9508

Stodulski, D., Kowalska, B., & Stankiewicz, C. (2006). Otogenic skull base osteomyelitis caused by invasive fungal infection. Case report and literature review. *Eur Arch Otorhinolaryngol,* Vol.263, No.12, (December 2006), pp. 1070-1076, ISSN 0937-4477

Subotic, U., Kluwe, W., & Oesch, V. (2011). Community-associated methicillin-resistant Staphylococcus aureus-infected chronic scalp wound with exposed dura in a 10-year-old boy: vacuum-assisted closure is a feasible option: case report. *Neurosurgery,* Vol.68, No.5, (May 2011), pp. E1481-1484, ISSN 0148-396X

Tattersall, R. (2002). Pott's puffy tumour. *Lancet,* Vol.23, No.359(9311), (March 2002), pp. 1060-1063, ISSN 0140-6736

Tumeh, SS., Aliabadi, P., Weissman, BN., & McNeil, BJ. (1986). Chronic osteomyelitis: bone and gallium scan patterns associated with active disease. *Radiology,* Vol,158, No.3, (March 1986), pp. 685-688, ISSN 0033-8419

Turk, JL. (1995). Syphilitic caries of the skull--the changing face of medicine. *J R Soc Med,* Vol.88, No.3, (March 1995), pp. 146-148, ISSN 0141-0768

Valainis, GT., Cardona, LM., & Greer, DL. (1991). The spectrum of Mycobacterium kansasii disease associated with HIV-1 infected patients. *J Acquir Immune Defic Syndr,* Vol.4, No.5, pp. 516-520, ISSN 1525-4135

Van Lente, F. (1982). The diagnostic utility of C-reactive protein. *Hum Pathol,* Vol.13, No.12, (December 1982), pp. 1061-1063, ISSN 0046-8177

Vogelsang, JP., Wehe, A., & Markakis, E. (1998). Postoperative intracranial abscess--clinical aspects in the differential diagnosis to early recurrence of malignant glioma. *Clin Neurol Neurosurg,* Vol.100, No.1, (March 1998), pp. 11-14, ISSN 0303-8467

Vourexakis, Z., Kos, MI., & Guyot, JP. (2010). Atypical presentations of malignant otitis externa. *J Laryngol Otol,* Vol.124, No.11, (November 2010), pp. 1205-1208, ISSN 0022-2151

Weinroth, SE,, Pincetl, P., & Tuazon, CU. (1994). Disseminated Mycobacterium kansasii infection presenting as pneumonia and osteomyelitis of the skull in a patient with AIDS. *Clin Infect Dis,* Vol.18, No.2, (February 1994), pp. 261-262, ISSN 1058-4838

Welsh, O., Salinas, MC., & Rodriguez, MA. (1995). Treatment of eumycetoma and actinomycetoma. *Curr Top Med Mycol,* Vol.6, pp. 47-71, ISSN 0177-4204

Witte, DA., Chen, I., Brady, J., Ramzy, I., Truong, LD., & Ostrowski, ML. (2000). Cryptococcal osteomyelitis. Report of a case with aspiration biopsy of a humeral lesion with radiologic features of malignancy. *Acta Cytol,* Vol.44, No.5, (September-October 2000), pp. 815-818, ISSN 0001-5547

Wood, RE., Nortje, CJ., Grotepass, F., Schmidt, S., & Harris, AM. (1988). Periostitis ossificans versus Garre's osteomyelitis. Part I. What did Garre really say? *Oral Surg Oral Med Oral Pathol,* Vol.65, No.6, (June 1988), pp. 773-777, ISSN 0030-4220

Yucel, OT., & Ogretmenoglu, O. (1998). Subdural empyema and blindness due to cavernous sinus thrombosis in acute frontal sinusitis. *Int J Pediatr Otorhinolaryngol,* Vol.15, No.46(1-2), (November 1998), pp. 121-125, ISSN 0165-5876

4

Chronic Non-Bacterial Osteitis/Chronic Recurrent Multifocal Osteomyelitis

Paivi M.H. Miettunen
Alberta Children's Hospital, University of Calgary, AB Canada

1. Introduction

Chronic non-bacterial osteitis (CNO) is a rare disease, which is a great mimic of infectious osteomyelitis (*Table 1*). It is currently classified as an autoinflammatory osteopathy. Autoinflammatory diseases are a group of disorders characterized by seemingly unprovoked inflammation in the absence of high-titer antibodies or antigen-specific T-cells. CNO primarily affects children, although it can be seen in any age group (Girschick, Raab et al. 2005). It is a disease of unknown etiology that was first recognized 4 decades ago as a disorder of non-infectious bone inflammation. It was initially described as "subacute and chronic symmetrical osteomyelitis," which affected multiple bones either simultaneously or sequentially with a recurrent pattern (Giedion, Holthusen et al. 1972). Later, similar non-infectious osteitis has been described as both multifocal and unifocal disorder, with recurrent or monophasic course, and in association with other inflammatory conditions such as ankylosing spodylitis, psoriasis, and inflammatory bowel disease. Recurrent episodes of painful swollen lesions of the bone are noted, elevated ESR can occur, and radiographic changes can be confused with bacterial osteomyelitis. Negative findings on culture are the rule, and no improvement is noted with antimicrobial therapy.

Chronic Non-Bacterial Osteitis (CNO) /
Chronic Recurrent Multifocal Osteomyelitis
CNO is a non-infectious auto-inflammatory osteitis
It is more common in children than in adults
It can mimic bacterial osteomyelitis
It can affect any bone
This chapter will cover
Epidemiology and etiology
Clinical manifestations
Laboratory, histopathological and radiological assessment
Proposed role of osteoclasts in CNO disorders
How to differentiate CNO from other "mimicking" bone disorders
Treatment modalities (including biologics and bisphosphonates)
Natural history and expected long-term outcome

Table 1. Synopsis of chronic non-bacterial osteitis and outline of the chapter

Historically, CNO disorders have been described by many names, such as chronic recurrent multifocal osteomyelitis (CRMO), SAPHO (synovitis, acne, pustulosis, hyperostosis and osteitis) syndrome, and diffuse sclerosing osteomyelitis affecting the mandible (DSO) (Soubrier, Dubost et al. 2001). In 2005, the term CNO was coined to describe all of these disorders, and the current understanding is that non-infectious inflammatory bone disorders present a clinical spectrum within which CRMO is the most severe form (Girschick, Raab et al. 2005). There have been further attempts to classify patients into defined groups (unifocal nonrecurrent, unifocal recurrent, multifocal nonrecurrent, multifocal recurrent) to establish diagnostic criteria and to find prognostic indicators, although such classification criteria have not been uniformly adapted (Beck, Morbach et al. 2010).

Because the clinical course of the patients may vary according to clinical subtype, in this chapter the term CNO will be used as an umbrella term to describe all of these inflammatory bone disorders, and the sub-categories of CRMO, SAPHO syndrome, DSO, etc. will be retained for subgroups of relevant CNO patients.

2. Epidemiology

Because CNO is a relatively new term, epidemiologic data is primarily available for the subcategory CRMO only. CRMO is recognized worldwide accounting for 2% to 5% of all osteomyelitis cases (Chun 2004). CRMO is primarily a disease of childhood, with the mean age at presentation around 10 years. The youngest age at CRMO presentation has been reported to be 6 months, and the oldest 55 years (Khanna, Sato et al. 2009). The true incidence and prevalence of CRMO remain unknown with more than 300 cases of classic CRMO reported in the literature. Several studies have demonstrated that the disorder is more common in girls than boys, with approximately 2:1 ratio. Although most of the initial reports of CRMO were from Scandinavian countries, later it has been recognized worldwide with no specific racial predilection (El-Shanti and Ferguson 2007).

There is only one existing study on the epidemiology of the general category of combined non-bacterial osteitis disorders. A recent German study reported an annual incidence of 0.4 per 100,000 children, with approximately 60 new patients diagnosed annually suggesting that this disorder is much more common than previously suspected (Jansson and Grote 2011).

3. Etiology and pathogenesis

Pathogenesis of CRMO/CNO continues to be poorly understood. It is not known what triggers the initial episode or why some patients have more persistent disease than others. Environmental, immunological, and genetic factors have been postulated as causative factors with varying evidence.

3.1 Environmental factors

Because of the intermittent nature of clinical symptoms, and clinical similarity to bacterial osteomyelitis, the search for infectious etiologies has been vigorous. Despite initial case reports suggesting that *Staphylococcus aureus, mycoplasma hominis, propionibacterium acnes, bartonella henselea* etc. could have been present in putative CRMO lesions, larger studies have not confirmed a common infectious agent using standard bacterial cultures. More elaborate techniques, such as polymerase chain reaction (PCR) technique for microbial testing, including examination for mycobacteria, have also failed to disclose a causative infectious agent in patients with CRMO (Girschick, Raab et al. 2005). The presence of negative cultures and failure of CRMO symptoms to improve with antibiotic therapy make an infectious etiology very unlikely.

3.2 Possible immune mediated etiology

A possible immune-mediated etiology has been speculated, but immunologic evaluations of cases have not revealed abnormalities in T-cell subsets, oxidative burst of phagocytic cells, mononuclear cell response to mitogens, neutrophil chemotaxis, or phagocytosis. Antinuclear antibody (ANA) and rheumatoid factor have rarely been reported in association with classic CRMO (Chun 2004). A recent pediatric series with 37 CNO patients reported that 51.3% of patients had a low titer ANA level (1:80), and 8.1% of patients had titres ≥ 1:160 (Beck, Morbach et al. 2010). However, these levels of ANA were not different when compared with a healthy control group of age-matched children. Both local and systemic increase of tumor necrosis factor alpha (TNF-α) has been documented in active CRMO (Jansson, Renner et al. 2007). Because of the clinical similarity of CNO to a syndrome presenting with neonatal onset of sterile multifocal bone inflammation with periostitis and skin pustulosis associated with a deficiency of IL-1 receptor antagonist (DIRA) (Aksentijevich, Masters et al. 2009), the role of interleukin-1 in CNO has also been speculated but not confirmed (Eleftheriou, Gerschman et al. 2010).

3.3 Genetic factors

More recently, genetic origin for at least the CRMO subtype has been suggested secondary to observation of disease in siblings and monozygotic twins. The susceptibility focus has been indentified at 18q21.3-22 (Khanna, Sato et al. 2009) . The genetic origin of CRMO is further supported by identification of the *LPIN2* gene in Majeed syndrome (Khanna, Sato et al. 2009). This is an autosomal-recessive syndrome characterized by bone lesions identical to CRMO, congenital dyserythropoietic anemia, and inflammatory dermatosis. The exact function of *LPIN2* is unknown, but it has been postulated that if *LPIN2* plays a role in the regulation of the innate immune system, a defect in the protein would lead to increased production of inflammatory signals (El-Shanti and Ferguson 2007). Spontaneously occurring mouse models of CRMO have been identified that show an autosomal-recessive gene defect localized to the murine *pstpip2* gene (Khanna, Sato et al. 2009). The mice develop destruction of caudal and spinal vertebrae by 3 to 4 weeks of age, tail kinks by 6 to 8 weeks of age and additional hindfoot deformities by 3 months of age (Ferguson, Bing et al. 2006). *PSTPIP2* is highly expressed in macrophages, but it is not known how it contributes to inflammatory bone changes. The human *PSTPIP2* is located on chromosome 18q21.1, but its role in human CNO disorders has not been confirmed so far. However, although these findings suggest a possible genetic predisposition in selected inflammatory bone disorders, it is not known how genes play a role in the etiology of the various CNO disorders, which appear to have heterogeneous clinical presentation. Despite some CNO patients progressing to a spondyloarthropathy, HLA-B27 is not more common in CNO patients than in the general population (Beck, Morbach et al. 2010).

4. Diagnosing CNO

CNO remains a syndromic disorder, defined and diagnosed by a unique pattern of clinical, radiological, and histopathological findings. For the diagnosis of classic CRMO, all of the following criteria should be met: (a) the presence of one or more clinically or radiographically diagnosed bone lesions; (b) a prolonged course of at least 6 months with characteristic exacerbations and remissions; (c) typical radiographic lytic lesions surrounded by sclerosis with increased uptake on bone scan; (d) a lack of response to parenteral antibiotic therapy of at least 1 month's duration to cover clinically suspected organisms; and (e) a lack of an identifiable etiology (King, Laxer et al. 1987).

The suggested diagnostic guidelines for the non-bacterial osteitis disorders in general are presented in *Table 2* (Jansson, Renner et al. 2007). According to these criteria, the general diagnosis of nonbacterial osteitis is reached if two major criteria or one major criterion plus three minor criteria are found (Jansson, Renner et al. 2007). Accordingly to the authors, the more criteria that are met the more likely the diagnosis is CRMO. Although this scheme of diagnosis is not yet universally adopted, no other standardized diagnostic criteria exist for the CNO disorders.

Major Diagnostic Criteria	Minor Diagnostic Criteria
Radiologically proven osteolytic/sclerotic bone lesion	Normal blood cell count and good general state of health
Multifocal bone lesions	CRP and ESR mildly to moderately elevated
PPP[α] or psoriasis	Course is longer than 6 months
Sterile bone biopsy with signs of inflammation and sclerosis	Hyperostosis
	Association with other autoimmune diseases other than PPP or psoriasis
	Grade I or II relatives with autoimmune or autoinflammatory disorders or with NBO[β]

[α]PPP = palmoplantar pustulosis, NBO[β] = non-bacterial osteitis
Two major criteria or one major criterion plus three minor criteria are required for the diagnosis of non-bacterial osteitis (Reproduced with permission from Jansson, Renner et al. Classification of Non-Bacterial Osteitis, Rheumatology 2007;46:154-160)(Jansson, Renner et al. 2007)

Table 2. Proposed major and minor diagnostic criteria for nonbacterial osteitis

4.1 Clinical features

4.1.1 Musculoskeletal manifestations

Patients typically present with insidious onset of localized bone pain, associated with soft tissue and bone swelling. Although most patients present with a single symptomatic site, other sites of disease become apparent at imaging or during follow-up. The average number of sites per patient at CNO diagnosis has been reported to be 5.0 by using whole body (WB) magnetic resonance imaging (MRI) (Beck, Morbach et al. 2010) but during disease course the number per patient can range from 1 to 18 (Khanna, Sato et al. 2009). The common sites of skeletal involvement include the long tubular bones and clavicle, but lesions have been described throughout the skeleton. Involvement of the lower extremity has been reported to be three times more common than disease in the upper extremity (Khanna, Sato et al. 2009).

4.1.2 Extra-bone and non-specific systemic manifestations

Arthritis is the most common extra bone manifestation, reported to occur in up to 80% of the patients over time in some large studies (Girschick, Raab et al. 2005). In a recent prospective German study of 37 pediatric CNO patients, arthritis was present in 38% initially (Beck, Morbach et al. 2010). Typically patients are systemically well with no additional features. However, 33% of children can have associated low grade fever and non-specific malaise (Schultz, Holterhus et al. 1999). Skin lesions are present in up to 30% of pediatric and adolescent patients with CNO and include pustulosis of the hands and feet, psoriatic skin lesions, severe pustular acne, Sweet syndrome, and pyoderma gangrenosum (Beretta-Piccoli, Sauvain et al. 2000). All the above-mentioned skin conditions share the common denominator of being aseptic lesions filled with neutrophils at some stage during the course of their development. The skin disease may precede or occur after the bone lesions, and the interval may be as long as 20 years (Azouz, Jurik et al. 1998). Inflammatory bowel disease is seen in association with CRMO in adult and pediatric patients in approximately 10% of cases and in the majority of cases, CRMO preceded the onset of inflammatory bowel disease by months to up to 5 years (Bousvaros, Marcon et al. 1999). Rarely, CRMO is seen in association with asymptomatic infiltration of the lung with pyogenic abscesses of the skin, cranial nerve lesions, Wegener's granulomatosis, and following leukemia diagnosis (Schultz, Holterhus et al. 1999).

4.2 Laboratory findings

4.2.1 Traditional laboratory tests

Unfortunately, traditional laboratory tests have been disappointing in CNO with no uniform criteria to detect active or remitted disease. For example, one can have clinically and radiologically active CNO with normal erythrocyte sedimentation rate (ESR) and C-reactive protein (CRP), so unfortunately "normal" values cannot be used to indicate "inactive disease"(Miettunen, Wei et al. 2009). However, because CNO is a diagnosis of exclusion, laboratory investigations can be used as supportive features for CNO diagnosis, and to help differentiate it from infectious or other etiologies. We recommend standard testing including blood count, ESR, CRP, serum ferritin, HLA-B27 and blood cultures. White blood cells may be minimally elevated. Very elevated ESR and CRP should prompt for a search for infectious osteomyelitis or a malignant process.

4.2.2 Novel laboratory tests

Based on the presence of osteolytic bone lesions on radiographs, increased osteoclasts in early CRMO lesions (Solau-Gervais, Soubrier et al. 2006), and beneficial effects of bisphosphonates, the role of osteoclasts seems intriguing in CNO disorders. In adult onset SAPHO syndrome, increased levels of serum osteocalcin have been observed in some patients, suggesting greater importance of bone resorption compared with bone formation in this disorder (Bjorksten and Boquist 1980; Mortensson, Edeburn et al. 1988; Rosenberg, Shankman et al. 1988; Yu, Kasser et al. 1989). At our center, we also utilize urinary N-telopeptide/urine creatinine ratio (uNTX/uCr) in selected cases. Urinary N-telopeptide is a marker of collagen-1 breakdown that is traditionally used to monitor treatment response to bisphosphonates in adult patients with bone diseases characterized by accelerated bone turnover, such as Paget's disease of bone (Solau-Gervais, Soubrier et al. 2006; Ralston, Langston et al. 2008). UNTX/uCr is measured from the "spot urine" (2nd void in the morning) (Miettunen, Wei et al. 2009). We have found it to be particularly helpful following bisphosphonate therapy to identify patients whose osteoclast function has returned to normal. At our center, no patients have relapsed while their uNTX/uCr level remained suppressed below age-and sex determined levels, but approximately 50% of those patients whose uNTX/uCr level had returned to normal range relapsed. However, interpretation of uNTX/uCr can be challenging. Unlike adult patients, who have a clearly defined upper level of normal for uNTX/uCr at 65 nmol/mmol creatinine, pediatric patients require plotting of the uNTX/uCr values on age and sex specific graphs (Fig. 1.)

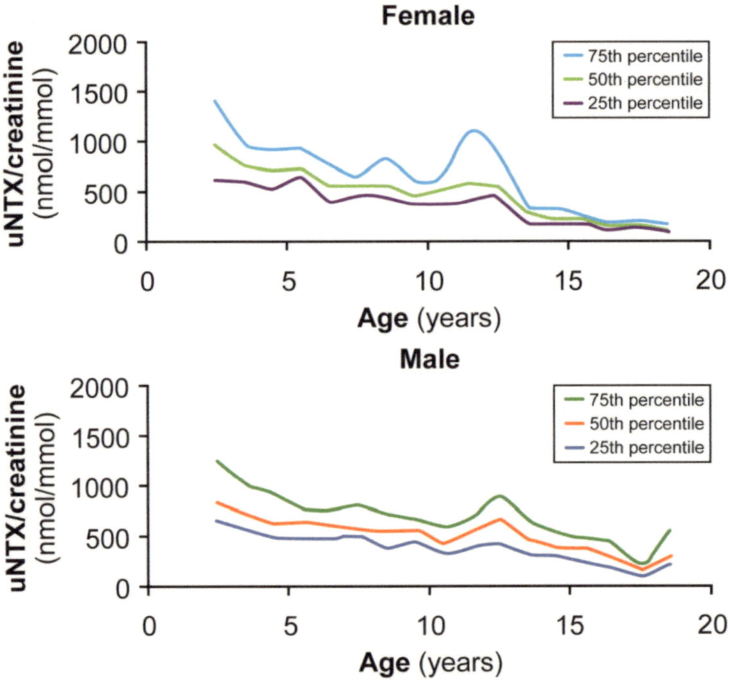

Fig. 1. Age and sex specific graphs for urinary N-telopeptide/urinary creatinine ratios (This figure and figures 10-13 are reproduced with permission from Miettunen, Wei, et al. "Dramatic pain relief and resolution of bone inflammation following pamidronate in 9 pediatric patients with persistent chronic recurrent multifocal osteomyelitisi (CRMO). Pediatr Rheumatol Online J 7:2)(Miettunen, Wei et al. 2009).

4.3 Histopathology

Because of similarity of radiographic appearance of CNO with bone infection or malignancy, we recommend a routine bone biopsy on all suspected cases. Histologically, bone lesions in all CNO categories (unifocal and multifocal, monophasic and recurrent) have similar acute and chronic features. Most commonly, an admixture of inflammatory cells, dominated by plasma cells and lymphocytes, with varying numbers of neutrophils and histiocytes, is present.

Increased osteoclasts and bone resorption can characterize early lesions (Chow, Griffith et al. 1999) (Giedion, Holthusen et al. 1972; King, Laxer et al. 1987; Rosenberg, Shankman et al. 1988). In chronic lesions, reparative changes of the osseous tissue (marrow fibrosis, trabecular osteoid apposition, periosteal hyperostosis) are present. Predominance of CD3 (+), CD45RO(+) T-cells which are mainly CD4 negative and CD8 positive has been reported (Girschick, Huppertz et al. 1999). CD68(+) macrophages or monocytes are common, while CD20(+) B cell infiltrates are uncommon (Girschick, Huppertz et al. 1999).

All these pathological changes, namely inflammatory infiltration of the marrow, active resorption of cortical lamellar bone and reactive woven bony deposition, are responsible for the radiographic picture of expansile and lytic areas occurring in conjunction with separate areas of sclerosis. Importantly, although bone biopsy can differentiate between a malignancy and CNO, histological examination alone cannot distinguish CNO from bacterial osteomyelitis (Girschick, Raab et al. 2005). Therefore extensive microbial investigation of the biopsy specimen with standard culture techniques to detect aerobic and anaerobic bacteria, mycobacteria, and fungi is mandatory. Additional studies using PCR to detect bacterial ribosomal DNA may be utilized.

4.4 Imaging

Radiological investigations have an important role in assessing the likelihood and confirming the extent of the disease and often include a combination of radiographs, isotope bone scans, computerized tomograms, and magnetic resonance imaging. Because the clinical presentation and radiological findings vary depending on the type of bone involved, this review first describes the general radiologic techniques and generalized findings, followed by a focused review of specific clinical and radiologic findings based on the type of bone involved.

4.4.1 Radiographs

The most common sites of disease are the metaphyses or metaphyseal equivalents, accounting for approximately 75% of all lesions in the series of Mandell et al (Mandell, Contreras et al. 1998). The sites of predilection are similar to those of acute hematogenous osteomyelitis in infants and children. The lesions are often but not always symmetric, round in appearance, are surrounded by thin sclerotic borders, and may be associated with periosteal new bone formation. Multifocal destructive bony changes in different stages of development and healing may be present, including lesions that are purely osteolytic, osteolytic and sclerotic, and purely sclerotic with or without periosteal elevation (Fig. 2.) (Khanna, Sato et al. 2009).

4.4.2 ^{99m}Technetium-phosphate bone scan

The findings on bone scan include mild to moderate increase in the uptake of the radionuclide in the lesion. The main contributions of a ^{99m}Technetium-phosphate bone scan are the ability to demonstrate activity at unsuspected sites, which are clinically silent at the time of scintigraphy, and the ability to detect lesions at sites which may be difficult to examine radiographically, e.g. in the spine or in the pelvic bones (Fig.3.) (Mortensson, Edeburn et al. 1988). Similar to all other imaging modalities, bone scan does not separate inflammatory from an infectious or malignant process. It is not a sensitive tool for assessing treatment response, as the bone scan can remain abnormal for months to years following an active CNO event.

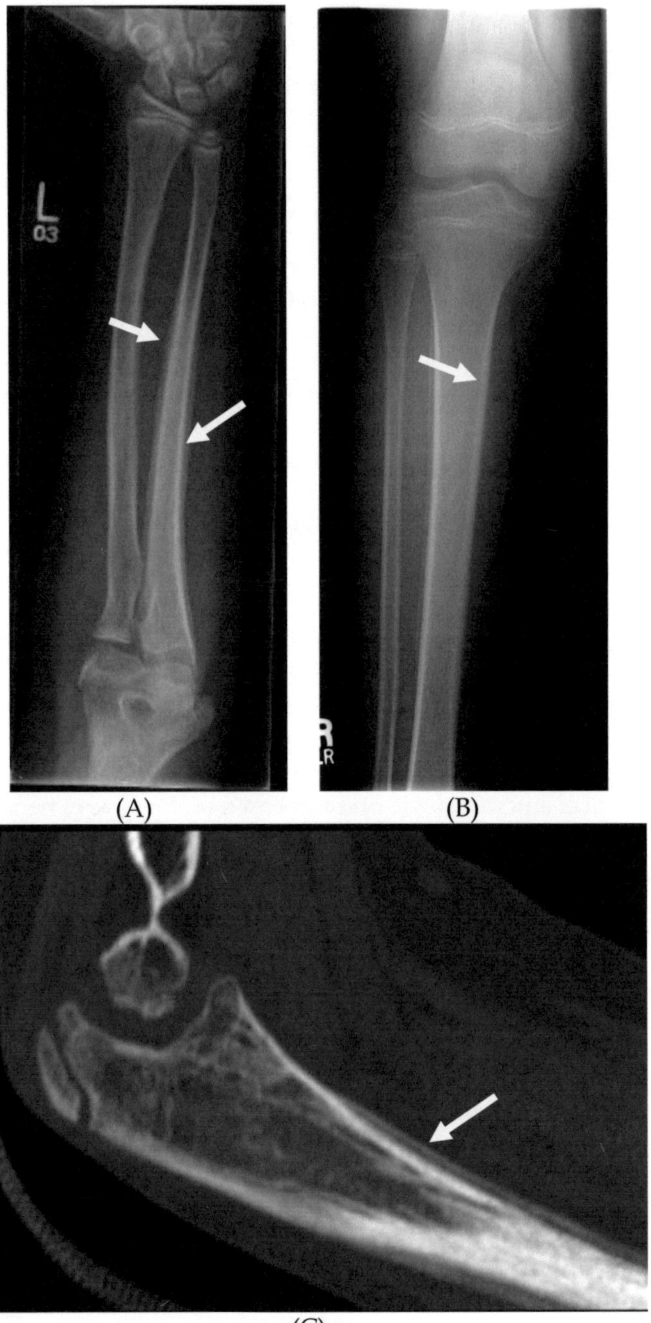

Fig. 2. **Anteriorposterior radiographs (A-B) and CT-scan (C)of a 12-year old boy with CRMO affecting the left ulna and right tibia**. Extensive single-layer subperiosteal reaction extends along the ulnar shaft (A) and tibial shaft (B) (arrows). The periosteal reaction affecting the left ulna is also nicely seen on CT (arrow). (This image and all subsequent images are reproduced with the written permission of the child/parents).

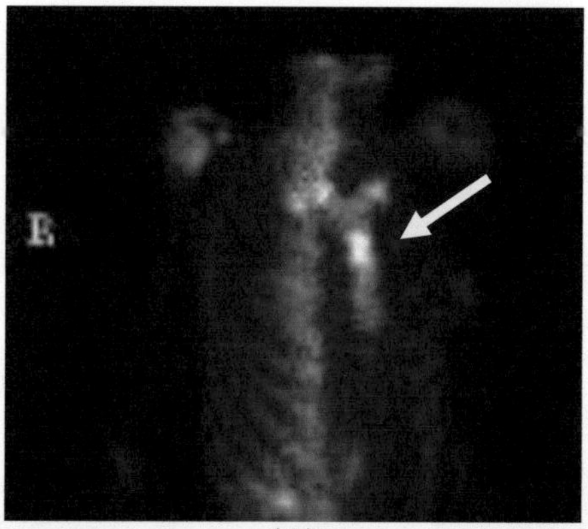

(A)

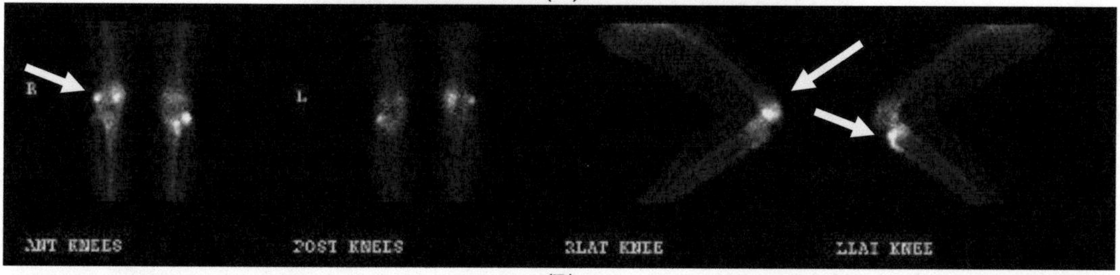

(B)

Fig. 3. **^{99m}Technetium-phosphate bonescan of a 19-year old female with multi-site CRMO.** (A). On delayed imaging, focused view of the chest wall reveals intense intake in the mid-sternal area (arrow). (B). Focused view of the knee area reveals additional intake in the right lateral femoral condyle, right patella and left tibial tubercle (arrows).

4.4.3 Computed tomography (CT)

CT-scan can be helpful as an initial step in differentiating an inflammatory process from a malignant one by showing a lack of soft-tissue mass and bone destruction in CNO. Because of radiation associated with CT, it is now used less often.

4.4.4 Magnetic resonance imaging (MRI)

MRI is emerging as the imaging modality of choice for initial diagnosis of CNO, and for monitoring its progress. It is a non-invasive imaging modality that is highly sensitive to active and remitted inflammatory lesions in bone and soft tissues in CRMO (Jurik and Egund 1997; Jurik 2004). In acute bone inflammation, an increased water content results in longer T1 and T2 relaxation times, and active CRMO lesions occur with increased signal intensity on short tau inversion recovery (STIR) or fat-saturated T2-weighted images and decreased signal intensity on T1-weighted images (Jurik 2004). Adjacent soft tissue edema can be present. MRI can detect abnormal bone marrow edema before changes are noted in x-ray of even bone scintigraphy (Fig.4.) (Girschick, Krauspe et al. 1998). Conversely, resolved CRMO is reflected by no signs of inflammation by MRI (Girschick, Raab et al. 2005).

While the classic MRI features of CNO/CRMO are indistinguishable from septic osteomyelitis, MRI can exclude abscess formation, sequestration, marrow infiltration, or

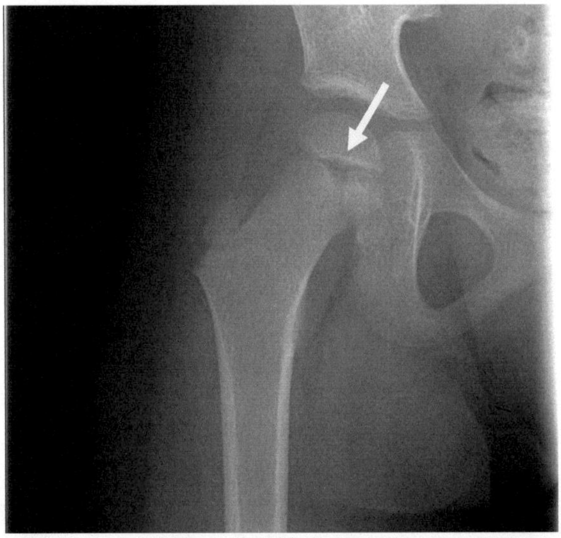

(A)

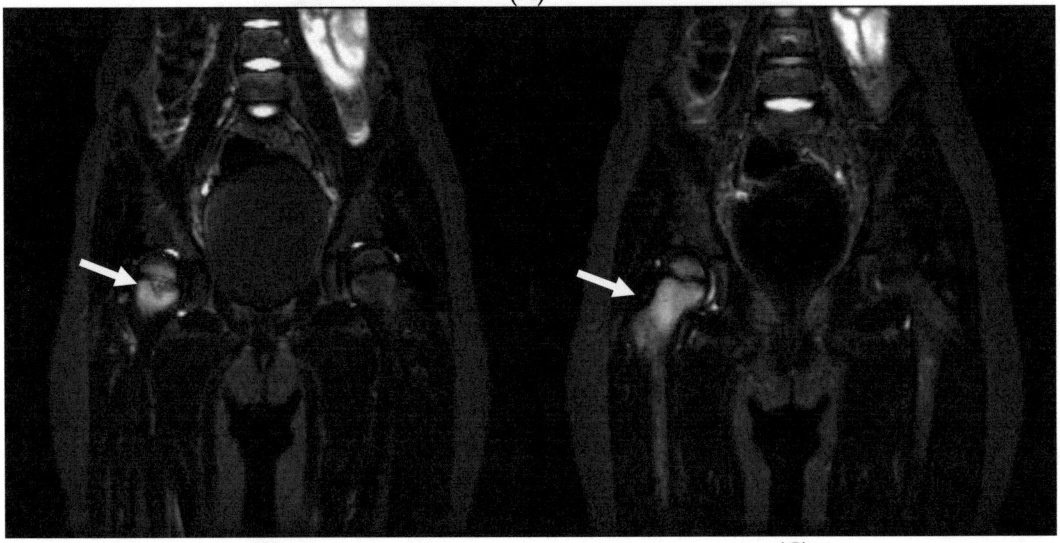

(B) (C)

Fig. 4. **Images of a 4.5-year old girl at CRMO diagnosis. (A).** Pre treatment right femoral radiograph: only subtle radiolucency is seen at the femoral metaphysis (arrow) despite severe hip pain. (B). Short-tau inversion-recovery (STIR) images of MRI performed at the same day confirms the focal lesion adjacent to the growth plate (B), but also shows extensive bone marrow edema in the proximal femur (C) (arrows).

sinus tracts, features commonly seen in chronic infective osteomyelitis (Robertson and Hickling 2001). MRI has been reported to be more specific and sensitive than plain radiography or isotope bone scan also in defining the extent of spinal lesions (Martin, Desoysa et al. 1996). Recently, whole body evaluation by MRI has been used to characterize all active CNO lesions at disease onset, and to systematically evaluate radiological treatment response (Beck, Morbach et al. 2010).

MRI can normalize relatively rapidly in inactive CRMO. From experience at this center, following initiation of bisphosphonate therapy, pelvic lesions can resolve within weeks, while vertebral and long bone lesions can persist longer and complete resolution may take 5-9 months after initiation of bisphosphonate therapy. At our center, whole-body MRI is restricted to patients with recalcitrant disease when bisphosphonates or biologic medications are contemplated, to better delineate the extent of bone involvement and to aid in deciding when to stop therapy.

4.5 Imaging appearances of specific bones affected by CNO/CRMO

4.5.1 Long bones

The most commonly affected sites in all CNO disorders involve the long bones, and the most frequent anatomic sites (two-thirds of patients) with bilateral bony changes include the distal femora or proximal tibiae (Mandell, Contreras et al. 1998). Patients present with "deep bone pain" that can be associated with palpable tenderness, bone enlargement, soft tissue erythema and swelling, and increased heat.

Radiographs reveal typically circular radiolucent lesions, periosteal elevation, and/or bone remodeling. With the older lesions abutting the joint space, localized growth abnormalities with premature epiphyseal fusion or overgrowth can be present. A peculiar finding can be a well-demarcated osteolytic lesion with a pyramidal shape, located in the metaphysis of the tubular bones adjacent to the physis (Fig. 5.) (Mortensson, Edeburn et al. 1988) . Over time, remodeling occurs and osteolytic lesions may heal completely (Giedion, Holthusen et al. 1972).

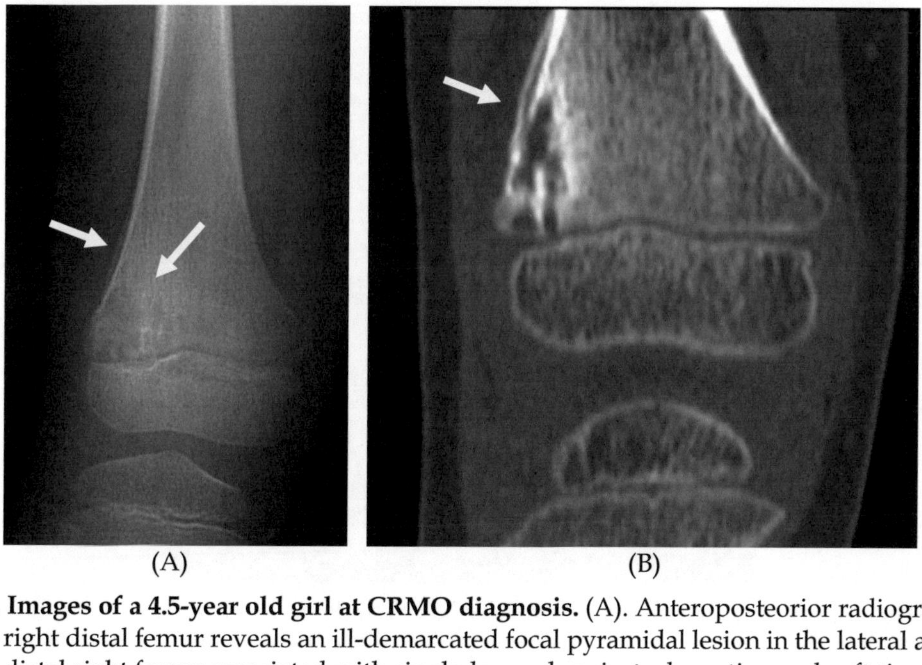

(A) (B)

Fig. 5. **Images of a 4.5-year old girl at CRMO diagnosis.** (A). Anteroposteorior radiograph of the right distal femur reveals an ill-demarcated focal pyramidal lesion in the lateral aspect of the distal right femur associated with single-layered periosteal reaction and soft-tissue edema. (B).A coronal reformat from CT images of the distal femur better delineates the bony changes.

4.5.2 Clavicle

Up to 30% of all CRMO lesions are located in the clavicle (Khanna, Sato et al. 2009). Clinically, the patients present with local swelling and pain, and may have associated restriction in the shoulder movement and thoracic outlet syndrome from nerve compression (Azouz, Jurik et al. 1998). Isolated clavicular area involvement is a well-described entity and is known as "sternocostoclavicular hyperostosis" (Azouz, Jurik et al. 1998). Clavicular hyperostosis is more common in adults, with the usual age at presentation being 30-50 years. In SAPHO syndrome, clavicular area involvement is characterized by osseous hypertrophy and soft-tissue ossification at the sternum, clavicle, and upper ribs. There seems to be a higher prevalence of clavicular disease in CRMO patients with palmoplantar pustulosis or acne fulminans (Khanna, Sato et al. 2009).

Radiographs initially reveal mixed lytic and sclerotic lesions, often with clavicular expansion that is located in the mid-portion. Periosteal reaction can be robust. Over time, the clavicle may remain sclerotic and thickened even in the absence of clinical symptoms (Giedion, Holthusen et al. 1972). In adults the disease course can be complicated by ligamentous ossification and bony bridging across the sternoclavicular joint and between the clavicle and the anterior part of the upper ribs (Azouz, Jurik et al. 1998). These changes are not seen in children. Bone scintigraphy can reveal a characteristic "bullhorn" pattern of increased uptake in the sternoclavicular region, with the sternoclavicular joints as the "horns" and the manubrium as the "head" (Sidhu, Andrews et al. 2003). MRI may not differentiate early clavicular CNO from Ewing's sarcoma, and can demonstrate robust soft tissue edema (Fig.6.).

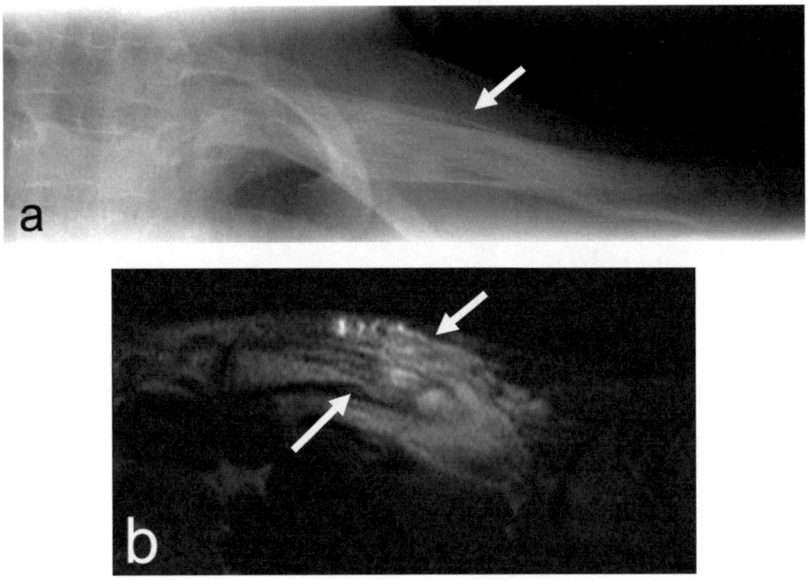

Fig. 6. **Images of CRMO lesion involving the left clavicle in a 7-year old girl.** (A). Plain radiograph of the left clavicle demonstrates periosteal new bone formation (arrow). (B). Axial (fat-saturated, T2-weighted MRI performed at the same time demonstrates hyper-intense T2 signal within the clavicle with marked soft tissue inflammation (arrows) (Miettunen, Wei et al. 2009).

4.5.3 Mandible

CRMO can involve the mandible in about 5% of cases (Khanna, Sato et al. 2009). Mandibular lesions are most often seen by dentists or oral and maxillofacial surgeons and in dental literature mandibular involvement is known by the name mandibular osteitis or diffuse sclerosing osteomyelitis (Suei, Tanimoto et al. 1995). Patients experience recurrent pain and swelling typically in one half of the mandible. Trismus and paresthesia can develop. Occasionally progression of the disease leads to involvement of the temporomandibular joint or temporal bone. Mandibular CNO can be difficult to treat, and the cosmetic deformity can be distressing to the patient (Fig. 7).

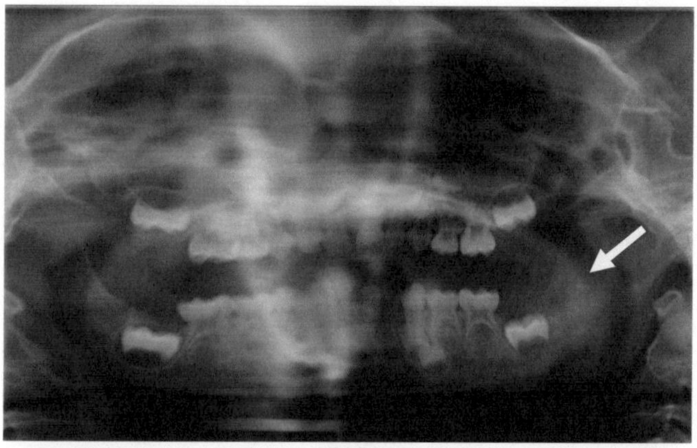

(A)

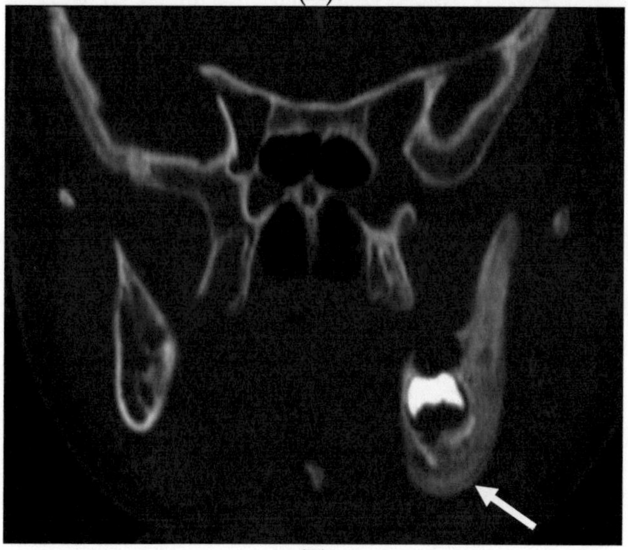

(B)

Fig. 7. **Imaging data of CNO lesion involving the left mandible in a 4-year old girl.** (A). Panorex of the mandible shows sclerosis and enlargement of the left mandibular angle and ramus (arrows). A few small focal lucencies are seen with the lesion. (B). A coronal reformat image of non-contrast CT scan confirm the findings on plain X-ray with additional finding of periosteal reaction (arrows).

Radiographs are commonly normal at disease onset. Early findings are discrete, thin zones of increased density parallel to the lower border of the mandible. Later, the radiographic appearance is characterized by mixed sclerotic and lytic lesions or by diffuse sclerosis (Soubrier, Dubost et al. 2001). At times local cortical bone deficit at the mandibular angle and/or shortening of roots are present. Radionucleide imaging can be helpful in early lesions, as the uptake of ^{99m} Tc is extremely intense, even if the radiographs are still normal. CT scan shows unilateral enlargement of the mandible, with thickening of cortical and trabecular bone. Subperiosteal bone formation and endosteal sclerosis are typically present (Van Merkesteyn, Groot et al. 1988).

4.5.4 Spine

Initial presentation with primary spinal involvement has been reported to occur in only about 3% of patients with classic CRMO (Anderson, Heini et al. 2003), but vertebral lesions accompany other bone lesions in up to 24% of CNO patients at initial presentation (Jansson and Grote 2011). Typically patients complain of localized back pain, but can also present with anterior chest pain from referred pain. Up to 40% may develop vertebral crush fractures (Jansson and Grote 2011).

Radiographs may demonstrate vertebral erosion, osteolytic lesions with "square outline" within the vertebral bodies, sclerosis and mild collapse with reduction of disc space (Mortensson, Edeburn et al. 1988; Kayani, Syed et al. 2004). Complete vertebral collapse (vertebra plana) is more rare (Schilling 2002). All vertebrae from the mid-cervical spine to the sacrum can be potentially affected. A characteristic MRI finding is a subchondral endplate fracture-like line associated with increase in signal in the vertebral marrow (Anderson, Heini et al. 2003). Multifocal disease is common, with spontaneous healing and new lesions presenting over a period of years. MRI is particularly useful in determining the activity of lesions, as healed lesions have abnormal contour but normal marrow, or show fatty replacement of normal red marrow (Fig. 8.). Spinal CNO can initially be confused with pyogenic vertebral osteomyelitis. However, unlike pyogenic vertebral osteomyelitis, CNO involving the vertebrae is not associated with involvement of the intervertebral disc, and typically several vertebral bodies are involved at different levels with one or several normal intervening vertebrae.

4.5.5 Pelvis

CNO of the pelvic bones can be difficult to diagnose, and its incidence is not known. It typically presents as insidious onset of deep pain localized to sacroiliac or other pelvic bone areas. The preferred sites in the pelvis include the metaphyseal equivalents—such as the ischiopubic synchondrosis and the sacroiliac joints. Initial radiographs may be normal. MR imaging shows edema in active lesions and occasionally demonstrates associated soft-tissue inflammation. Additionally, lytic lesions or sclerosis of the iliac wings can be present (Fig.9.). CRMO of the pelvic synchondrosis tends to heal without sequalae (Khanna, Sato et al. 2009). Sacroiliac joints should be assessed carefully for asymmetry, as patients with CRMO may evolve into a spondyloarthropathy with unilateral or less commonly, bilateral sacroiliitis.

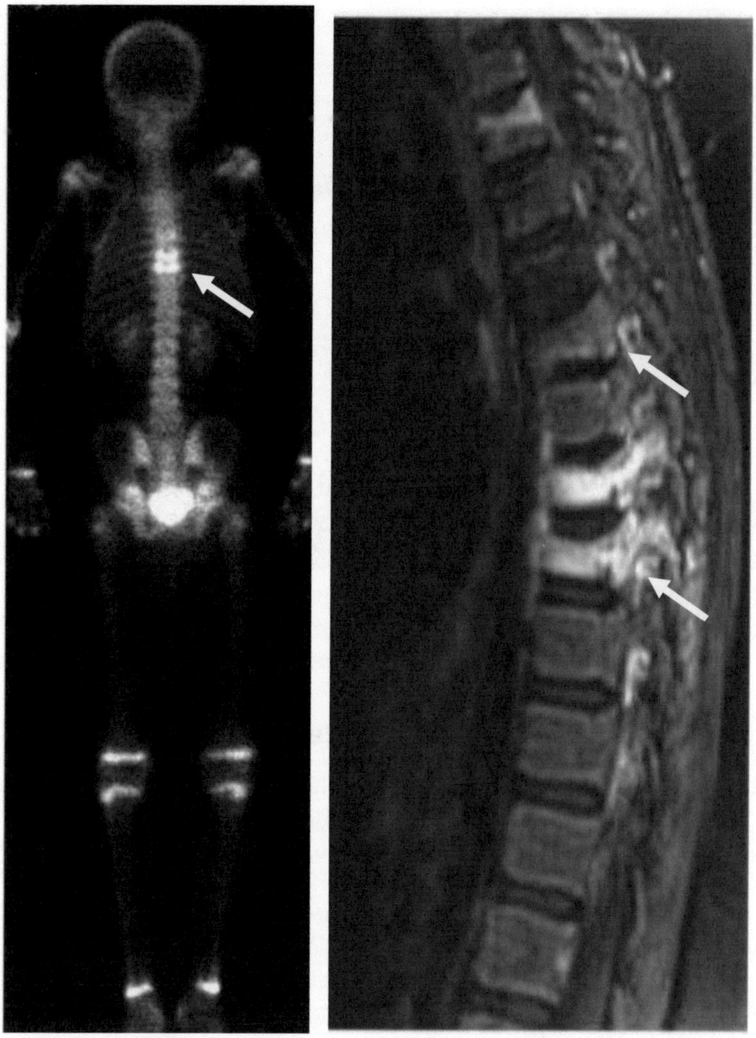

(A) (B)

Fig. 8. **Imaging data of a 13-year old boy with CRMO involving multiple vertebrae.** (A). ^{99m} Tc Bone Scan demonstrates increased uptake in several thoracic vertebrae (arrow). (B). MRI with gadolinium demonstrates abnormal enhancement in several vertebrae consistent with inflammation along with vertebral collapse (arrows).

4.5.6 Hands and feet

CRMO is more common in the small bones of the feet than those in the hands. Typical sites of involvement in the feet include tarsal bones such as the calcaneous and talus, which are metaphyseal equivalents, or the metatarsals and phalanges which are short tubular bones. The radiographic findings are similar to those in other sites of the disease with lytic lesions with surrounding sclerosis, periosteal reaction and soft tissue swelling. Patients may develop localized growth abnormalities as a result of premature physeal closure with metatarsal and phalangeal involvement (Khanna, Sato et al. 2009).

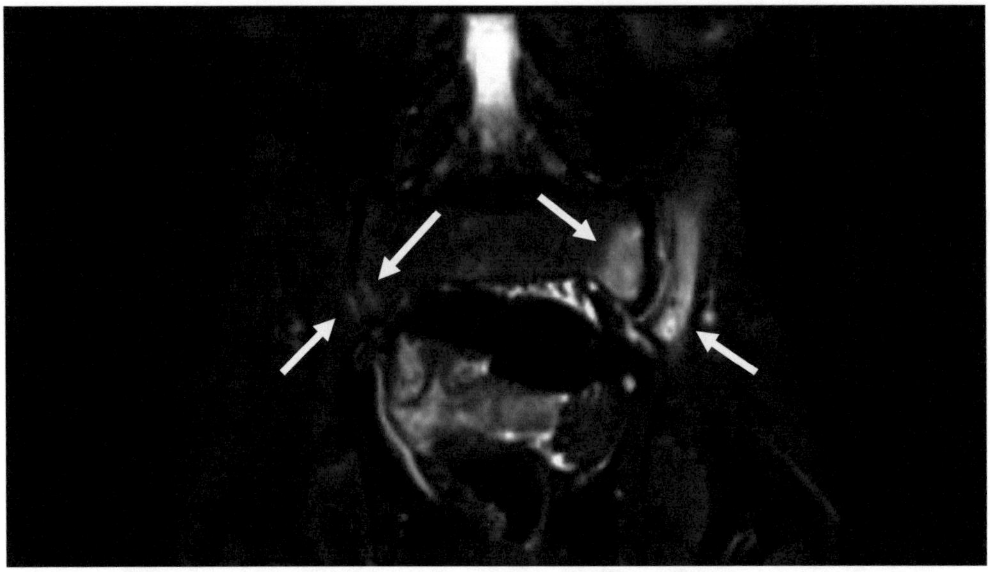

Fig. 9. **Pelvic MRI of a 6-year old girl with multisite CRMO.** On T2-weighed images with fat saturation, there are bilateral increased T2 signal intensities involving the periarticular region of the sacroiliac joints as well as the iliac bones mainly noted on the left side (arrows).

5. Differential diagnosis and related disorders

The differential diagnosis of CNO disorders includes other diseases that produce either bone swelling or osteolysis. Bone swelling is produced by Caffey's disease (infantile cortical hyperostosis), Camurati-Engelmann disease (progressive diaphyseal dysplasia), mono-ostotic Paget's disease, and fibrous dysplasia (Kaftori, Kleinhaus et al. 1987). By virtue of the combination of expansile, destructive, or regenerative bony changes, CNO can produce radiologic changes simulating neoplasia, such as osteoid osteoma, Ewing's sarcoma, osteosarcoma, osteoblastoma, leukemia, non-Hodgins lymphoma, Langerhans histiocytosis, and metastasis. Their diagnosis requires bone biopsy. Finally, it should be emphasized that even though chronic inflammation constitutes the common histopathologic change in both CNO and infectious osteomyelitis, CNO is not associated with abscess formation, fistula, or sequestra (*Table* 3).

6. Treatment

The treatment of CNO remains empiric due to the lack of controlled studies. Because there are no generally accepted treatment protocols available, the treatment approach depends on the severity of pain, location of bone lesions, and the perceived risk for long term complications if the inflammation is not controlled.

While in the past, treatment used to focus on symptom control, the availability of MR imaging to detect active and remitted lesions has made it clear that some CNO lesions truly remit while others remain persistently active. Thus the treatment focus is shifting to achieving clinical and radiologic remission (Beck, Morbach et al. 2010). These new goals have generated an interest in the development of outcome measures tools for CNO

Variable	Chronic non-bacterial osteitis	Bacterial Osteomyelitis
Clinical features		
Bone pain +/- localized soft tissue swelling	+++	+++
Unifocal bone involvement	+	+++
Multifocal bone involvement	+++	<4%
Recurrent symptoms	+++	-
Systemic features		
Fever	+	+++
Arthritis adjacent to affected bone	+	+
Skin disease (psoriasis, etc)	≤10%	-
Inflammatory bowel disease	≤10%	-
Laboratory investigations		
Elevated ESR and CRP	+	+++
Elevated white blood cells	+	+++
Blood culture reveals organism	-	+++
Culture of bone biopsy reveals organism	-	+++
Imaging		
Radiographs Periosteal elevation, osteolysis, sclerosis	+++	+++
^{99m}Technetium-phosphate bone scan Increased uptake at affected areas	+++	+++
Magnetic Resonance Imaging (MRI)		
Abscess, fistula or sequestra	-	+
Contiguous vertebral body involvement with intervening disc involvement	-	+
Treatment response		
Nonsteroidal anti-inflammatory agents	50-70% response	-
Antibiotics	-	+++ (Practical pearl: CRP is expected to decrease by approximately one half each day following successful antibiotic therapy)

- = Typically not present
+ = low-grade to moderate, but exact incidence is not known
+++ = high grade, present in > 50% of cases
ESR = erythrocyte sedimentation rate, CRP = C-reactive protein

Table 3. Description of similarities and differences between chronic non-bacterial osteitis and bacterial osteomyelitis.

disorders. One ongoing prospective study, which follows newly diagnosed patients with CNO with serial MRIs at predetermined points over 5 years (Beck, Morbach et al. 2010), has utilized a novel scoring system for assessing CNO activity and severity. It comprises of newly defined pediatric CNO core set (PedCNO), laboratory analysis, and sequential whole-body MRI. This study aims to capture the clinical and radiological treatment response over time in patients who are treated with the currently acceptable sequence of medications, namely initially with naproxen, and in recalcitrant cases with a short course of oral steroids and addition of sulfasalazine as a disease modifying anti-rheumatic drug. The preliminary results of the study after 1 year are presented below in the section on non-steroidal anti-inflammatory agents. The ultimate results of this study will be important in helping identify poor prognostic indicators at disease presentation for more persistent disease.

The suggested scoring system by Beck *et al* is comprehensive, and we recommend its use in clinical practice, although it may need to be modified as new knowledge about pathogenesis of CNO becomes available. The five items that comprise the CNO core set are presented in *Table 4*. The definition of improvement is analyzed as follows: for the PedCNO30 (PedCNO50, PedCNO70) score, at least 30% (50%, 70%) improvement in at least three out of five core set variables, with no more than one of the remaining variables deteriorating by more than 30% is required. The current short-coming of the proposed core set reflects the lack of specific laboratory markers in CNO, and therefore the inclusion of ESR in the core-set may not reflect true disease activity in CNO. From this author's point of view, it is essential to include MRI evaluation at least in clinical trials, as it can be difficult or impossible to assess disease activity on radiographs or bone scintigraphy, which do not differentiate between an active inflammatory bone lesion and chronic damage from previously active lesions.

Item
Erythrocyte sedimentation rate (ESR)
Number of radiological lesions
Severity of disease estimated by the physician on 10-cm visual analogue scale (VAS), "0" = no disease activity, "10" = the most severe activity possible
Severity of disease estimated by the patient or parent on 10-cm VAS
Childhood health assessment questionnaire (CHAQ)[a]

[a]CHAQ is the most widely used functional status measure in pediatric rheumatology

Table 4. PedCNO (pediatric chronic non-bacterial osteomyelitis) core set (Beck, Morbach et al. 2010).

6.1 Traditional medications

6.1.1 Non-Steroidal Anti-Inflammatory Agents (NSAIDs)

NSAIDs currently are the first choice for the treatment of initial CNO episodes and relapses. The most common NSAID is naproxen (10-15 mg/kg/day in 2 divided doses), which has been reported to be effective in up to 70% of patients regarding symptom control (Schultz, Holterhus et al. 1999). However, there are new emerging data that suggest that NSAIDs rarely induce true remission in CNO. The data from a recent prospectively followed cohort of 37 children with CNO indicate that naproxen induces a clinically asymptomatic state in 43% of patients after 6 months, and in 51% at 12 months. However, the corresponding percentages for radiologic resolution using serial WB MRIs were much lower, at 14% at 6 months and 27% at 12 months (Beck, Morbach et al. 2010). New lesions occurred in 41% of patients during the first year despite anti-inflammatory treatment. The authors concluded that NSAIDs were not able to reach remission (radiologically defined) in the majority of patients during/after 1 year.

6.1.2 Corticosteroids

Corticosteroids have been used with variable success. Currently, corticosteroids are recommended as "bridging" therapy only when NSAIDs have failed, and use of disease modifying drugs is initiated. One recommended schedule consists of oral glucocorticoids for 1 week at 2 mg prednisone/kg/day, followed by discontinuation stepwise by 25% every 5 days (Girschick, Zimmer et al. 2007). Intravenous methylprednisolone pulses have been reported to be effective in selected refractory cases but no uniform treatment protocol exists (Holden and David 2005).

6.1.3 Disease Modifying Anti-Rheumatic Drugs (DMARDs)

Methotrexate, sulfasalazine (20 mg/kg/day), colchicine, etc. have been tried with varying success in recalcitrant CNO. Traditionally DMARDs have been reserved for patients with frequent relapses or if NSAIDs must be discontinued because of ineffectiveness or side effects (Girschick, Zimmer et al. 2007). However, because of the recent evidence that NSAIDs fail to induce radiologic remission in the majority of the patients, use of DMARDs may increase as information becomes available regarding risk factors for non-response to NSAID therapy. The only currently known indicator for resistance to NSAID therapy includes multifocal lesions at presentation (Catalano-Pons, Comte et al. 2008). Beck *et al* have suggested that NSAIDs be augmented by DMARDs already at diagnosis for such patients (Beck, Morbach et al. 2010). However, no recommendations exist which DMARD would be the most beneficial.

6.2 Novel treatment modalities

6.2.1 Bisphosphonates

Bisphosphonates are anti-osteoclastic agents and their beneficial effect in CNO/CRMO is postulated to be secondary to their ability to inhibit bone resorption, to have pain modifying effect, and to suppress proinflammatory cytokines, such as TNF-α, interleukin (IL)-6, and IL-1(Miettunen, Wei et al. 2009). They are usually recommended if the above treatment approaches with NSAIDs, bridging treatment with oral corticosteroids, and addition of DMARD(s) are not successful. Pamidronate is the most commonly used bisphosphonate in pediatric CNO patients, although some patients have also received alendronate (Eleftheriou, Gerschman et al. 2010).

6.2.1.1 Bisphosphonate treatment protocol

The total number of patients treated with bisphosphonates remains small worldwide, and no generally accepted treatment protocols are available. At our center, we have treated 12 pediatric patients with pamidronate with excellent clinical and radiological response. Our pre-pamidronate work-up and suggested monitoring during treatment are presented in

Table 5. We do not use bisphosphonates if the spine z-score is above "0" because of the potential for making bones less flexible with risk for secondary fractures. Renal investigations are performed because of the potential nephrotoxicity of bisphosphonates.

Base line Investigation/monitoring	During follow-up
Radiological	
MRI[α] of the affected lesion	One month after pamidronate is completed, and then at time of suspected flare
DEXA[β] scan for bone density	Annually during pamidronate treatment, and before re-treatment is considered
Renal ultrasound	No, unless clinically indicated
Laboratory	
Bone specific markers	
uNTX/uCr[μ] ratio (spot urine, using the 2nd void sample of the morning), serum alkaline phosphatase	On day 3 of the 1st treatment, preceding each treatment, and at time of suspected flare
Other laboratory investigations	
ESR[π], CRP[§], complete blood count	At monthly intervals during pamidronate treatment
Serum calcium	Preceding each treatment, and at time of completion of each infusion
Other suggested monitoring	
PedCNO[∞] core set	At monthly intervals during pamidronate treatment, and at time of suspected flare
Screening for extra-skeletal manifestations: *palmoplantar pustulosis, psoriasis, or inflammatory bowel disease*	At each follow-up visit
Dental examination	Yearly during pamidronate treatment

[α] MRI= magnetic resonance imaging; [β]DEXA = dual-energy X-ray absorptiometry; [μ]uNTX/uCr = urinary N-telopeptide/urinary creatinine; [π]ESR = erythrocyte sedimentation rate; [§]CRP= C-reactive protein ; [∞] PedCNO core set = pediatric chronic non-bacterial osteomyelitis core set

Table 5. Pre-pamidronate workup, and investigations/monitoring during pamidronate treatment

A specific treatment protocol, presented in *Table 6*, is in use at our center, but it needs to be emphasized that these guidelines have not been validated in clinical trials. Because "the minimally effective dose" of pamidronate is not known, and because of potential associated side effects, our current treatment protocol is aimed to ameliorate pain, to improve radiologic lesions, and to have the ability to re-treat if the patient relapses. For the initial course of pamidronate, if there is complete pain resolution after 4 months of treatment, no

Medication	Subsequent doses	Suggested duration of treatment
Pamidronate		
Initial 3-day cycle:	*1-day infusion monthly:*	Initially 4 months, then re-assess
Day 1: 0.5mg/kg/day (up to 30mg/day) Days 2-3:1mg/kg/day (up to 60mg/day)	1mg/kg/day (up to 60mg/day)	
Calcium	500-1000 mg of elemental calcium/day	During pamidronate treatment
Vitamin D	400-800 international units/day	During pamidronate treatment

Table 6. Suggested pamidronate treatment protocol

further pamidronate is given. In case of whole-body MRI confirmed CNO flare, those patients with only single active lesion receive one day pamidronate treatment only, and patients with ≥ 2 lesions receive once monthly 1-day pamidronate. All patients are re-imaged with whole body MRI after 3 months to determine potential need for further treatment. The total yearly dose of pamidronate is limited to ≤ 9mg/kg/year. If the spine z-score improves to above "0" during follow-up, we do not give further pamidronate.

6.2.1.2 Side effects associated with bisphosphonates

Approximately 30-60% of patients may develop fever, myalgia, and bone pain, which occur with the first infusion only. These are felt to reflect the standard acute phase response with bisphosphonate therapy, and the symptoms respond to regular Tylenol and resolve within 12-48 hours (Miettunen, Wei et al. 2009). Some patients may develop acute phlebitis within 12-24 hours at the intravenous cannula site, and this can mimic acute infection. Serum calcium is measured just preceding each infusion, and one hour after completion of infusion to monitor for possible bisphosphonate induced hypocalcemia.

Patients are counseled regarding the potential long term side effects involved in the use of bisphosponates, including the theoretical risk for fetal bone formation in future pregnancies, and the potential for jaw necrosis. Although there have been no pediatric cases of jaw necrosis, we recommend no elective dental extractions or braces during pamidronate treatment, and preferably during 18-months following the final pamidronate treatment. All patients undergo a dental examination prior to starting bisphosphonates, and at 6-12-monthly intervals during treatment (Miettunen, Wei et al. 2009).

6.2.1.3 Expected clinical and MRI response

There are now reports in the literature confirming the efficacy of bisphosphonates in several adult patients with inflammatory osteitis (Kerrison, Davidson et al. 2004; Solau-Gervais, Soubrier et al. 2006), in pediatric and adult onset SAPHO syndrome (Compeyrot-Lacassagne, Rosenberg et al. 2007), in pediatric patients with chronic inflammatory lesions of the mandible (Gleeson, Wiltshire et al. 2008; Simm, Allen et al. 2008), and in several cases of CRMO (Bjorksten and Boquist 1980). Vertebral re-modeling has been reported in

3 pediatric CRMO patients including improvement of kyphosis in one patient who presented with vertebral fractures pre-pamidronate (Gleeson, Wiltshire et al. 2008). The improvement in pain and resolution/decrease in associated soft tissue swelling is expected to occur within the first week following the first 3-day pamidronate treatment. MRI documented improvement in CNO lesions lags behind the pain response, and occurs within weeks to months (Figs. 10., 11., and 12.) (Miettunen, Wei et al. 2009). By current reports, approximately 70% of CNO patients have long lasting symptom control following pamidronate. The exact rate of relapse is not known, but is reported between 30-100% (Kerrison, Davidson et al. 2004; Miettunen, Wei et al. 2009). The time to relapse has varied from 9 to 17 months following completion of the initial course of pamidronate, and most relapsed patients have responded equally well to re-treatment with pamidronate (Kerrison, Davidson et al. 2004; Compeyrot-Lacassagne, Rosenberg et al. 2007; Miettunen, Wei et al. 2009). However, pamidronate has not been uniformly effective in all patients, or in all CNO lesions in individual patients (Gleeson, Wiltshire et al. 2008; Eleftheriou, Gerschman et al. 2010).

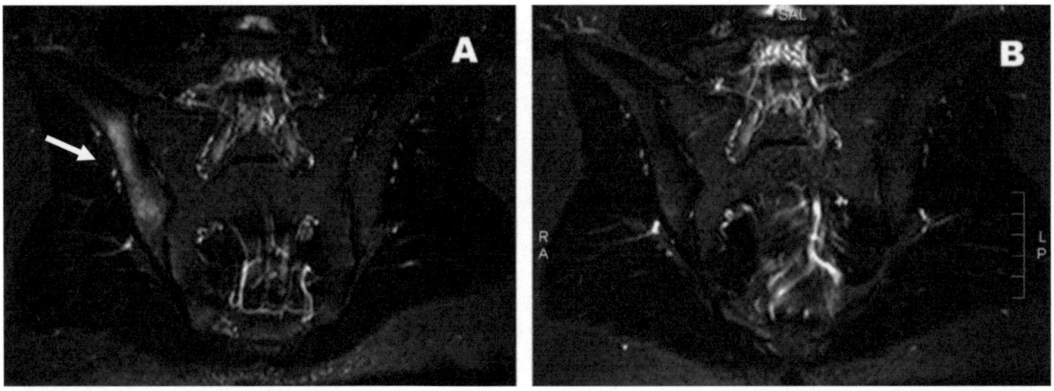

Fig. 10. (A). Pre-pamidronate treatment (MRI) with gadolinium demonstrates enhancement consistent with inflammation in the right sacroiliac area. (B). Post treatment MRI with Gadolinium 6 weeks after first treatment with pamidronate: No enhancement (Miettunen, Wei et al. 2009).

6.2.1.4 Expected response of bone remodeling markers following bisphosphonates

There is only one existing report regarding bone remodeling markers in pediatric CRMO patients (Miettunen, Wei et al. 2009). At our center, we did not show generalized increase in bone resorption markers or in markers of bone formation compared to age-specific norms. Although four out of nine patients in our series had baseline uNTX/uCr values above the 75th % percentile for age, we hypothesized that this increase most likely reflected the on-set of puberty, rather than increase from CRMO related osteolysis.

All patients had an expected decrease in uNTX/uCr following pamidronate, and interestingly no patient relapsed while his/her bone turnover remained suppressed below age and sex-specified norms (Miettunen, Wei et al. 2009) (Fig. 13). It is therefore tempting to speculate that bone and adjacent soft tissue inflammation may require functioning osteoclasts for clinical manifestations. However, further studies are required on the role of osteoclasts and on the potential use of uNTX/uCr in pediatric and adult CNO disorders.

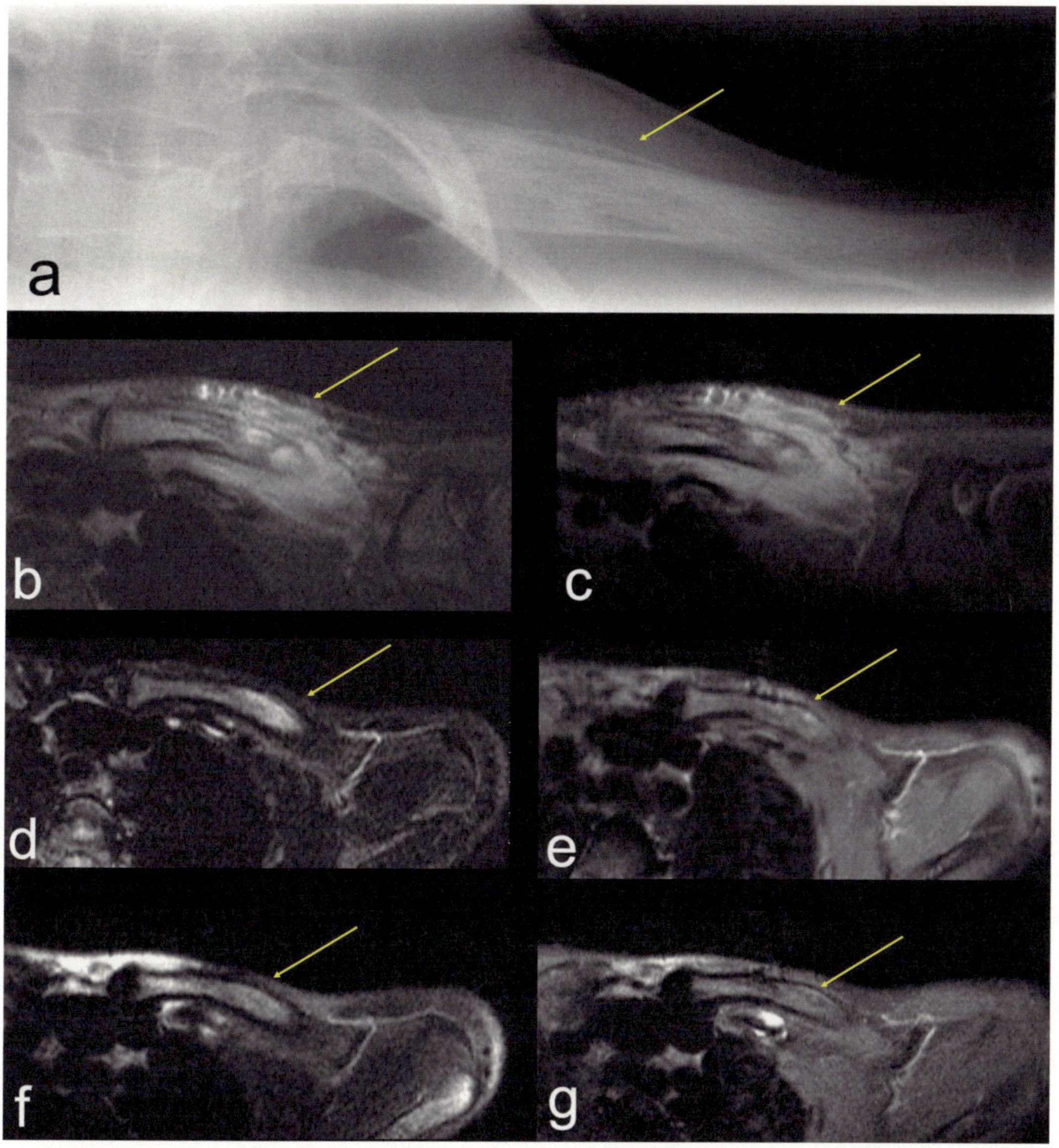

Fig. 11. **Imaging data of CRMO lesion involving left clavicle in a 7-year old girl pre- and post pamidronate treatment**. (A). Pre-treatment imaging. Radiograph of the left clavicle demonstrates periosteal new bone formation (arrow). (B -C). Pre-treatment MRI: (B) Axial (fat-saturated, T2-weighted) and (C) post gadolinium MRI: Hyper-intense T2 signal with post-contrast enhancement is seen within the clavicle (arrow) with marked soft tissue inflammation (arrow). (D-E). Post-treatment MRI (5 months after initiation of treatment with pamidronate) with the same technique as B and C, respectively. The intra-osseous abnormal signal has significantly improved, and marked soft tissue abnormality has almost completely resolved. (F-G). Post-treatment MRI (8 months after initiation of treatment with pamidronate) with the same technique as B and C, respectively, reveals complete resolution of the intra-osseous abnormal signal (Miettunen, Wei et al. 2009).

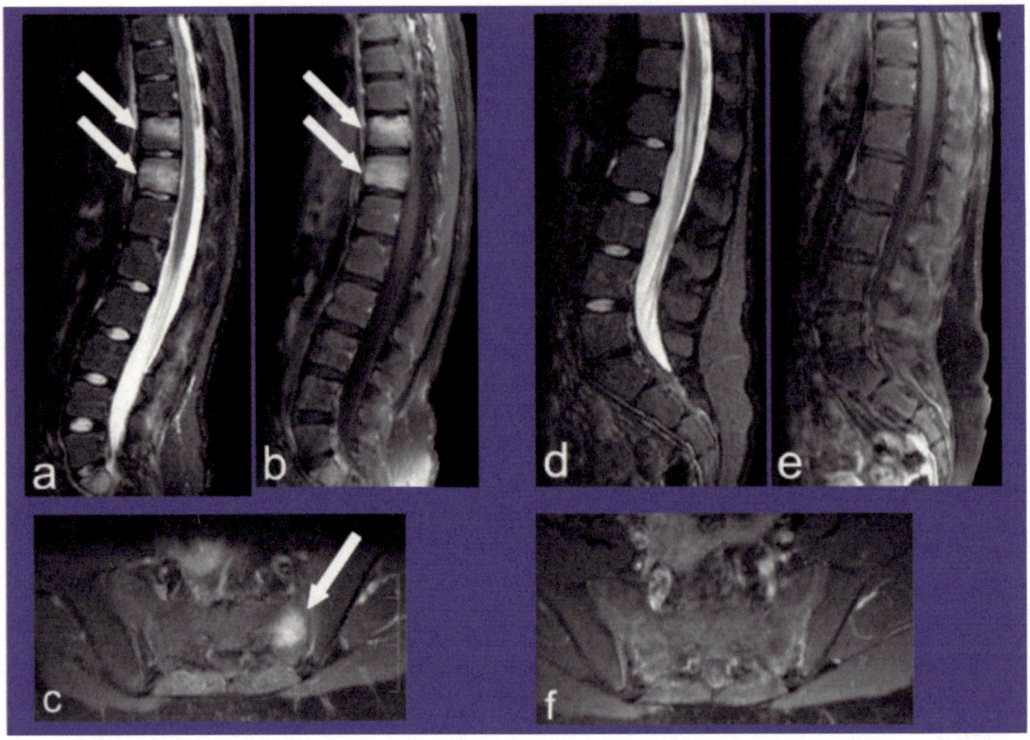

Fig. 12. **CRMO involving the spine in a 10-year old girl. (A-C)**. MR images at sagittal plane (A and B) and axial plane (C) using STIR (Short TI inversion recovery) sequence (A) and post-contrast spin-echo T1-weighted sequence (B and C) reveal abnormal signal in vertebral bodies of T10, T11, and S1 (arrows), as well as sacral ala (arrow). **(D-F)**. MR images using the same technique obtained 5-months later. Complete resolution of the previously seen abnormal signal (Miettunen, Wei et al. 2009).

6.2.1.5 Current recommendations for bisphosphonates

At the present time, we reserve the use of bisphosphonates to patients who have severe pain or functional limitation which fails to respond to traditional medications. In addition, because up to 40% of patients with vertebral CNO have associated crush fracture(s), we recommend that such patients are considered for pamidronate therapy early after diagnosis, especially if severe pain and incipient fractures are present.

6.2.2 Biologic therapy

The principle behind the use of biologic therapy in CNO is based on the observation that there is increased TNF expressed locally and systemically in CNO disorders (Eleftheriou, Gerschman et al. 2010). There are no controlled trials so far, and the results have been more encouraging in adults. Overall, TNF-alpha (TNF-α) blocking agents seem to have the most beneficial effect. TNF is a proinflammatory cytokine that has a wide range of effects, including granulocyte recruitment and activation, induction of edema, activation of coagulation, induction of granuloma formation, and activation of T and B cells (Carpenter, Jackson et al. 2004).

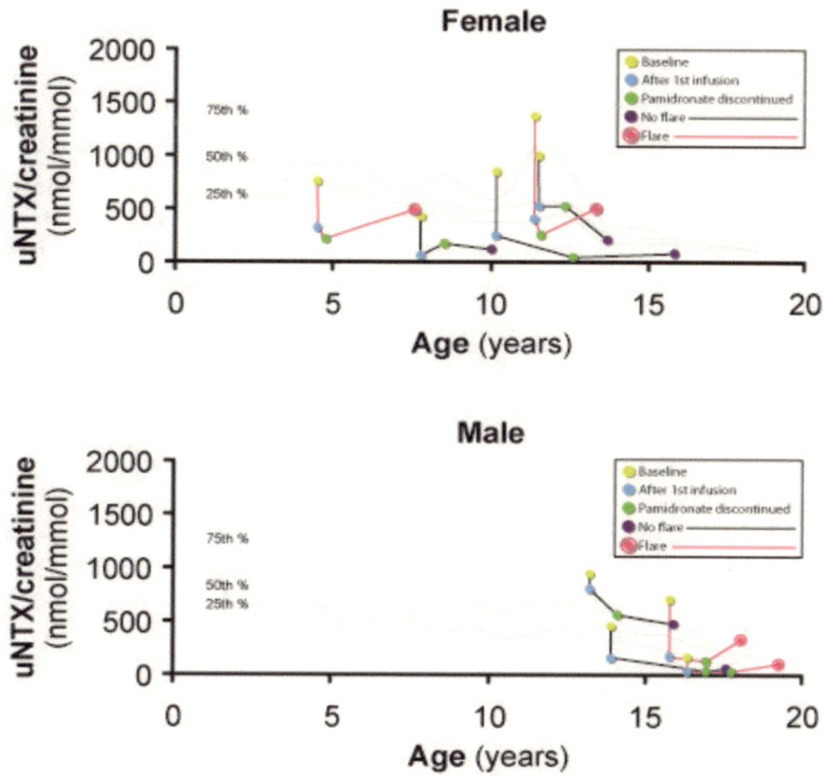

Fig. 13. **Urinary N-telopeptide/urinary creatinine ratio (uNTX/uCr) in girls (*upper panel*) and in boys (*lower panel*).** Data is shown for each individual patient prior to the first intravenous pamidronate treatment; just after the first treatment; at the time of pamidronate discontinuation; and either at the time of last follow-up for patients who did not flare or at the time of CRMO flare. Continuous lines represent the 75th (*top*), 50th (*middle*), and 25th (*bottom*) percentile, respectively, of the reference range for healthy subjects (Miettunen, Wei et al. 2009).

6.2.2.1 Biologic treatment protocol(s)

There are no specific CNO treatment protocols for biologic agents, and the dosing regimens and pre-treatment work-up have typically followed the existing ones for other inflammatory diseases, such as rheumatoid arthritis or inflammatory bowel disease. Because of the risk of re-activating tuberculosis while on biologic therapy, the minimum pre-biologic work-up includes Mantoux skin test and chest radiograph in selected cases. The reader is encouraged to follow the specific local guidelines for pre-biologic work-up, as geographic variations exist.

6.2.2.2 Side effects to biologic medications

Infections remain the most worrisome side effect from biologic therapy, and patients are encouraged to seek medical attention urgently if they developed fever, systemic symptoms, or are otherwise unwell. Autoimmune diseases, such as systemic lupus erythematosus, can rarely develop following biologic therapy. In recent years, a concern has been raised about potential increased risk of malignancies but so far the data are inconclusive (Horneff, Foeldvari et al. 2010).

6.2.2.3 Expected clinical response

In adults, there are at least 20 patients with various CNO disorders who have experienced a beneficial effect from anti TNF-α blockers. Infliximab, a chimeric monoclonal IgG1k antibody directed against TNF-α, has resulted in clinical and at times radiologic improvement in sternal hyperostosis, clavicular osteitis, and SAPHO syndrome (Eleftheriou, Gerschman et al. 2010). Infliximab has also resulted in remission of Crohn's disease associated CRMO (Carpenter, Jackson et al. 2004). The improvement in symptoms occurred within 2 weeks in most patients, although some patients had loss of efficacy with ongoing treatment, and others experienced relapse of symptoms within 6 months after infliximab withdrawal. Only 4 pediatric patients have so far been reported in detail, and all of these patients had received adjunctive therapy that could have contributed to some of the reported efficacy. Infliximab (given at a dose of 6 mg/kg followed by infusions at weeks 2, 6 and then every 8 weeks) was partially helpful in 3 patients, although therapy was discontinued due to suspected fungal skin infection in one patient, and the remaining 2 patients required infliximab every 4 weeks because of symptom recurrence with every 8-weekly infusions (Eleftheriou, Gerschman et al. 2010). Adalimumab (a fully humanized IgG1 anti-TNF-α monoclonal antibody) was helpful in 1 pediatric SAPHO patient with sustained response to at least 15 months. Anakinra (a recombinant IL-1 receptor antagonist) resulted in good symptom control in one patient at 6 weeks, with gradual loss of treatment efficacy by 12 months with new bone lesions and psoriasis-like rash (Eleftheriou, Gerschman et al. 2010).

6.2.2.4 Current recommendations for biologic medications

The current recommendations for biologic therapy in pediatric CNO include consideration of anti-TNF therapy for recalcitrant CNO that is refractory to bisphosphonates (Eleftheriou, Gerschman et al. 2010). The role of anti-IL-1 therapy remains unclear.

6.3 Surgery

Surgical decortications of the affected bone can result in symptom relief (Carr, Cole et al. 1993). However, symptoms often recur, and repeated surgical procedures are required.

7. Course of the disease and prognosis

7.1 Natural history

CNO has a relapsing and remitting course with a variable prognosis. Although majority of patients with CNO have resolution of symptoms post-pubertally, the bone pain in active disease is severe. In addition, long-term studies reveal that up to a quarter of patients have persistent disease, with risk for poorer quality of life, and difficulty in achieving vocational goals (Huber, Lam et al. 2002). Some patients may have up to 25 years of ongoing pain, and without treatment, the episodes of pain vary between months to years. Currently, despite traditional treatment, about 7-25% of patients develop long term sequelae including growth retardation caused by premature closure of epiphyses, bone deformities, premature osteoarthritis, kyphosis, and thoracic outlet syndrome (Schultz, Holterhus et al. 1999). Up to

40% of pediatric patients with vertebral lesions develop vertebral crush fractures (Jansson and Grote 2011).

7.2 Risk factors for persisting disease

Very few studies have analyzed predictive factors for persistent evolution of CRMO. There is one existing study on long term outcome of 40 patients with childhood onset CRMO which suggests that young patients at the onset of the disease with a high number of bony sites seem to be at risk for persistent disease (Catalano-Pons, Comte et al. 2008).

7.3 Extra-bone manifestations

Between 30-80% of CNO patients develop arthritis, including seronegative spondyloarthropathy, over the years. Extra-skeletal inflammatory disorders may emerge, the most common manifestations being palmoplantar pustulosis and psoriasis (30-80% of patients), and inflammatory bowel disease (10% of patients).

8. Conclusions

Clinicians caring for children should be familiar with CNO because it typically occurs during childhood and is a diagnostic mimic of infectious osteomyelitis and malignancies. CNO should be included in the differential diagnosis of patients presenting with suspected unifocal osteomyelitis. Because other sites of bone involvement may be asymptomatic, a bone scan is recommended for patients with negative bacterial cultures of bone biopsy and poor response to antimicrobial agents. Prompt diagnosis of CNO will allow patients to avoid the risks associated with lengthy courses of antibiotic therapy and repeat bone biopsies. NSAIDs are recommended as the first-line agent; DMARDs and short courses of oral steroids are then tried; and bisphosphonates should be considered when vertebral or treatment-resistant CNO is present. Biologic treatment may be considered in selected cases. However, because of the recent discovery that persistent CNO may be more common than previously suspected (Beck, Morbach et al. 2010), the suggested treatment paradigms may well change. The focus of future research will be on the etiology of CNO, with the ultimate goal of developing therapies that can result in true remission. Validation of the proposed pediatric CNO disease activity core set is required, along with the development of tools to identify poor prognostic indicators for persistent disease.

Currently, there is no cure for CNO. Although the individual case series on effects of bisphosphonates and of biologic therapy suggest that clinical and radiologic remission is possible in selected patients with these medications, these results are uncontrolled and observational. There is now a great need for a randomized controlled trial, with participation of many centers, to help define the place of these newer treatment modalities in the management of pediatric CRMO and other CNO disorders.

9. Acknowledgment

I would like to thank Dr Xing-Chang Wei (Radiologist, Alberta Children's Hospital, Calgary, Canada) for assisting with the image preparation and Greg Stephenson for editorial assistance. I also want to thank my patients without whom this work would not have been possible.

10. References

Aksentijevich, I., S. L. Masters, et al. (2009). "An autoinflammatory disease with deficiency of the interleukin-1-receptor antagonist." N Engl J Med 360(23): 2426-37.

Anderson, S. E., P. Heini, et al. (2003). "Imaging of chronic recurrent multifocal osteomyelitis of childhood first presenting with isolated primary spinal involvement." Skeletal Radiol 32(6): 328-36.

Azouz, E. M., A. G. Jurik, et al. (1998). "Sternocostoclavicular hyperostosis in children: a report of eight cases." AJR Am J Roentgenol 171(2): 461-6.

Beck, C., H. Morbach, et al. (2010). "Chronic nonbacterial osteomyelitis in childhood: prospective follow-up during the first year of anti-inflammatory treatment." Arthritis Res Ther 12(2): R74.

Beretta-Piccoli, B. C., M. J. Sauvain, et al. (2000). "Synovitis, acne, pustulosis, hyperostosis, osteitis (SAPHO) syndrome in childhood: a report of ten cases and review of the literature." Eur J Pediatr 159(8): 594-601.

Bjorksten, B. and L. Boquist (1980). "Histopathological aspects of chronic recurrent multifocal osteomyelitis." J Bone Joint Surg Br 62(3): 376-80.

Bousvaros, A., M. Marcon, et al. (1999). "Chronic recurrent multifocal osteomyelitis associated with chronic inflammatory bowel disease in children." Dig Dis Sci 44(12): 2500-7.

Carpenter, E., M. A. Jackson, et al. (2004). "Crohn's-associated chronic recurrent multifocal osteomyelitis responsive to infliximab." J Pediatr 144(4): 541-4.

Carr, A. J., W. G. Cole, et al. (1993). "Chronic multifocal osteomyelitis." J Bone Joint Surg Br 75(4): 582-91.

Catalano-Pons, C., A. Comte, et al. (2008). "Clinical outcome in children with chronic recurrent multifocal osteomyelitis." Rheumatology (Oxford) 47(9): 1397-9.

Chow, L. T., J. F. Griffith, et al. (1999). "Chronic recurrent multifocal osteomyelitis: a great clinical and radiologic mimic in need of recognition by the pathologist." Apmis 107(4): 369-79.

Chun, C. S. (2004). "Chronic recurrent multifocal osteomyelitis of the spine and mandible: case report and review of the literature." Pediatrics 113(4): e380-4.

Compeyrot-Lacassagne, S., A. M. Rosenberg, et al. (2007). "Pamidronate treatment of chronic noninfectious inflammatory lesions of the mandible in children." J Rheumatol 34(7): 1585-9.

El-Shanti, H. I. and P. J. Ferguson (2007). "Chronic recurrent multifocal osteomyelitis: a concise review and genetic update." Clin Orthop Relat Res 462: 11-9.

Eleftheriou, D., T. Gerschman, et al. (2010). "Biologic therapy in refractory chronic non-bacterial osteomyelitis of childhood." Rheumatology (Oxford) 49(8): 1505-12.

Ferguson, P. J., X. Bing, et al. (2006). "A missense mutation in pstpip2 is associated with the murine autoinflammatory disorder chronic multifocal osteomyelitis." Bone 38(1): 41-7.

Giedion, A., W. Holthusen, et al. (1972). "[Subacute and chronic "symmetrical" osteomyelitis]." Ann Radiol (Paris) 15(3): 329-42.

Girschick, H. J., H. I. Huppertz, et al. (1999). "Chronic recurrent multifocal osteomyelitis in children: diagnostic value of histopathology and microbial testing." Hum Pathol 30(1): 59-65.

Girschick, H. J., R. Krauspe, et al. (1998). "Chronic recurrent osteomyelitis with clavicular involvement in children: diagnostic value of different imaging techniques and therapy with non-steroidal anti-inflammatory drugs." Eur J Pediatr 157(1): 28-33.

Girschick, H. J., P. Raab, et al. (2005). "Chronic non-bacterial osteomyelitis in children." Ann Rheum Dis 64(2): 279-85.

Girschick, H. J., C. Zimmer, et al. (2007). "Chronic recurrent multifocal osteomyelitis: what is it and how should it be treated?" Nat Clin Pract Rheumatol 3(12): 733-8.

Gleeson, H., E. Wiltshire, et al. (2008). "Childhood chronic recurrent multifocal osteomyelitis: pamidronate therapy decreases pain and improves vertebral shape." J Rheumatol 35(4): 707-12.

Holden, W. and J. David (2005). "Chronic recurrent multifocal osteomyelitis: two cases of sacral disease responsive to corticosteroids." Clin Infect Dis 40(4): 616-9.

Horneff, G., I. Foeldvari, et al. (2010). "Report on malignancies in the German juvenile idiopathic arthritis registry." Rheumatology (Oxford) 50(1): 230-6.

Huber, A. M., P. Y. Lam, et al. (2002). "Chronic recurrent multifocal osteomyelitis: clinical outcomes after more than five years of follow-up." J Pediatr 141(2): 198-203.

Jansson, A., E. D. Renner, et al. (2007). "Classification of non-bacterial osteitis: retrospective study of clinical, immunological and genetic aspects in 89 patients." Rheumatology (Oxford) 46(1): 154-60.

Jansson, A. F. and V. Grote (2011). "Nonbacterial osteitis in children: data of a German Incidence Surveillance Study." Acta Paediatr 100(8): 1150-7.

Jurik, A. G. (2004). "Chronic recurrent multifocal osteomyelitis." Semin Musculoskelet Radiol 8(3): 243-53.

Jurik, A. G. and N. Egund (1997). "MRI in chronic recurrent multifocal osteomyelitis." Skeletal Radiol 26(4): 230-8.

Kaftori, J. K., U. Kleinhaus, et al. (1987). "Progressive diaphyseal dysplasia (Camurati-Engelmann): radiographic follow-up and CT findings." Radiology 164(3): 777-82.

Kayani, I., I. Syed, et al. (2004). "Vertebral osteomyelitis without disc involvement." Clin Radiol 59(10): 881-91.

Kerrison, C., J. E. Davidson, et al. (2004). "Pamidronate in the treatment of childhood SAPHO syndrome." Rheumatology (Oxford) 43(10): 1246-51.

Khanna, G., T. S. Sato, et al. (2009). "Imaging of chronic recurrent multifocal osteomyelitis." Radiographics 29(4): 1159-77.

King, S. M., R. M. Laxer, et al. (1987). "Chronic recurrent multifocal osteomyelitis: a noninfectious inflammatory process." Pediatr Infect Dis J 6(10): 907-11.

Mandell, G. A., S. J. Contreras, et al. (1998). "Bone scintigraphy in the detection of chronic recurrent multifocal osteomyelitis." J Nucl Med 39(10): 1778-83.

Martin, J. C., R. Desoysa, et al. (1996). "Chronic recurrent multifocal osteomyelitis: spinal involvement and radiological appearances." Br J Rheumatol 35(10): 1019-21.

Miettunen, P. M., X. Wei, et al. (2009). "Dramatic pain relief and resolution of bone inflammation following pamidronate in 9 pediatric patients with persistent chronic recurrent multifocal osteomyelitis (CRMO)." Pediatr Rheumatol Online J 7: 2.

Mortensson, W., G. Edeburn, et al. (1988). "Chronic recurrent multifocal osteomyelitis in children. A roentgenologic and scintigraphic investigation." Acta Radiol 29(5): 565-70.

Ralston, S. H., A. L. Langston, et al. (2008). "Pathogenesis and management of Paget's disease of bone." Lancet 372(9633): 155-63.

Robertson, L. P. and P. Hickling (2001). "Chronic recurrent multifocal osteomyelitis is a differential diagnosis of juvenile idiopathic arthritis." Ann Rheum Dis 60(9): 828-31.

Rosenberg, Z. S., S. Shankman, et al. (1988). "Chronic recurrent multifocal osteomyelitis." AJR Am J Roentgenol 151(1): 142-4.

Schilling, F., Fedlmeier, M., Eckardt, A., Kessler, S. (2002). "Vertebral Manifestation of Chronic Recurrent Multifocal Osteomyelitis (CRMO)." Fortschr Rontgenstr 174: 1236-1242.

Schultz, C., P. M. Holterhus, et al. (1999). "Chronic recurrent multifocal osteomyelitis in children." Pediatr Infect Dis J 18(11): 1008-13.

Sidhu, G., G. Andrews, et al. (2003). "Residents' corner. Answer to case of the month #89. Chronic recurrent multifocal osteomyelitis as a presentation of SAPHO syndrome." Can Assoc Radiol J 54(3): 189-91.

Simm, P. J., R. C. Allen, et al. (2008). "Bisphosphonate treatment in chronic recurrent multifocal osteomyelitis." J Pediatr 152(4): 571-5.

Solau-Gervais, E., M. Soubrier, et al. (2006). "The usefulness of bone remodelling markers in predicting the efficacy of pamidronate treatment in SAPHO syndrome." Rheumatology (Oxford) 45(3): 339-42.

Soubrier, M., J. J. Dubost, et al. (2001). "Pamidronate in the treatment of diffuse sclerosing osteomyelitis of the mandible." Oral Surg Oral Med Oral Pathol Oral Radiol Endod 92(6): 637-40.

Suei, Y., K. Tanimoto, et al. (1995). "Possible identity of diffuse sclerosing osteomyelitis and chronic recurrent multifocal osteomyelitis. One entity or two." Oral Surg Oral Med Oral Pathol Oral Radiol Endod 80(4): 401-8.

Van Merkesteyn, J. P., R. H. Groot, et al. (1988). "Diffuse sclerosing osteomyelitis of the mandible: clinical radiographic and histologic findings in twenty-seven patients." J Oral Maxillofac Surg 46(10): 825-9.

Yu, L., J. R. Kasser, et al. (1989). "Chronic recurrent multifocal osteomyelitis. Association with vertebra plana." J Bone Joint Surg Am 71(1): 105-12.

Part 3

Methods of Approach to Treat the Disease

5

Photodynamic Therapy in the Treatment of Osteomyelitis

João Paulo Tardivo[1] and Mauricio S. Baptista[2]
[1]*Faculdade de Medicina do ABC, São Paulo*
[2]*Departamento de Bioquímica, Instituto de Química da USP, São Paulo*
Brazil

1. Introduction

Osteomyelitis is a bone infection that may initiate due to a local trauma or infection or it may originate due to infections occurring elsewhere in the body (microorganisms are transported by the bloodstream in this case). The bone may be predisposed to infection because of trauma or because of a medical condition like diabetes. The microorganisms responsible for the infection are usually pyogenic bacteria. The most frequent infectious agents are in order of prevalence *Staphylococcus aureus*, *Streptococcus* (groups A and B), *Haemophilus influenzae*, and *Enterobacter species* [1].

Osteomyelitis is highly prevalent in patients with diabetes (extremity bones), patients with fractured and exposed bones and with bone systems that have continuous internal or external trauma/aggression/inflammation (vertebrae in adults). In theory any bone may develop the disease. Extremity bones (arms and legs, especially in children) and spine (vertebral column, especially in adults) are the most affected. In diabetic patients, a large percentage of the patients who have foot ulcers developed osteomyelitis in extremity bones (feet and toes) [1].

Patients with diabetes usually have chronic diseases in the lower ends because they have a higher incidence of vascular failure and reduced sensitivity to pain (diabetic neuropathy). Consequently, they may have skin lesions called skin ulcers that grow in length and in depth, often without the patient realizing it, due to the absence of pain. These ulcers greatly increase the chance of other complications, like soft-tissue infection, tissue infection that may culminate in osteomyelitis and some sort of amputation due to infection that installs both in soft and bone tissues. It is known that diabetic patients have lower immunity responses than the population in general and added with the poor peripheral blood circulation, become more vulnerable to infections, which are more difficult to respond to the treatment. 10% of diabetic patients will develop some sort of foot ulcers followed by amputation. 85% of amputations are preceded by a foot ulcer and 70-100% of the ulcers show signs of peripheral neuropathy associated with various degrees of commitment of the peripheral vasculature [2].

The mortality rate is usually low, unless sepsis occurs. The severity of the disease increases with the dissemination of the infection to surrounding tissues and articular cavity; evolution to chronic osteomyelitis, amputation of the involved extremity, generalized infection or sepsis. It is a disease that can only be treated with long-term systemic and local antiobiotics treatments [1,3]

Photodynamic therapy (PDT) is a promising clinical modality for the management of various tumors and nonmalignant diseases, due to two main effects that are induced by photo-activation of specific drugs called photosensitizers: cell killing properties [4-12] and its ability to modulate the immune response [13, 14]. PDT is based on an excited-state process called photosensitization (see below), which is a combination of a photosensitizer that is selectively localized in the target tissue and illumination of the lesion with visible light, resulting in photodamage and subsequent cell death (microbial killing). The first time the photodynamic effect shown was in the area of microbiology. Raab conducted in-vitro experiments showing the killing of paramecium parasites by PDT [15]. Several other papers were published showing the photo-induced killing of microorganisns [4]. However, development in this area was bunged for several decades because of the discovery of penicillin. With the growing problem of bacterial antibiotic resistance in the last 15 years, there was a resurge in the research focusing in the anti-microbial application of PDT. Currently, PDT is a potential approach to treat localized infectious diseases mainly due microbial resistance. Numerous worldwide clinical studies have shown that PDT represents an effective and safe modality for various types of diseases [4-9], including osteomyelitis [10-12].

2. Mechanisms and drug development in PDT

The cell killing mechanism of PDT is based on the process called photosensitization (Figure 1), which involves a molecule that absorbs light and gets excited from the ground-state (PS) into singlet excited state ($^1PS^*$), which is short-lived ($\cong 10^{-9}$ seconds) and can be quickly deactivated by radiative and non-radiave processes before it has time to react. A good photosensitizer (PS) will undergo a photophysical process called intersystem crossing, which converts the singlet state to a triplet state ($^3PS^1$). Triplet states cannot relax efficiently having a higher tendency to donate or accept electrons, being therefore both stronger reducing and oxidant agents compared to the ground state. Triplets also have a large tendency to engage in energy transfer reactions especially with oxygen. When triplet states are disabled by electron transfer reactions, it originates radical species, in mechanisms that are called type I. These radicals can initiate radical chain reactions leading to damage in lipids, proteins and nucleic acids. In oxygenated environments the photosensitizers can undergo type II photochemical process that involves energy transfer between the excited triplet state of the photosensitizer and stable triplet oxygen ($^3O_2$), producing short lived and highly reactive singlet oxygen ($^1O_2$) [15-17].

Therefore, one can separate the mechanisms of PDT in two classes. The mechanism TYPE I: light energy passes from triplet excited molecules to biomolecules by electron transfer reactions (radical mechanism) that culminates in direct damage to biomolecules or the formation of reactive oxygen species. TYPE II mechanism in the excitation energy is transferred to molecular oxygen, resulting in the formation of singlet oxygen ($^1O_2$), which is highly electrophilic and capable of causing damage to membranes, proteins and DNA [16-18]. The actual chemical mechanism that takes place in cells will depend on the specific microenvironment of the photosensitizer, and clearly depend on specific interactions with membranes and proteins [18-24]. Although most photosensitizer can bind DNA and can

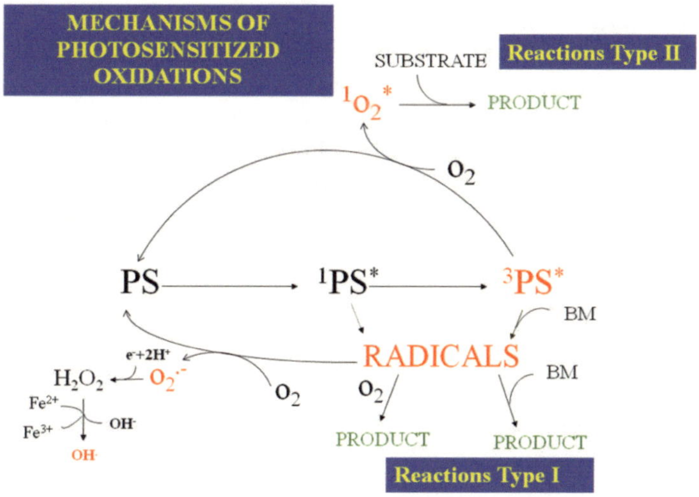

Fig. 1. Photosensitization mechanisms where PS is a photosensitizer that absorbs light going to the first singlet state ($^1PS^*$), converting into a triplet state ($^3PS^*$) by intersystem crossing. The excited species, specially $^3PS^*$ can react by electron transfer forming radical species (Type I mechanism) and starting radical chain reactions or react with oxygen by energy transfer forming Singlet oxygen (Type II mechanism).

photo-damage it in *in-vitro* solution-based experiments, the charged photosensitizers in use do not enter and do not accumulate in cell nuclei, decreasing the possibility of mutagenesis. Adjuvants like hydrogen peroxide can increase the photodynamic efficiency by allowing better uptake of the photosensitizer [25]. Also, nanoparticle platforms have a great potential to control the mechanisms and efficiency of photodynamic action [26-30].

Penetration of light through the skin is dependent on the characteristics of the treated tissue, the absorption by endogenous chromospheres and the scattering of the skin tissues. Wavelengths shorter than 600 nm are absorbed mainly by hemoglobin and other skin choromophores, whereas vibration overtones of water and other molecules induce absorption at wavelengths longer than 950 nm. Tissue scattering, which decreases as the wavelength increases, hinders light penetration of shorter wavelength photons. Forward directed scattering allows for penetration even in high absorbing and scattering tissues. By considering all these processes one can explain light penetration depth (10-20 mm) inside the tissue in the therapeutic window, which is light wavelength from 600 to 950 nm [16]. Therefore, one should choose a photosensitizer that absorbs in the therapeutic window in order to treat internal tissues by PDT. The light dose, which is usually given in joules per square centimeter, is empirical and varies widely. For interstitial applications, radiant exposures between 20 and 300 J/cm2 are needed [5-10, 16].

As mentioned above the first report of PDT action was of a dye (Acridine), which was used to kill a microorganism (paramecium) under illumination [15, 31]. Just few years after the experiment of Raab, the photodynamic concept was applied to dermatology using another dye (eosin) [31]. In 1912 Friedrich Betz Meyer published results of an experiment he did on himself, by injecting himself with a mixture of porphyrin oligomers and showed that he only had erythema reaction in tissues that were illuminated with light, proving that the photodynamic effect depends on light and on photosensitizer [31, 32].

In the 70´s-80´s the protocols developed by Dougherty and his group used a photosensitizer similar to the one Meyer injected himself with, which was called hematoporphyrin derivative (HPD, later called PhotofrinR, Figure 2D). HPD showed great potential to treat tumors, leading to the PDT approval by FDA as a treating modality for head and neck cancers [5, 33]. The protocols developed by Dougherty´s group rely on expensive laser systems, being restricted to only very few research centers in the world. PhotofrinR targets mainly the leakage vasculature of tumor tissues [33, 34]. Intracellular photosensitizers were subsequently tested clinically and have shown to be potentially more efficient. Oseroff and co-workers were the first to propose the strategy of targeting intracellular organelles instead of the tumor vasculature [35].

In the clinical realm, new generation photosensitizers were designed to have intracellular targets. A successful example was Foscan (Tetra-meso hydroxyphenyl chlorin, Figure 2F), which is a powerful intra-cellular photosensitizer. Its high photodynamic efficiency has been explained by the photooxidation of intracellular targets, because the quantum yields of singlet oxygen production is comparable or inferior to other relevant photosensitizers [36, 37]. The intracellular generation of protoporphyrin IX by administration of its metabolic precursors (ALA), was another successful example that helped to expand the applications of PDT (Figure 2E). Today almost any dermatologist around the world knows and uses PDT with ALA to treat a variety of skin diseases.

It is important to mention that although being more efficient than the initial protocols, the available PDT treatments are still very expensive and consequently are nor very useful in terms of public health, especially for developing and under-developed countries. In fact, during three decades of clinical PDT, most of the treating protocols were based on the use of hematoporphyrin and its derivatives, irradiated with lasers or very sophisticated non-coherent light sources [5,16]. The combination of inexpensive photosensitizers and light sources have allowed the development of new PDT protocol that are inexpensive, safe and efficient [6-10]. Therefore, we can conclude that there is a great potential for the widespread use of PDT even in underserved populations.

The concept of photodynamic cell killing was soon extended to treat infectious diseases, i.e., its photoantimicrobial action [4, 38]. The effect of the generation of large amounts of radicals and non-radicals oxidizing species on microbials is extremely destructive for two main reasons: lack of effective microbial defenses against these species and multiple sites of attack. Although cells have several natural defenses against reactive species, the level of redox imbalance inflicted by PDT is several orders of magnitude larger than the level or protection allowed by enzymatic and molecular antioxidants within the cell. Besides that, bacteria can defend itself against superoxide radical and hydrogen peroxide, but hydroxyl radical and singlet oxygen cannot be naturally deactivated. Consequently, an important advantage of PDT is the absence of microbial resistance [4, 38].

The development of improved drugs in any pharmaceutical application depends on the knowledge of structure activity-relationships and of the action mechanisms involved. We and others have invested a lot of efforts on solving these issues related with PDT [6,16-25]. New molecular structures, nanoparticles or nanoemulsions are being investigated in order to develop new and more efficient photo-active drugs [18-30]. Several medical conditions were treated by different protocols and depending on the medical condition, specific molecules and delivery systems were designed [5-10]. There are several low-cost options to

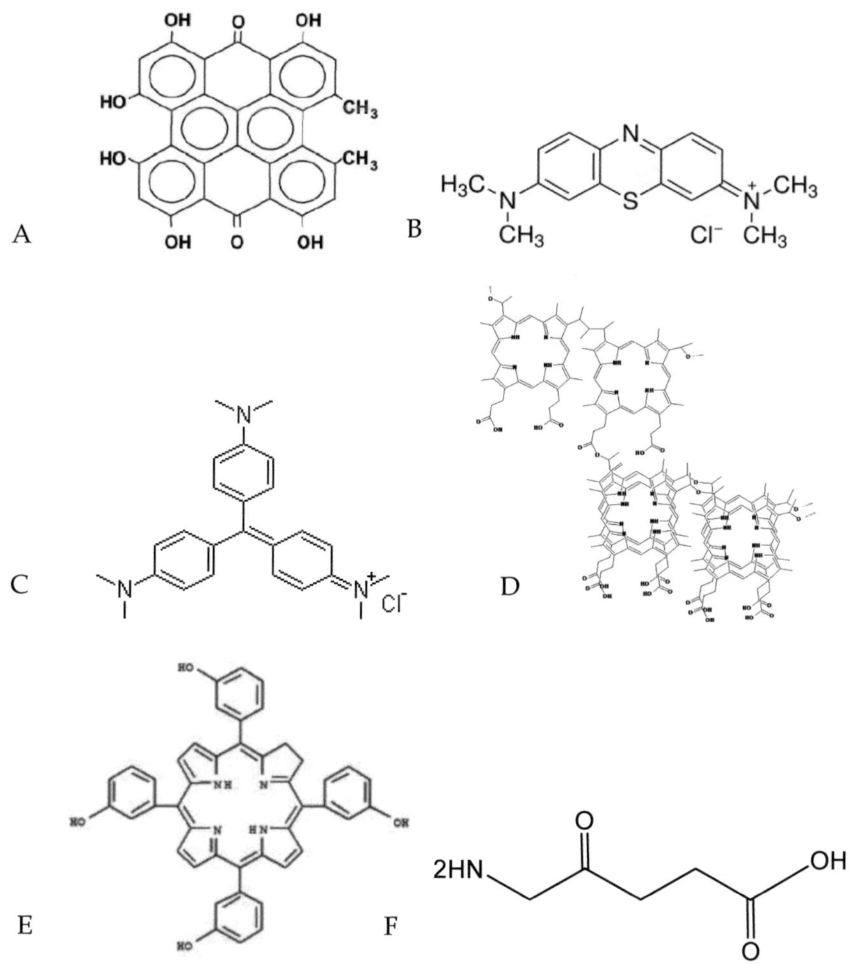

Fig. 2. Examples of photosensitizers used in PDT, from A to E, hypericin, methylene blue, crystal violet, hematoporphyrin derivative and tetra-meso-hydroxyphenyl-chlorin (FoscanR). Compound labeled F is 5-aminolevulinic acid (ALA), which is a pro-drug that is metabolized in the intra-cellular environment to the actual photosensitizer that is Protoporphyrin IX.

be considered as photosensitizers in PDT, which include hypericin, methylene blue and other phenothiazines, crystal violet and other tryarilmethanes (Figure 2A-C).

3. PDT in the case of osteomyelitis

The classical treatment of osteomyelitis requires surgical removal of the diseased tissue and high doses of antibiotics, which are often nephrotoxic, further compromising the health of patients. In-vitro and animal studies in the laboratory have shown the potential of PDT for causing efficient cell death of infecting bacteria as well as treating animals with the disease [11,12]. Low-cost PDT protocols were also tested with success in diabetic patients with osteomyelitis [10].

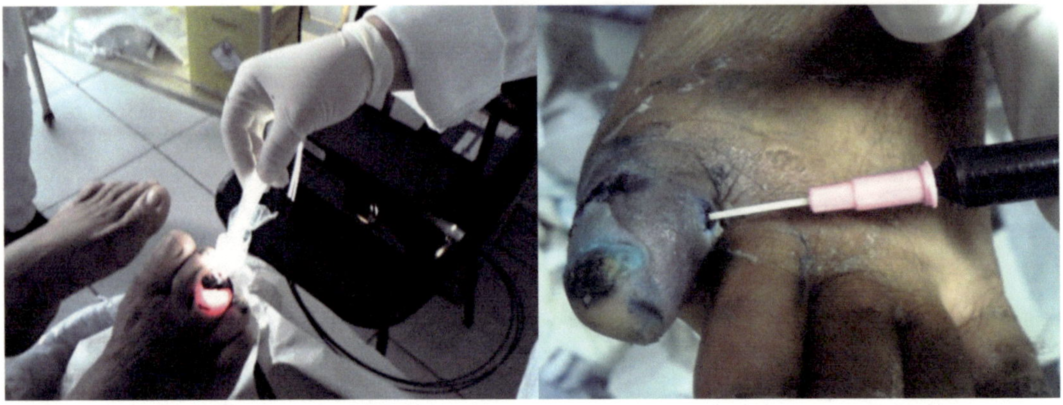

Fig. 3. Two osteomyelitis patients that were selected in the clinical studies conducted by JP Tardivo in the Hospital da Fundação ABC. The picture in the left shows how Methylene Blue solution is injected in the bone through the fistula. In the right the illumination with optical fiber conducted by the continuous white-light source (FASA).

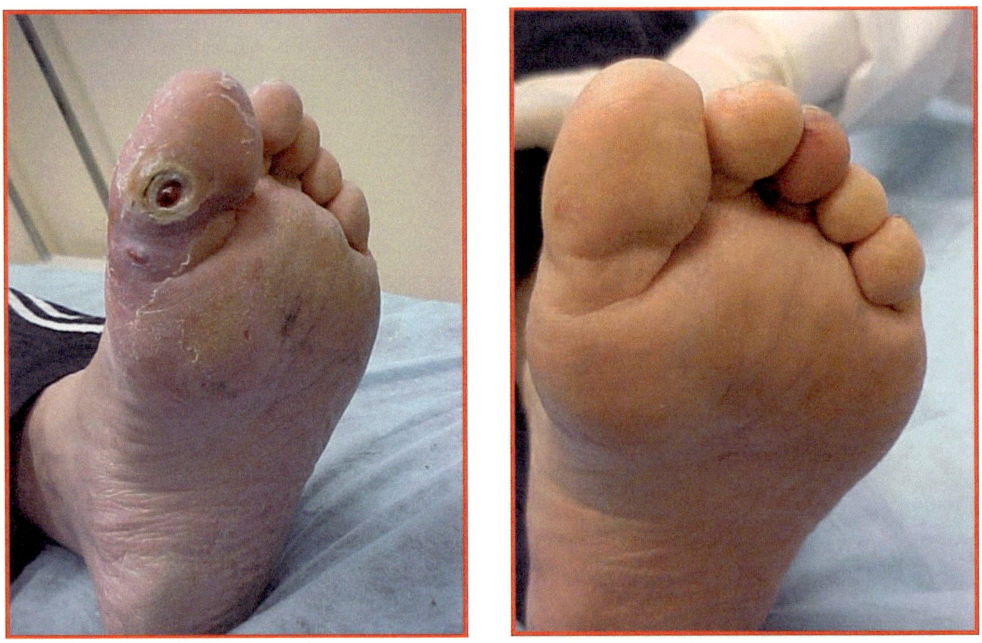

Fig. 4. Plantar region of the thumb of a diabetic patient with osteomyelitis pre and post treatment with PDT. A 1:1 mixture of MB 2% and TB 2% was injected into the patient's great toe. Further details of treatment and conditions are described in **Reference 10**.

PDT in osteomyelitis is intended to eliminate any micro-organism that is installed in bone tissue. In order to combat infection in the bone and soft tissue a photosensitizer solution has to be introduced in the lesion tissue that must be subsequently illuminated (Figures 3, 4). Usually this can be easily realized by administrating the photosensitizer by the drainage of the skin fistulas, which reaches the bone (Figure 3). Illumination should be conducted for around 10 minutes to allow a light dose of around ~20-30 J/cm2, by internal and external irradiation. Internal irradiation is obtained by introducing optical fibers delivering light directly in the bone and external irradiation with non-coherent polychromatic light sources (Figures 3 and 4). Patients are only accompanied in the ambulatory throughout the treatment, which usually lasts for several weeks. In that period, spontaneously removal of bone fragments was observed by radiographies, fistulas were healed and patient were considered cured (Figures 3 and 4). In the clinical studies conducted so far, 12 patients were treated with success and 8 are being treated. The patients selected in this clinical study had not responded well to usual antibiotic therapy and had had indication of amputation.

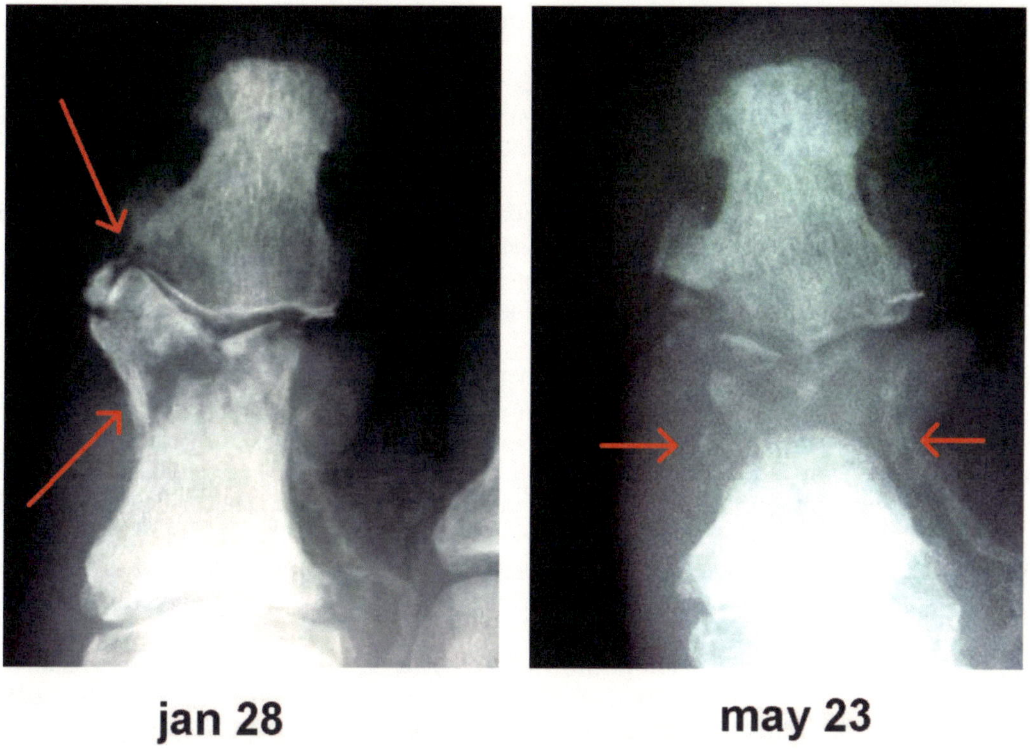

Fig. 5. Radiography of great toe of P1 before (A) and after (B) PACT treatment. Arrows in A: fractures in distal and proximal phalanges. Arrows in B: bone fragments spontaneously removed after treatment. A 1:1 mixture of MB 2% and TB 2% was injected into the patient's great toe. Further details of treatment and conditions are described in **Reference 10**.

4. Conclusions

Photodynamic therapy reduces the risk of amputation, causing cell death to microorganisms that are infecting bone tissues and consequently accelerate healing of osteomyelitis lesions. It also reduces inflammation and pain in the tissue ulcers. PDT provides an efficient and quick treatment that helps avoiding amputations. The physiological/cosmetic outcomes are impressive with small side effects (small pain during treatment is sometimes reported). Besides all these benefits, PDT may be performed in office or clinic and low-cost protocols are available. Consequently, PDT can clearly help to improve the quality of life of diabetic patients.

5. References

[1] Lew, D.P.; Waldvogel, F.A. Osteomyelitis. *N Engl J Med* 1997, 336, 999-1007.

[2] Diabetic Foot, International Consensus, 2003; http://www.iwgdf.org.

[3] Calhoun, J.H.; Mader, J.T. Treatment of Osteomyelitis With a Biodegradable Antibiotic Implant. Clin *Orthop Related Res* 1997, 341, 206-214.

[4] Wainwright, M. Photodynamic antimicrobial chemotherapy (PACT). *J Antimicrob Chemother* 1998, 42, 13-28.

[5] Dougherty T.J. Photochemistry in the treatment of cancer in *Advances in Photochemistry,* Vol. 17, Eds. D.H. Volman, G.S. Hammond and D.C. Neckers, 275-311, Wiley: New York, 1992.

[6] Tardivo, J.P.; Del Giglio, A.; Oliveira, C.S.; Gabrielli, D.S.; Junqueira, H.C.; Tada, D.B.; Severino, D.; Turchiello, R., Baptista, MS. Methylene Blue in Photodynamic Therapy: From Basic Mechanisms to Clinical Applications *Photodiag Photodyn Ther* 2005, 2/3, 175-191.

[7] Tardivo JP; Del Giglio A; Paschoal LH; Baptista MS; A New PDT protocol to treat AIDS-related Kaposi's sarcoma, *Photomed Laser Surg* 2006, 24 (4), 528-531.

[8] Tardivo, J.P., Del Giglio A., Paschoal, L.H.C., Ito A.S., Baptista, M.S., "Treatment of Melanoma Lesions Using Methylene Blue And RL50 Light Source" *Photodiag Photodyn Ther* 2004, 1, 345-346.

[9] Baptista, M.S.; Wainwright, M. Photodynamic antimicrobial chemotherapy (PACT) for the treatment of malaria, leishmaniasis and trypanosomiasis *Braz J Med Biol Res* 2011, 44(1) 1-10.

[10] Tardivo, J.P.; Baptista, M.S. Treatment of Osteomyelitis in the Feet of Diabetic Patients by Photodynamic Antimicrobial Chemotherapy *Photomed Laser Surg* 2009, *27,* 145-150.

[11] Bisland, S.K.; Chien, C.; Wilson, B.C.; Burch, S. Pre-clinical *in vitro* and *in vivo* studies to examine the potential use of photodynamic therapy in the treatment of osteomyelitis *Photochem. Photobiol. Sci.*, 2006, *5*, 31–38.

[12] Goto, B.; Iriuchishima, T.; Horaguchi, T.; Tokuhashi, Y. Nagai, Y.; Harada, T.; Saito, A.; Aizawa, S.Therapeutic Effect of Photodynamic Therapy Using Na-Pheophorbide a on Osteomyelitis Models in Rats. *Photomed Laser Surg* 2011, *29*, 183–189.

[13] Pawel, M.; Huang, Y.-Y.; Hamblin, M.R. "Photodynamic therapy for cancer and activation of immune response." Biophotonics and Immune Responses V. Ed. Wei R. Chen. San Francisco, California, USA: SPIE, 2010. 756503-8.

[14] Ana P. Castano, A.P.; Mroz, P.; Hamblin, M.R. Photodynamic therapy and anti-tumour immunity *Nat Rev Cancer* 2006, 6(7): 535–545.

[15] Raab, O. Action of fluorescent materials on infusorial substances *Zeitschrift fuer Biologie* 1900, 39, 524-546.

[16] Ochsner M. Photophysical and photobiological processes in the photodynamic therapy of tumors. *J Photochem Photobiol B* 1997, 39:1-18.

[17] Castano, A.P.; Demidova, T.N.; Hamblin, M.R. Mechanisms in photodynamic therapy: Part three—Photosensitizer pharmacokinetics, biodistribution, tumor localization and modes of tumor destruction *Photodiag. Photodyn. Ther.* 2005, *2*, 91-106.

[18] Baptista, M.S.; Indig, G.L. Effect of BSA Binding on Photophysical and Photochemical Properties of Triarylmethane Dyes *J Phys Chem B* 1998, *102*, 4678-4688.

[19] Junqueira, H. C.; Severino, D.; Dias, L.G.; Gugliotti, M. ; Baptista, M. S. "Modulation of the Methylene Blue Photochemical Properties Based on the Adsorption at Aqueous Micelle Interfaces" *Phys Chem Chem Phys* 2002, 4, 2320-2328.

[20] Gabrieli, D.; Belisle, E.; Severino, D.; Kowaltowski, A.J.; Baptista, M.S. Binding, aggregation and photochemical properties of methylene blue in mitochondrial suspensions *Photochem. Photobiol.* 2004, 79, 227-232.

[21] Engelmann, F. M.; Mayer I.; Gabrielli, D.; Araki, K.; Toma H. E.; Kowaltowski, A.; Baptista, M. S. Interactions of Cationic *Meso*-Porphyrins with biomembranes *J Bioenerg Biomembr* 2007, 39(2), 175-185.

[22] Engelmann, F.M.; Mayer, I.; Araki, K.; Toma, H.E.; Baptista, M.S.; Maeda, H.; Osuka, A.; Furuta, H. "Photochemistry of Doubly N-confused porphyrin bond to non-conventional high oxidation state Ag(III) and Cu(III) ions" *J. Photochem.Photobiol.A: Chemistry* 2004, 163, 403-411.

[23] Pavani, C.; Uchoa, A.F.; Oliveira, C.S; Iamamoto, Y.; Baptista, M.S. Effect of zinc insertion and hydrophobicity on the membrane interactions and PDT activity of porphyrin photosensitizers *Photochem. Photobiol. Sci.* 2009, *8*, 233–240.

[24] Uchoa, A.F., Oliveira, C.S., Baptista, MS Relationship between structure and photoactivity of porphyrins *J Porph Phthaloc* 2010, 14: 832–845.

[25] Garcez, *A.S;* Núñez, *S.C.* Baptista, *M.s.;* Daghastanli, *N.A.;* Itri, *R;* Hamblin, M.R.; Ribeiro, M.S Antimicrobial mechanisms behind photodynamic effect in the presence of hydrogen peroxide *Photochem. Photobiol. Sci.* 2011, 10, 483–490, 483-490.

[26] Tada, D.B.; Rossi, L.M.; Leite, C.A.P.; Itri, R.; Baptista, M.S.. Nanoparticle platform to modulate reaction mechanism of phenothiazine photosensitizers *J Nanosci Nanotech* 2010, 10, 3100-3108.

[27] Engelmann, F.M.; Rocha, S.V.O.; Toma, E.; Araki, K.; Baptista, M.S. Determination of *n*-octanol/water partition coefficients and membrane binding of cationic porphyrins. *Int J Pharm* 2007, 329, 12-18.

[28] Tada, D.; Vono, L.L.R.; Duarte, E.Itri, R.; Kiyohara, P.K.; Baptista, M.S.; Rossi, L.M Methylene blue-containing silica coated magnetic particles: a potential magnetic carrier for photodynamic therapy, *Langmuir* 2007, *23*, 8194-8199.

[29] Rossi, L.M.; Silva, P.R.; Uchoa, A.F., Tada, D.B.; Baptista, M.S Protoporphyrin IX nanoparticle-carrier: preparation, optical properties and singlet oxygen generation. *Langmuir* 2008, *24*, 12534-12538.

[30] Deda, D.K.; Caritá, E.; Baptista, M.S.; Toma, H.E., Araki, K. A New Polymeric Nanocapsule Formulation with Potential Applications for thePDT Treatment of Skin Cancer *Int J Pharm* 2009, 376, 76-83.

[31] Roberts, D.J., Cairnduff, F. Photodynamic therapy of primary skin cancer: a review. *Brit. J. Plast. Surg.* 1995, *48*, 360-370.

[32] Meyer-Betz F. Untersuchungen uber die bioloische (photodynamische) wirkung des hamatoporphyrins und anderer derivative des blut-und gallenfarbstoffs. *Dtsch Arch Klin Med.* 1913, *112*, 476-503.

[33] Dougherty, T.J.; Kaufman, J.E.;.Goldfarb, A.; Weishaupt, K.R.; Boyle, D. Mittleman, A. Photoradiation Therapy for the Treatment of Malignant Tumors. *Cancer Res* 1978, *38*, 2628.

[34] Dougherty, T.J. Photodynamic therapy (PDT) of malignant tumors *Critical Reviews in Oncology/hematology* 1984, *2*(2):83-116.

[35] J.S. Modica-Napolitano, J. L. Joyal, G. Ara, A.R. Oseroff and J.R. Aprille Mitochondrial toxicity of cationic photosensitizers for photochemotherapy *Cancer Res* 1990, 50, 7876-7881.

[36] H. J. Jones, D. I. Vernon, S. B. Brown, Photodynamic therapy effect of *m*-THPC (Foscan®) *in vivo*: correlation with pharmacokinetics *Brit. J. Cancer* 2003, 89, 398–404.

[37] M-H.Teiten, L.Bezdetnaya, P.Morliere, R.Santus, F.Guillemin, Endoplasmic reticulum and Golgi apparatus are the preferential sites of Foscan® localisation in cultured tumour cells *British J. Cancer* 2003, 88, 146-152.

[38] Wainwright, M *Photosensitizers in Biomedicine*, 1ed. Oxford:Wiley, 2009.

6

Antibiotic Loaded Acrylic Bone Cement in Orthopaedic Trauma

Sumant Samuel
Department of Orthopaedics (III), Christian Medical College, Vellore India

1. Introduction

Local antibiotic delivery with antibiotic loaded acrylic bone cement has been used extensively in the management of chronic osteomyelitis and implant related infections. It is considered the gold standard for treatment of musculoskeletal infections (Nelson, 2004; Hanssen, 2005; Samuel et al., 2010). The critical factors in the treatment of any orthopaedic infection are adequate surgical debridement, integrity of the host immune system, and adequate antibiotic levels (Brien et al., 1993). Antibiotic loaded bone cement **(ALBC)** is popular as it is a proven way to deliver high concentrations of the drug locally, even to avascular areas that are inaccessible by systemic antibiotics. Another advantage of local antibiotic delivery is that the high concentrations of the drug achieved locally would be effective against organisms that are resistant to drug concentrations achieved by systemic antibiotics. Finally, its use results in only low serum antibiotic concentrations and hence less toxicity than that associated with systemic administration. It is perceived that with future developments local antibiotic delivery systems will likely supplant the traditional use of systemic antibiotics for the treatment of musculoskeletal infections(Hanssen, 2005). This chapter will review the role of antibiotic loaded acrylic bone cement in orthopaedic trauma

2. Historical background

The novel concept of local antibiotic delivery by incorporation of gentamicin into acrylic bone cement was introduced by Buchholz et al in the 1970s (Buchholz et al., 1981). Their pioneering work initiated the concept of local drug delivery by antibiotic loaded bone cement thus beginning a new era in the treatment of musculoskeletal infections. One of the first confirmatory laboratory studies was done by Marks et al who showed that Oxacillin, cefazolin, and gentamicin elutes in a microbiologically active form from palacos and Simplex bone cements (Marks et al., 1976). In another early study, Elson et al showed that when antibiotic loaded acrylic bone cement is placed next to cortical bone, dense cortical bone is penetrated by the eluted antibiotic and its concentration in the bone is much higher than that can be achieved safely by systemic administration(Elson et al., 1977). This was followed by in vivo animal studies of Schurman et al and Wahlig et al confirming the elution of pharmacologically active gentamicin from acrylic bone cement (Schurman et al., 1978; Wahlig et al., 1978). Wahligs report also stated their experience with gentamicin loaded bone cement in forty-one patients with infection of either bone or soft tissue, mainly of the lower limb. They reported that high concentrations of gentamicin were measurable in the exudate from the wound and that this form of treatment was well tolerated (Wahlig et al., 1978). In 1981, Bucholz published his landmark article on the treatment of infected total joint replacement. Though many orthopaedic surgeons doubted its efficacy till then, his work was well received and established the principle of using antibiotic loaded bone cement (Nelson, 2004; Buchholz et al., 1981).

3. Rationale for use

Musculoskeletal infection presents when bone or orthopaedic implants are colonized by micro-organisms by hematogenous seeding, direct inoculation or airborne contamination (Nelson, 2004). These micro-organisms are planktonic in nature to begin with. Over time and on attachment to implants, they become sessile, reduce their metabolic rate, and become covered by biofilm. Biofilm is an extracellular polymeric glycocalyx. Once formed, this biofilm protects the micro-organism from antimicrobials, opsonization, and phagocytosis (Nelson, 2004). To effectively eliminate bacteria in a biofilm, local antibiotic concentrations achieved must be 10 to 100 times the usual bactericidal concentration. This usually cannot be achieved by safe doses of parenteral antibiotics; therefore, systemic antibiotic treatment of sessile bacterial infections is often ineffective (Nelson, 2004). Antibiotic loaded bone cement is a proven way to deliver high concentrations of the drug locally, particularly in the case of poorly vascularized tissues (Brien et al., 1993; Cerretani et al., 2002; Baleani et al., 2008). Its use also results in a low serum antibiotic concentration and less toxicity than that associated with systemic administration (Cerretani et al., 2002).

Acrylic bone cement was primarily developed as a fixation device for arthroplasty. When used for prosthesis fixation, mechanical properties of the antibiotic loaded acrylic cement need to be considered (Baleani et al., 2008; Persson et al., 2006). Because mechanical performances are not a major concern for spacers or cement beads (they are temporary solutions and in these cases the bone cement is not significantly loaded mechanically), the cement may in these cases can contain high antibiotic concentrations considering only its elution properties, microbiological efficiency, and safety (Baleani et al., 2008).

Sensitivity of bacteria is currently determined on the basis of effective serum levels achievable by systemic antibiotics. Most bacteria defined as resistant by these criteria might be sensitive when exposed to significantly high local tissue levels, as is possible with local antibiotic delivery (Hanssen, 2005; Brien et al., 1993; Hanssen and Spangehl, 2004). For successful antimicrobial treatment, it is essential to re-classify the etiologic micro-organism as sensitive or resistant based on antibiotic levels locally achievable (Hanssen, 2005; Brien et al., 1993). And so, it has been stressed that the traditional methods of antibiotic sensitivity cannot be extrapolated simply for this method of treatment (Hanssen, 2005). This point is best exemplified by Bucholz's work where the antibiotic placed in the bone cement did not often correlate with the sensitivity of the organisms being treated (Buchholz et al., 1981).

4. Mechanism of action

Elution of antibiotics from PMMA beads follows a biphasic pattern, with an initial rapid phase and a secondary slow phase(Thonse and Conway, 2007). It is now well known that only a small portion of the antibiotic incorporated in bone cement is released. The mechanism by which these drugs are released is still debated. Early on it was thought that the elution of antibiotics from bone cement, though dependent on many factors, was mainly by diffusion(Buchholz et al., 1984). Bayston and Milner studied the release of gentamicin sulphate, sodium fusidate and diethanolamine fusidate from Palacos and CMW cements. They subscribed to the theory of diffusion of drugs through solid matrices and on the basis of their results, were convinced that antibiotics are released from the cement by a process of diffusion(Bayston and Milner, 1982). The diffusion theory relies on the presence of pores and connecting capillaries in bone cement, through which the circulating medium penetrates and dissolves the incorporated antibiotics which then slowly diffuse outwards(van de Belt et al., 2001). However, others have argued that a critical review of the data they presented does not support this conclusion(Masri et al., 1995).

The most commonly accepted theory is that the elution of antibiotics occurs from the surface of the bone cement and also from the pores and cracks in its matrix(van de Belt et al., 2001; Masri et al., 1995). In support of this theory, elution is improved with increasing surface area and porosity of the cement. Numerous studies have shown that that elution of antibiotics is a surface phenomenon that is related to pores and cracks within the bone cement matrix(Marks et al., 1976; Masri et al., 1995; Wroblewski, 1977; Baker and Greenham, 1988). Van de Belt et al studied the release of gentamicin as a function of time from six different gentamicin-loaded bone cements and related it to surface roughness, porosity and wettability of the cements. They concluded that the release kinetics of gentamicin from bone cements is controlled by a combination of surface roughness and porosity and suggested that the initial release antibiotic from bone cement was mainly a surface phenomenon, while sustained release over several days was a bulk diffusion phenomenon(van de Belt et al., 2000). This theory best accounts for the biphasic release characteristics of antibiotic bone cement.

5. Ideal antibiotic, dose and bone cement

The ideal local antibiotic delivery system has not been created and the search is still on for both the ideal delivery vehicle and the ideal antibiotic (Nelson, 2004). In most situations today, the use of antibiotic loaded bone cement for treatment of established infection still requires hand-mixing of higher dosages of various antibiotics into bone cement by the treating physician as a clinician directed application (Hanssen, 2005). Self- made antibiotic loaded bone cement beads are cheaper, antibiotic specific and have no availability issues (Samuel et al., 2010).

The traditional attributes for an antibiotic to be acceptable for mixing with bone cement in the operating room are that it must be safe, thermostable, water-soluble, hypoallergenic, bactericidal with a broad spectrum of activity, and in powder form (Brien et al., 1993). There still is no agreement concerning the choice or dose of the antibiotic to be mixed with the cement (Cerretani et al., 2002), as can be seen from the numerous published reports concerning vancomycin (Brien et al., 1993; Cerretani et al., 2002; Baleani et al., 2008), gentamicin, tobramycin (Brien et al., 1993)cephalosporins, clindamycin, ticarcillin, ciprofloxacin, amikacin, meropenem (Baleani et al., 2008), imipenem - cilastin(Cerretani et al., 2002) daptomycin and several others (Hanssen and Spangehl, 2004). Increasing bacterial resistance against common antibiotics, especially gentamycin, has lead to a demand for alternative drugs (Brien et al., 1993; Baleani et al., 2008; Hanssen and Spangehl, 2004; Hanssen, 2004).

The optimum dosing of antibiotics in bone cement with regards to safety and efficacy has yet to be determined (Springer et al., 2004). Many authors recommend an antibiotic proportion of 3 to 6% (Buchholz et al., 1981). Higher antibiotic doses are being recommended when the indication is therapeutic, which is the case when acrylic cement is used as beads or spacers (Hanssen and Spangehl, 2004; Springer et al., 2004). Hanssen classified antibiotic loaded bone cement into high dose (>2 g antibiotic per 40 g of cement) and low dose (<2 g antibiotic per 40 g of cement) and recommended high dose for use as beads or spacers and low dose for prosthesis fixation (Hanssen, 2004). It is possible to introduce as much as 10 to 12 g of antibiotics per 40-gram batch of bone cement and still accomplish cement polymerization. It is postulated that mixing high doses of powdered antibiotics creates considerable cement porosity and facilitates increased elution of antibiotics for at least 4 weeks (Hanssen and Spangehl, 2004)

The addition of two antibiotics to acrylic bone cement has been shown to increase the elution of the antibiotics (Cerretani et al., 2002; Baleani et al., 2008). Studies have shown that that the addition of meropenem increases the elution of Vancomycin (Baleani et al., 2008). This phenomenon has been reported previously for combinations of vancomycin with other antibiotics (Cerretani et al., 2002) and is referred to as passive opportunism (Baleani et al., 2008). The second positive effect of dual antibiotic loaded bone cement is the broadening of antibacterial spectrum (Cerretani et al., 2002; Baleani et al., 2008).

One of the many factors that affect the release of antibiotics from bone cement is the type of cement used (Cerretani et al., 2002; Hanssen, 2004). Palacos cement has been shown to be most effective for the purpose of antibiotic delivery in many studies(Elson et al., 1977; Bayston and Milner, 1982; Wininger and Fass, 1996). Marks et al. proved that, in vitro, Palacos R elutes larger amounts of oxacillin, gentamicin, and cefazolin for a longer period of time than Simplex P bone cement. They showed that scanning electron microscopy studies reveal a larger pore size in Palacos R bone cement compared with Simplex P bone cement. Based on this they concluded that their observation of improved elution with Palacos R bone cement was related to the increased pore size which in turn leads to an increase in the microscopic overall surface area of exposed bone cement(Marks et al., 1976). Increased pore size in palacos cement may be related to the fact that palacos cement contains polymethymethacrylate as a copolymer 'filler" in contrast with other brands of acrylic bone cement.

6. Drawbacks and adverse effects

The use of antibiotic bone cement results in low serum antibiotic concentrations and hence systemic toxicity is not a significant issue. However, as was stressed in the earlier section, the present trend is to use high doses of antibiotics in beads and spacers when the indication is therapeutic. Springer et al studied the systemic safety and potential adverse effects of using a high-dose antibiotic- impregnated cement spacer after resection arthroplasty of 36 infected total knee replacements in 34 patients. Spacers placed by them contained an average total dose of 10.5 g of vancomycin and 12.5 g of gentamicin and they found that the use of high-dose vancomycin and gentamicin antibiotic spacers seems to be clinically safe (Springer et al., 2004). However, reports do exist in literature where patients have developed systemic toxicity (renal failure) attributable to local antibiotic delivery through bone cement(Dovas et al., 2008; van Raaij et al., 2002; Curtis et al., 2005; Patrick et al., 2006). All these case reports describe this complication in elderly patients who had been implanted aminoglycoside loaded bone cement. Therefore, though systemic toxicity in uncommon, the use of high dose antibitic loaded bone cement in elderly patients warrants careful follow-up of renal function.

One of the most common concerns about the clinical efficacy of antibiotic-releasing bone cements is the debate over their role in causing antibiotic resistance in micro-organisms(van de Belt et al., 2001). Like any other biomaterial, PMMA also attracts infectious micro-organisms. These cause the surface of the bio-material to form a micro-ecosystem in which they thrive in a slime-enclosed biofilm. Various in vitro studies have shown the adherence and growth of bacteria on antibiotic-loaded bone cement. As micro- organisms adhere to and grow on these antibiotic-loaded bone cement beads, they are exposed to prolonged periods of low doses of the incorporated antibiotic and eventually become resistant to them(van de Belt et al., 2001; Neut et al., 2003).

Anagnostakos et al evaluated this problem by bacteriologically examining 18 chains of antibiotic-loaded beads (11 gentamicin-loaded, 7 gentamicin-vancomycin-loaded) that had been implanted for the treatment of orthopedic infections. In 4 cases (3 with S. epidermidis and one with MRSA), they found persistence of bacterial growth on the beads. While S. epidermidis strains persisted only on gentamicin-loaded beads, MRSA could grow on gentamicin-vancomycin impregnated cement. They observed the emergence of gentamicin-resistant S. epidermidis strain in one case despite the fact that preoperative samples of S. epidermidis of the patient had been susceptible to the antibiotic. Their study shows that the persistence of bacterial growth on bone cement remains a practical problem and that adherence of bacteria to cement can lead to emergence of bacterial resistance to antibiotics resulting possibly in clinical recurrence of infection(Anagnostakos et al., 2008).

Most of the clinical situations in orthopaedic trauma that require local antibiotic delivery for treatment or prophylaxis of infection also require stimulation of the process of bone regeneration. Classic examples include local antibiotic delivery for prophylaxis of infection in open fractures and treatment of infected non-unions(Thonse and Conway, 2007). There is concern that high concentrations of local antibiotics might affect osteoblast function and subsequent bone regeneration(Hanssen, 2005; Thonse and Conway, 2007). The quinolone class of antibiotics have in particular been shown to have an adverse effect on fracture at the low levels achieved with systemic administration and so it seems that these should be used with caution as systemic therapy or local therapy when bone regeneration is an important aspect of the treatment plan(Hanssen, 2005; Thonse and Conway, 2007). Keeping in mind that a possibility of local toxicity with regard to bone regeneration exists, investigation to determine the ideal dose of locally administered antibiotics to negotiate the balance between eradicating infection without excessively inhibiting the processes of bone regeneration is still required.

One of the main drawbacks of antibiotic bone cement beads is that it requires removal. This means a second surgical intervention solely dedicated for its removal, especially if further procedures are not required for a given case(Hanssen, 2005). The advise to remove antibiotic bone cement beads is based on the possibility that the cement beads would act as a foreign substance suitable for bacterial colonisation after the antibiotic has been depleted(Sener et al., 2010). In practise, after 4 to 6 weeks, beads become surrounded by dense scar tissue and the ability to identify and remove them can become extremely difficult(Hanssen, 2005).

7. Practical considerations

Local antibiotic delivery with antibiotic loaded acrylic bone cement beads has been used extensively in the management of osteomyelitis, infected non-unions and implant related infections **(Fig 1)**.

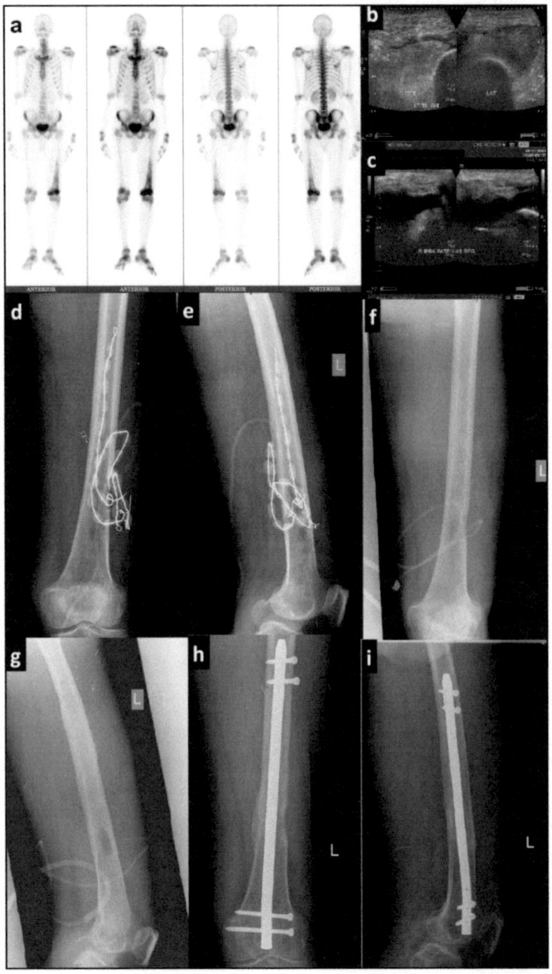

Fig. 1. A 55-year old diabetic male presented to us with fever and painful swelling of left distal femur for a period of 2 weeks. Radiographs at presentation were normal. **(a):** Tc99m MDP bone scan revealed increased tracer activity in the left distal femur suggestive of osteomyelitis. **(b and c):** Ultrasonography showed a collection of approximately 50ml around the knee and supra-patellar compartment. Pus culture identified the infecting organism as Burkholderia pseudomallei. **(d and e):** Following decompression and debridement, based on culture sensitivity report, Meropenem loaded acrylic bone cement beads were placed in-situ for local antibiotic delivery. **(f and g):** Complete clinical resolution of infection was noted and the antibiotic cement beads were removed 12 weeks later. **(h and i):** However, the patient sustained a pathological fracture of the distal femur following trivial trauma a few months later which necessitated operative stabilisation. The fracture healed well and the patient was infection free at final follow-up 18 months later.

Though newer drug delivery vehicles are being investigated, it remains the most widely used local antibiotic delivery vehicle in orthopaedic surgery. Self- made antibiotic loaded bone cement beads are cheaper, antibiotic specific and have no availability issues **(Fig 2)**. However they have been shown to elute less effectively than commercial antibiotic loaded cement beads(Zalavras et al., 2004). In this section, several tips and their rationale for increasing the elution and effectiveness of antibiotic loaded bone cement in clinical practice are discussed.

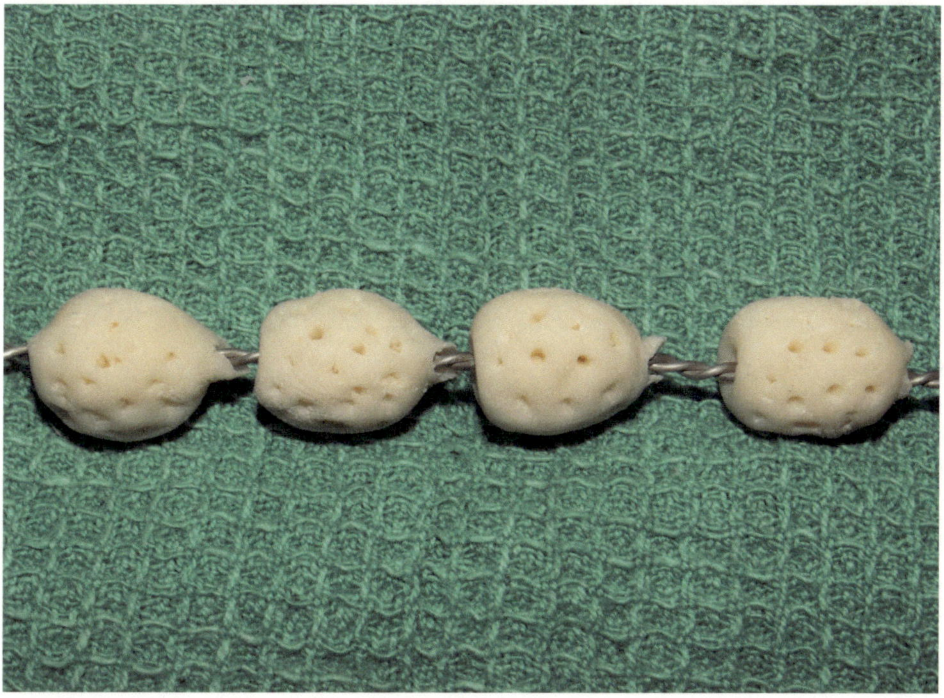

Fig. 2. Self-made antibiotic loaded bone cement beads strung on braided stainless steel wire.

#1: The liquid monomer is added to methyl- methacrylate powder in an inert bowl with a spatula as per the manufacturer's instructions, and hand mixing is commenced. At the early 'dough' phase, immediately after wetting the cement, antibiotic powder of appropriate weight for the desired concentration is added and thoroughly mixed with the Cement mixture in a standard fashion of one revolution per second to obtain a homogeneous compound.

The usual method advocated for making antibiotic loaded bone cement is mixing the antibiotic powder to the cement powder after which the liquid monomer is added. High volumes of the antibiotic powder make mixing difficult by this method as much of the liquid monomer is lost in dissolving the antibiotic powder. Instead one could first mix the polymethylmethacrylate monomer and cement powder together to form the liquid cement to which the antibiotic powder is added(Samuel et al., 2010).

#2: The choice of the antibiotic is determined by pre-operative culture report if present. Two antibiotics are chosen in the presence of mixed infections. When pre-operative culture reports are unavailable, for the treatment of infection, it is desirable to provide broad spectrum Gram-positive and negative coverage with two antibiotics. I use 2 gm

each of meropenem and vancomycin for a 40 gm batch of bone cement in such situations (total antibiotic concentration: 10%).

Successful therapy depends on achieving high local antibiotic concentrations. Hanssen classified antibiotic loaded bone cement into high dose (> 2 g antibiotic per 40 g of cement) and low dose (< 2 g antibiotic per 40 g of cement) and recommended high dose for use as beads or spacers and low dose for prosthesis fixation (Hanssen, 2004). It is postulated that mixing high doses of powdered antibiotics considerably increases cement porosity and facilitates increased elution of antibiotics (Samuel et al., 2010).

Secondly, the porosity of bone cements depends on the viscosity of the cement, higher viscosity cements possessing a higher porosity than low viscosity ones(van de Belt et al., 2001). I currently use high viscosity CMW1 bone cement to make antibiotic beads. The added advantage of using high-viscosity cement is that it gives a long working time to make the beads. The addition of two antibiotics to acrylic bone cement has been shown to increase the elution of antibiotics possibly by increasing its porosity(Samuel et al., 2010; Cerretani et al., 2002; Baleani et al., 2008). The second positive effect of dual antibiotic loaded bone cement is the broadening of antibacterial spectrum (Cerretani et al., 2002; Baleani et al., 2008).

#3: Prior to mixing of the antibiotic bone cement, two to three strings of braided stainless steel wires are made. These are made by holding a pair of 22 or 24 gauge stainless steel wires with a clamp in one end and a vise in the other end and twisting them in order to braid them.

Removal of antibiotic loaded bone cement after control of infection is desirable. However removal of these beads may be difficult because they are encased in dense fibrous tissue. Many a times, during bead removal, traction is exerted on the stainless steel wires. The use of braided stainless steel wires provides a better hold on the beads when compared to a single smooth stainless steel wire and decreases the chance of the beads from slipping out of the stainless steel wire(Samuel et al., 2010).

#4: The cement beads are made as small as possible (about 8 mm) and strung on to the braided stainless steel wires. It is essential to ensure that adjacent beads have a free gap between each other and are not in contact.

The elution of antibiotics occurs from the surface of the bone cement and also from the pores and cracks in its matrix (Masri et al., 1995). Elution is improved with increasing surface area and porosity of the cement exposed to liquid medium (Masri et al., 1995). Given the time consideration, It is difficult to make symmetrical spheres as advised and the beads end up being more oval. It is more important to ensure that the beads are kept small in size and the beads are so strung on the stainless steel wire that there is a gap between adjacent beads (Masri et al., 1995; Zalavras et al., 2004).

#5: A further attempt to increase the surface area is made by making multiple pits on the surface of the cement beads using a 1.5 mm Kirschner wire as it starts to set.

The use of Kirschner wires to make multiple pits on the surface of the beads to increase the surface area aids better elution of the antibiotic(Samuel et al., 2010).

#6: After setting, the antibiotic beads are placed in vivo. It is desirable to not only be in as close proximity as possible to the focus of infection but to also span it.

Antibiotic loaded acrylic bone cement delivers antibiotics locally but there is not much literature to reveal how far from the beads effective antibiotic levels will be maintained. Though this would depend on the local milieu, it has been suggested that it is no more than 2-3 cm (Samuel et al., 2010). Hence it would seem rational to assume that it is essential to be in as close proximity as possible to the focus of infection and also to span it.

#7: The wound is closed meticulously in layers over a suction drain. This suction drain is however kept closed. The drain is opened every 6 to 8 hours for only 15 minutes to allow periodic drainage of the wound

The antibiotic elutes from the cement beads into the postoperative wound haematoma which acts as a transport medium. The placement of a drain would lead to the removal of collected haematoma and with it the eluted antibiotic and is hence not recommended(Zalavras et al., 2005). Practical considerations however necessitate a drain after debridement. The above method allows the collected haematoma with the eluted antibiotic to act locally before being drained out periodically. Drain removal is done when the drainage level decreases in 48-72 hours as usual.

8. Clinical experience

The use of antibiotic loaded bone cement in orthopaedic trauma can be considered under the following sections:

- Use of antibiotic loaded bone cement for prophylaxis of infection in open fractures.
- Use of antibiotic loaded bone cement for treatment of infected non-unions and osteomyelitis.
- Use of antibiotic loaded bone cement for treatment of infected implants.

8.1 Use of antibiotic loaded bone cement for prohylaxis of infection in open fractures

An open fracture is characterized by soft tissue violation resulting in communication of the fracture site and haematoma with the external environment(Zalavras et al., 2005). Infection is the most dreaded complication of open fractures with higher Gustilo types having a higher incidence of this complication(Zalavras et al., 2005; Ostermann et al., 1995). Microbial growth in open fractures is enhanced by a variety of factors like impaired vascularity, devitalized bone and soft tissue, and loss of skeletal stability(Henry et al., 1993).It is now well recognized that integrity of soft tissue is essential for an uncomplicated course of fracture healing(Henry et al., 1993). Current principles in the management of open fractures include wound irrigation, serial radical debridement, early systemic administration of a short course of broad-spectrum antibiotics, stabilisation of the bone and early soft-tissue coverage(Zalavras et al. 2005; Ostermann et al., 1995). Prevention of infection is one of the main goals of open fracture management. It has been shown that about 65% of patients with open fractures have wound contamination with micro-organisms at the outset(Zalavras et al. 2005). Therefore it can be said that antibiotics are not just for prophylaxis but rather for treatment of wound contamination per se(Zalavras et al. 2005). The use of local antibiotics to achieve therapeutic tissue levels in target areas as an alternative to systemic route which requires high serum levels of potentially toxic and costly antibiotics is an attractive and viable option(Ostermann et al., 1995). Aminoglycosides are the most frequently chosen antibiotic because of their broad anti-bacterial spectrum, thermostability and low allergenicity(Zalavras et al. 2005). The prophylactic use of local antibiotic delivery has been shown to reduce the risk infection in open fractures(Zalavras et al. 2005; Ostermann et al., 1995; Ostermann et al., 1989).

Ostermann et al descibed the 'antibiotic bead pouch' technique for the management of severe compound fractures as early as 1989(Ostermann et al., 1989). Their initial report was on the management of 21 type II and III open tibial fractures treated by external fixation augmented by the bead pouch technique. The results of this small series were encouraging with only one deep infection and no case of osteomyelitis. In this technique the patient undergoes a thorough debridement after adequate extension of the wound margins and all avascular, necrotic, and contaminated tissue is removed. This is followed by copious irrigation of the fracture site. A lavage is then performed with normal saline solution and bacitracin solution. The fracture is then reduced and stabilized. In patients with significant soft-tissue injuries in whom closure is not possible at the time of the initial debridement, one or more chains of antibiotic beads are placed in the open wound. A suction drain is brought out through normal intact skin. The soft-tissue defect is covered with an adhesive porous polyethylene wound film (Opsite). This establishes a "closed" bead - hematoma - fracture environment containing high local levels of antibiotic at the fracture site. The drain is used only for overflow purposes and suction is not used. The “bead pouch” dressing and the beads are completely changed every 48 to 72 hours in the operating room under sterile conditions to ensure high levels of antibiotic elution. Wound closure is accomplished by either delayed primary suture closure, split-thickness skin grafts, or flap coverage when further debridements are not required.

The antibiotic bead-pouch technique has numerous advantages. Firstly as expected, high local concentration of antibiotic is achieved in the target area, which is often 10 to 20 times higher than with systemic administration thereby decreasing the need for systemic use of antibiotics and its associated side effects. The most useful indication for this technique is for the management of severe open fractures with Grade III wounds. Secondly, sealing of open fracture site from the external environment by the semipermeable barrier prevents secondary contamination by nosocomial microbes. In this “closed” bead-hematoma-fracture environment, the bone is kept in a moist warm, sterile soft-tissue compartment. This technique facilitates multiple debridements and the dead space is temporarily adequately filled with antibiotic beads extending the available period for soft tissue transfers. In addition, an aerobic wound environment is established which aids in avoiding catastrophic anaerobic infections. The entire process is patient friendly as it avoids frequent painful dressing changes(Henry et al., 1993; Ostermann et al., 1989).

Henry et al reported on the efficacy of antibiotic bead pouch for prophylaxis of deep and soft tissue infection following open fractures. They reviewed 404 open fractures, 334 of which had received bead pouch treatment along with intravenous antibiotics. This group was compared to a historical control of 70 open fractures treated with a protocol of systemic antibiotics alone. The rate of wound infection was 2.7% in the antibiotic bead pouch group as compared to 11.4% in the group treated with antibiotics alone. The rate of chronic osteomyelitis was 2.4% and 14.3%, respectively, in favour of the bead pouch group. They concluded that the antibiotic bead pouch technique was responsible for the reduction of the infection rate. However, there are some concerns with the interpretation of the study results. The wound management protocol in the two groups differed with a high proportion of the group treated without a bead pouch having immediate wound closure at the time of initial debridement, a practice that probably influences the infection rate(Henry et al., 1990).

In a subsequent study, Henry et al described a consecutive series of 704 compound fractures wherein 227 open fractures in 204 patients were managed with the antibiotic bead pouch technique. Fluid sampled from the bead pouch was shown to contain therapeutic levels of tobramycin with very low serum levels. They reported a wound infection rate of 0% for Grade I open fractures, 1.2% for Grade II compound fractures, and 8.6% for Grade III open fractures. The osteomyelitis rate was 0% in Grade I compound fractures, 2.4% in Grade II open fractures, and 5.5% in Grade III compound fractures. They observed that the bead pouch technique decreased the incidence of infection and permitted a staged wound closure of severe open fractures(Henry et al., 1993).

In another report by the same group, Ostermann et al. compared two groups of open fractures, with 157 receiving prophylactic systemic antibiotics and another group of 547 having antibiotic bead pouch in addition. Comparison of overall infection rates demonstrated a rate of 17% in the group treated with antibiotics alone compared to 4.2% in the bead pouch group. Subdivision of results based on injury severity Gustilo grading revealed statistically significant difference only in grade IIIb injuries. Once again, the wound management protocol between the two groups was not similar raising concerns about the study results. They concluded that that the prophylactic use of antibiotic-laden cement beads in addition to systemic antibiotics was of benefit in preventing infectious complications, particularly in Type IIIB open fractures(Ostermann et al., 1993).

In a follow-up landmark article, Ostermann et al described their experience in treating 1085 consecutive compound limb fractures treated in 914 patients(Ostermann et al., 1995). Of these fractures, 240 received only systemic antibiotic prophylaxis and 845 were managed by the supplementary tobramycin loaded bone cement beads. Other therepeutic interventions like copious wound irrigation, meticulous debridement and skeletal stabilisation remained identical in both groups but wound management and the use of antibiotic bone cement beads depended on the surgeon's individual preference and there was no randomisation. In the group treated with local antibiotics 49.5% wounds were primarily closed over beads, 45.1% severe soft-tissue defects were managed by the 'antibiotic-bead-pouch' technique and 5.4% of the wounds were loosely closed over beads as a temporary measure until final wound closure could be achieved. In contrast to the group of patients treated with systemic antibiotics alone which had an overall infection rate of 12% , the infection rate was only 3.7% in the group of patients who were treated with local antibiotic delivery ($p < 0.001$). Both acute infection and local osteomyelitis showed a decreased incidence in the later group which was statistically significant in Gustilo type-IIIB and type-IIIC fractures for acute infection, and in type-II and type-IIIB fractures for chronic osteomyelitis. The drawbacks of the article are that the study was retrospective and the groups were not randomized. The choice of treatment was dependent on the preference of the attending surgeon and the wound treatment was not identical between the two groups with 95% of wounds in the antibiotic bead pouch group being either closed primarily or sealed. Therefore, the relative contribution of the local antibiotic delivery versus the sealing of the wound cannot be determined(Ostermann et al., 1995).

Keating et al studied the efficacy of antibiotic bead pouch in the management of open tibial fractures stabilized by reamed intra-medullary nail. They found that this technique decreased the deep infection rate in open tibial fractures from 16% to 4% in their practice. Though the differences observed did not achieve statistical significance, they suggested that the addition of the bead pouch to the wound management protocol was associated with a worthwhile reduction in deep infection rate(Keating et al., 1996).

Moehring and colleagues compared the efficacy of antibiotic loaded beads with conventional intravenous antibiotics for open fractures in a randomized prospective study(Moehring et al., 2000). The infection rate was lower (5.3%) in the antibiotic bone cement group compared to the conventional systemic antibiotic group (8.3%). However, the study was unable to achieve statistical significance and the data could only suggest that antibiotic bone cement beads are useful in preventing infection in open fractures. The use of local antibiotic delivery with antibiotic loaded acrylic bone cement has now emerged as an efficacious treatment protocol for the prophylaxis of infection in open fractures. However it must be recognized that the question of whether local antibiotics alone is sufficient and systemic antibiotics can be altogether be avoided in these cases is yet to be answered(Ostermann et al., 1995).

8.2 Use of antibiotic loaded bone cement for treatment of infected non-unions and osteomyelitis

Although there are variable definitions, infected nonunion has been defined as a failure of union with persistence of infection at the fracture site for a period of 6 to 8 months(Struijs et al., 2007). The management of this entity is challenging due to the dual problems of controlling infection and providing stability needed for fracture union.(Thonse and Conway, 2007). Treatment protocols may be a single stage revision surgery or a staged strategy where eradication of infection is the primary focus initially and union of the fracture in the later stage(Struijs et al., 2007; Thonse and Conway, 2007). Numerous studies have shown the efficacy of staged strategy using antibiotic bone cement beads for the eradication of infection in infected non-unions though the level of evidence is low. Union rates ranging from 93% to 100% with persistence of infection in 0% to 18% has been reported and is considerabley higher than single stage revision surgery or other staged surgery protocols(Struijs et al., 2007; Chan et al., 2000; Ueng et al., 1999, 1997; Ueng et al., 1996). In a randomized controlled trial by Calhoun et al, 4 weeks of intravenous antibiotics was compared with antibiotic beads in 52 patients with infected nonunions having debridement and reconstructive surgery. Patients in the antibiotic bead group also received perioperative (2 to 5 days) systemic antibiotic therapy. The success rate for treating the infection was 83% (20 of 24 patients) in the systemic antibiotic group and 89% (25 of 28 patients) in the antibiotic bead group, suggesting that long-term systemic antibiotic therapy can be substituted by local antibiotic therapy in infected non-unions(Calhoun et al., 1993).

Patzakis et al compared antibiotic loaded bone cement beads (supplemented with as much as 5 days of systemic antibiotics) to systemic antibiotic therapy in 33 patients with chronic osteomyelitis and bone defects. The infection control rate was 100% (12 of 12 patients) in the Septopal group and 95% (20 of 21 patients) in the systemic antibiotic group. Bony union was accomplished in all patients(Patzakis et al., 1993).

The efficacy of local antibiotic therapy has been reported in several clinical studies on open fractures and osteomyelitis. The use of antibiotic bone cement beads for bone and soft tissue defects after debridement for dead space management and local antibiotic delivery is now an accepted treatment protocol especially if reoperation is needed (second-look debridement, soft tissue coverage, bone grafting).

Intra-medullary infections in long bones may be encountered after infection of intra-medullary nails and usually involves the entire medullary canal. These can be difficult to treat with antibiotic cement beads because of difficulties in not only placing but also in retrieving them(Madanagopal et al., 2004). Of late there is considerable interest in the use of antibiotic bone cement coated intra-medullary nails for the treatment of infected non-unions of long bones(Thonse and Conway, 2007; Madanagopal et al., 2004; Shyam et al., 2009). Thonse and Conway described their experience in the management of infected non-unions in a series of 20 patients with a antibiotic cement-coated interlocking intramedullary nail prepared in the operating room(Thonse and Conway, 2007). They achieved the goal of bony union in 85% and infection control in 95% of the patients. However, they noted cement debonding in all the four patients in whom nail removal was done. Shyam et al also reported on their experience with the use of antibiotic impregnated nail for control of infection in cases of infected non-union with bone defect. They prospectively studied 25 cases of infected non-union with varying bone defects and found that this technique was useful for infection control in cases with bone defect <6 cm(Shyam et al., 2009). Antibiotic coated nails not only provide antibiotic delivery but also provide some fracture stability(Madanagopal et al., 2004). It also provides for a more intimate contact with the entire medullary canal and elution of antibiotic to the endosteal surface which is the primary seat of infection in these cases. Though cement debonding and nail breakage may be encountered, these devices are easier to retrieve than traditional cement beads(Madanagopal et al., 2004).

8.3 Use of antibiotic loaded bone cement for treatment of infected implants

Infections in the setting of orthopaedic implants is a particularly serious problem(Sener et al., 2010; Diefenbeck et al., 2006). In orthopaedic trauma, infection of osteosynthetic devices results in considerable morbidity due to prolonged hospitalisation, poor functional status and sepsis. Staphylococcus aureus is a common organism that causes deep wound infection after orthopaedic operations and is capable of producing a protective exopolysaccharide biofilm. Other micro- organisms responsible include Staphylococcus epidermidis, Pseudomonas and other Gram-negative rods(van de Belt et al., 2001). Treatment protocol for this challenging problem is usually a combination of thorough surgical debridement including the removal of necrotic tissue, bone sequesters and often the implant itself, and local and systemic antibiotic therapy(Diefenbeck et al., 2006).

In additional to surgical considerations, this situation presents a microbiological problem as well. It is recognized that bacteria adhering to implant surfaces change their biological behavior. They produce a biofilm that creates a protective microenvironment against antibiotics(Diefenbeck et al., 2006). More importantly, these micro-organisms reduce their metabolic activity and increase their generation times. As antibiotics act on growing bacteria, the minimum inhibitory concentrations (MIC) of micro-organisms with reduced metabolic activity is increased(Diefenbeck et al., 2006). Systemic antibiotics are ineffective as they cannot reach such a high concentration at the local site. Local antibiotic delivery is therefore a very viable option for this clinical problem, especially if retention of stable implants is planned.

Sener et al studied the effectiveness of antibiotic loaded bone cement in the trreatment of implant-related infection in 32 Wistar albino rats in whom deep infection was established after intra- medullary stabilisation of fresh fractures(Sener et al., 2010). They studied the efficacy of three treatment modalities in this randomised study and the 4 treatment groups included: no treatment, surgical débridement, antibiotic-loaded bone cement and antibiotic-loaded autogenous bone. In terms of reduction of microbiological colonies, the antibiotic-loaded bone cement group revealed superior results compared with the other groups. However, they noted that three animals in the bone cement group revealed extensive infection, which was not seen in the debridement only group. Therefore, although antibiotic-loaded bone cement showed superiority over other treatment modalities, they concluded that it should be employed only after unsuccessful trials of débridement because of the risk of extensive infection(Sener et al., 2010). If the infection cannot be eradicated by débridement and the initial rapid phase of antibiotic elution, then the cement beads may provide a suitable environment for the spread of infection and development of resistance to antibiotics(Sener et al., 2010).

9. Recommendations for the antibiotic bone cement for different clinical situations in orthopaedic trauma

9.1 Open fractures where primary wound closure is feasible

In open fractures with contamination, the use of antibiotic loaded bone cement to prevent infection is a viable option **(Fig 3)**. Antibiotic beads can be placed in-situ after a thorough debridement and stabilisation of the fracture. The duration of implantation is usually 4-6 weeks and depends on the timing of subsequent planned procedures like bone grafting.

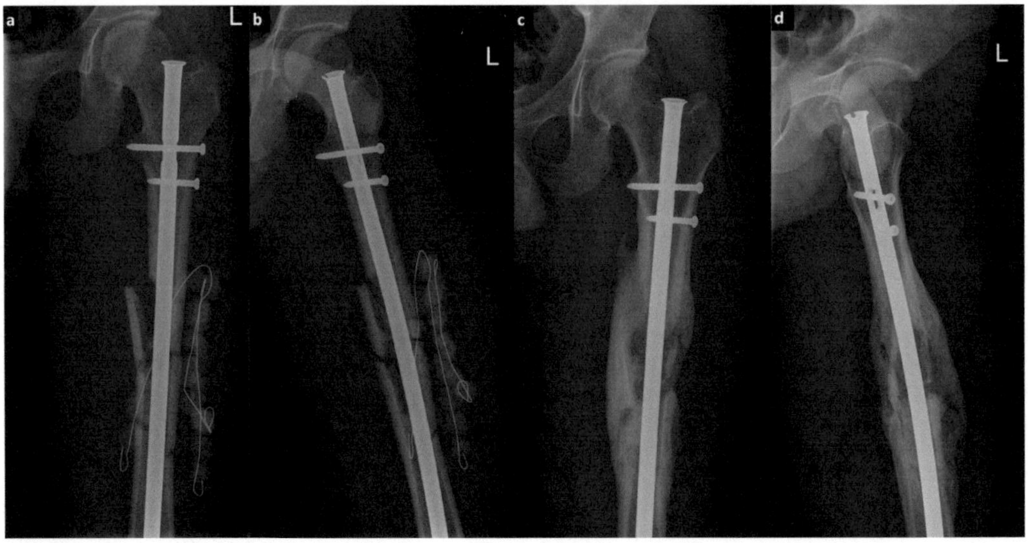

Fig. 3. **(a and b):** AP and Lateral radiographs of 19-year old man who underwent debridement, intra-medullary nailing for a 24-hour old open contaminated comminuted left femur fracture. Vancomycin and Meropenem loaded acrylic bone cement beads were prophylactically placed in-situ. A bead exchange procedure was done 4 weeks later. **(c and d):** The beads were removed 6 weeks later. At last follow-up at 12 months, the fracture had united and the patient was free from infection.

9.2 Open fractures where primary wound closure is not feasible

When confronted with a situation of an open fracture where primary wound closure is not feasible, the antibiotic bead pouch technique may be used. This technique allows for dead space management, periodic wound inspection and soft-tissue coverage as an elective procedure.

9.3 Acute infection after plate osteosynthesis

When acute infection complicates plate osteosyntheis, then early surgical intervention can be very successful. The standard procedure for this situation is an exploration of the surgical site, thorough debridement and necrectomy, copious irrigation followed by a course of systemic antibiotics. Local antibiotics with antibiotic loaded acrylic bone cement is extremely useful in this situation. The treatment of early infection by this technique can result in complete eradication of infection when the micro-organisms are still in the planktonic stage. The antibiotic bead chain can be removed during implant removal or bone grafting if the fracture fails to unite. In situations where infection is not cured but only suppressed by the use of antibiotic bone cement beads, radiological evidence of the same will manifest. This situation can be can be managed by periodic debridement and change of antibiotic bone cement beads with an aim to suppress infection till fracture union. Alternatively if the implant loosens over time, then a spanning fixator to temporarily stabilize the bone till infection is eradicated becomes necessary.

9.4 Infected non-unions

The protocol that can be followed for this situation would be a thorough debridement of all infected tissue, removal of unstable hardware, necrectomy, stabilization of the fracture and antibiotic bone cement beads for local antibiotic delivery. An external fixator is usually used in this situation either for temporary or definitive stabilization of the fracture **(Fig 4)**. Local antibiotic delivery with antibiotic bone cement beads has proven to be an effective way to combat these chronic infections. After control of infection, secondary surgical procedures like bone grafting and definitive fracture stabilization may be done as required **(Fig 5)**. Widespread intra-medullary infection which usually occurs following an infected intra-medullary nail osteosynthessis is especially amenable to antibiotic bone cement coated intra-medullary nails.

9.5 Chronic osteomyelitis with a stable skeleton

In this situation, a thorough debridement, sequestrectomy and removal of implants if present usually suffices **(Fig 6)**. In resistant cases, especially when avascularity of the bone or soft tissue complicates the situation, local antibiotic bone cement beads can be used.

10. Conclusion

The concept of local antibiotic delivery aimed at achieving high concentrations of the drug at target areas, even to avascular areas that are inaccessible by systemic antibiotics, with less toxicity than that associated with systemic administration, is physiologically and economically sound. Since the introduction of this concept by Buchholz et al in the 1970s,

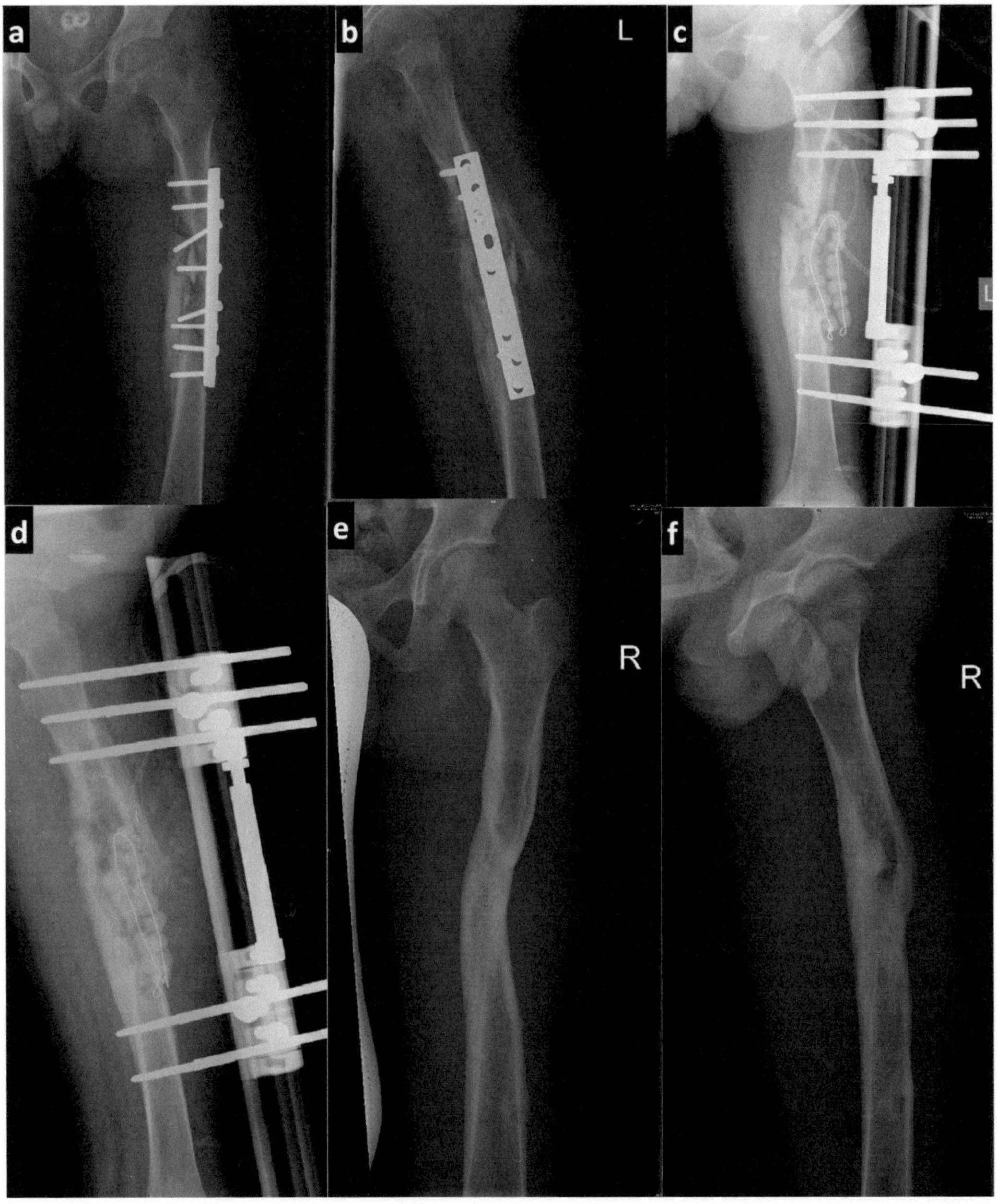

Fig. 4. **(a and b):** AP and Lateral radiographs of a 15-year old boy who presented to us with purulent discharge from his left thigh 8 months following open reduction internal fixation of open left femur fracture. Cultures identified the infecting micro-organism to be Methicilin resistant Staphylococcus aureus. **(c and d):** He underwent hardware removal, debridement and fracture stabilisation with a monolateral rail external fixator. Based on culture sensitivity report, Vancomycin loaded acrylic bone cement beads were placed in-situ. **(e and f):** The beads were removed 5 weeks later. At final follow-up 13 months later, the fracture had united and the patient was free from infection.

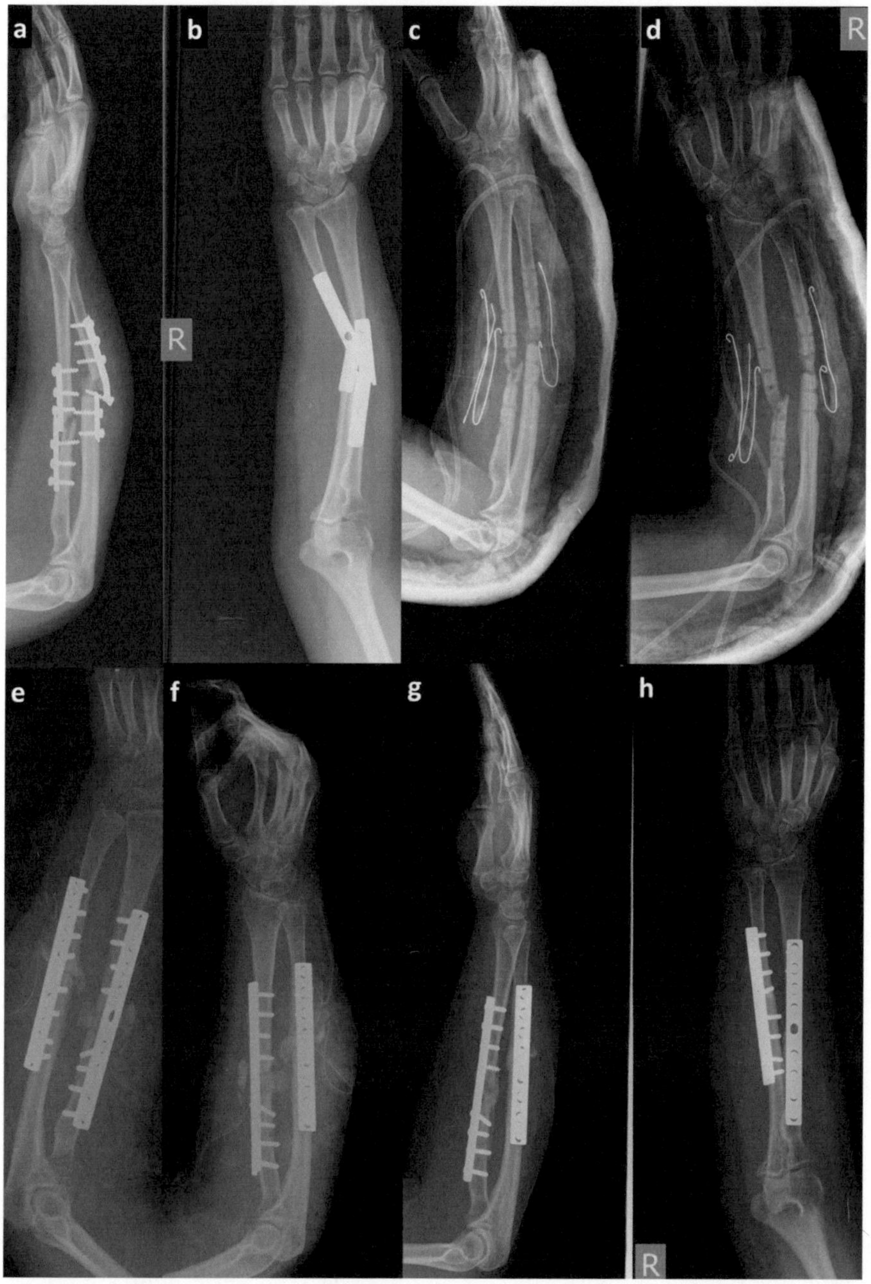

Fig. 5. **(a and b):** AP and Lateral radiographs of a 34-year old woman who presented to us with infected non-union of the right forearm with broken implants in-situ. **(c and d):** She underwent hardware removal and debridement. Vancomycin and meropenem loaded acrylic bone cement beads were placed in-situ. **(e and f):** 8 weeks later, the beads were removed and the patient underwent open reduction internal fixation of both forearm bones with dynamic compression plates. **(g and h):** At final follow-up 18 months later, the fracture had united and the patient was free of infection.

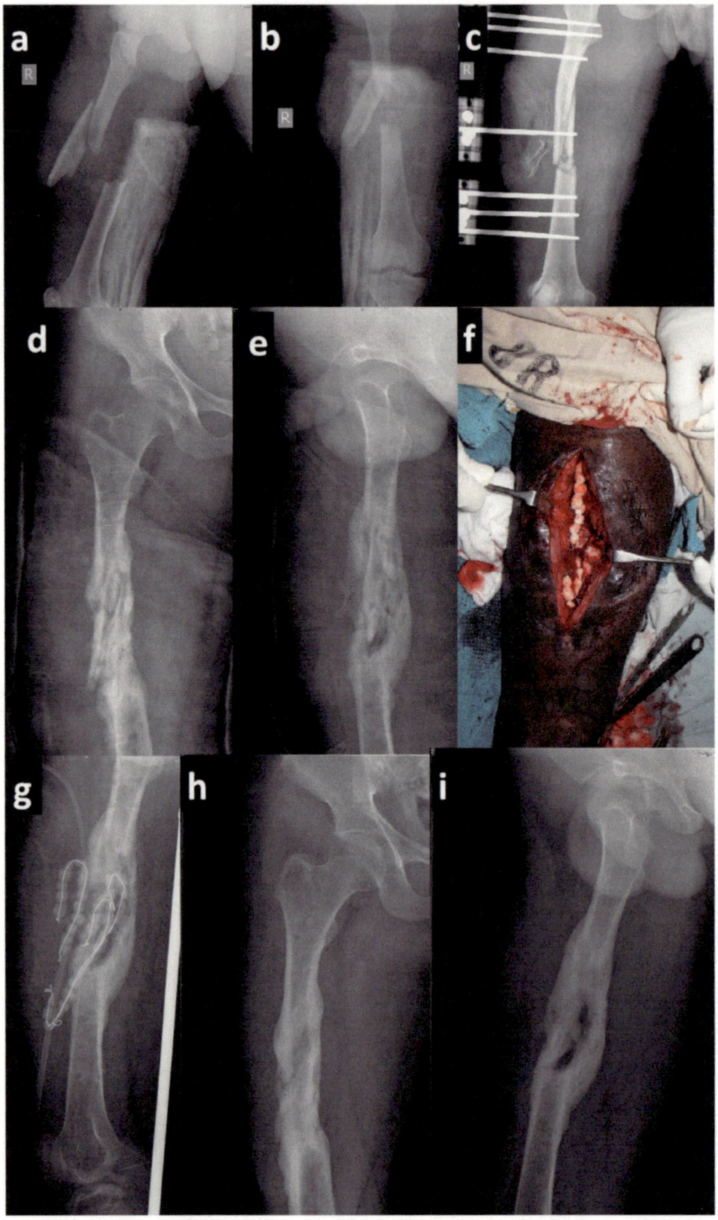

Fig. 6. **(a and b):** AP and Lateral radiographs of a 22-year old male with compound type 3B segmental fracture of the left femur who presented to us 5 days after injury with a contaminated wound. **(c):** After adequate debridement, the fracture was stabilized with a monolateral rail external fixator. **(d and e):** Though the fracture united, the entire middle segment sequestrated and the patient developed purulent discharge. The infecting micro-organism was identified to be Proteus mirabilis which was multi-drug resistant. **(f and g):** Debridement and removal of the the dead bone was done and the wound was packed with meropenem loaded acrylic bone cement. **(h and i):** At final follow-up 14 months later, the patient was free from infection

antibiotic loaded acrylic bone cement has been used extensively for the prevention and management of orthopaedic infections. Its role in different clinical situations like open fractures, acute and chronic osteomyelitis, infected non-unions and implant related infections has been documented. Though not without drawbacks, it remains the most widely used local drug delivery system in orthopaedics and represents the current gold standard for treatment of musculoskeletal infections. The elution of antibiotic from self-made acrylic bone cement beads, which are cheap, antibiotic specific and have no availability issues, can be improved by attention to detail.

11. Acknowledgement

The author thanks Dr. Ravichand Ismavel, Department of Orthopaedics (III), Christian Medical college, Vellore, India for photographic assistance.

12. References

Anagnostakos K, Hitzler P, Pape D, Kohn D, Kelm J. Persistence of bacterial growth on antibiotic-loaded beads: is it actually a problem? Acta Orthop 2008 Apr;79(2):302-307.

Baker AS, Greenham LW. Release of gentamicin from acrylic bone cement. Elution and diffusion studies. J Bone Joint Surg Am 1988 Dec;70(10):1551-1557.

Baleani M, Persson C, Zolezzi C, Andollina A, Borrelli AM, Tigani D. Biological and biomechanical effects of vancomycin and meropenem in acrylic bone cement. J Arthroplasty 2008 Dec;23(8):1232-1238.

Bayston R, Milner RD. The sustained release of antimicrobial drugs from bone cement. An appraisal of laboratory investigations and their significance. J Bone Joint Surg Br 1982;64(4):460-464.

van de Belt H, Neut D, Schenk W, van Horn JR, van der Mei HC, Busscher HJ. Infection of orthopedic implants and the use of antibiotic-loaded bone cements. A review. Acta Orthop Scand 2001 Dec;72(6):557-571.

van de Belt H, Neut D, Uges DR, Schenk W, van Horn JR, van der Mei HC, Busscher HJ. Surface roughness, porosity and wettability of gentamicin-loaded bone cements and their antibiotic release. Biomaterials 2000 Oct;21(19):1981-1987.

Brien WW, Salvati EA, Klein R, Brause B, Stern S. Antibiotic impregnated bone cement in total hip arthroplasty. An in vivo comparison of the elution properties of tobramycin and vancomycin. Clin. Orthop. Relat. Res 1993 Nov;(296):242-248.

Buchholz HW, Elson RA, Engelbrecht E, Lodenkämper H, Röttger J, Siegel A. Management of deep infection of total hip replacement. J Bone Joint Surg Br 1981;63-B(3):342-353.

Buchholz HW, Elson RA, Heinert K. Antibiotic-loaded acrylic cement: current concepts. Clin. Orthop. Relat. Res 1984 Nov;(190):96-108.

Calhoun JH, Henry SL, Anger DM, Cobos JA, Mader JT. The treatment of infected nonunions with gentamicin-polymethylmethacrylate antibiotic beads. Clin. Orthop. Relat. Res. 1993 Oct;(295):23-27.

Cerretani D, Giorgi G, Fornara P, Bocchi L, Neri L, Ceffa R, Ghisellini F, Ritter MA. The in vitro elution characteristics of vancomycin combined with imipenem-cilastatin in acrylic bone-cements: a pharmacokinetic study. J Arthroplasty 2002 Aug;17(5):619-626.

Chan YS, Ueng SW, Wang CJ, Lee SS, Chen CY, Shin CH. Antibiotic-impregnated autogenic cancellous bone grafting is an effective and safe method for the management of small infected tibial defects: a comparison study. J Trauma 2000 Feb;48(2):246-255.

Curtis JM, Sternhagen V, Batts D. Acute renal failure after placement of tobramycin-impregnated bone cement in an infected total knee arthroplasty. Pharmacotherapy 2005 Jun;25(6):876-880.

Diefenbeck M, Mückley T, Hofmann GO. Prophylaxis and treatment of implant-related infections by local application of antibiotics. Injury 2006 May;37 Suppl 2:S95-104.

Dovas S, Liakopoulos V, Papatheodorou L, Chronopoulou I, Papavasiliou V, Atmatzidis E, Giannopoulou M, Eleftheriadis T, Simopoulou T, Karachalios T, Stefanidis I. Acute renal failure after antibiotic-impregnated bone cement treatment of an infected total knee arthroplasty. Clin. Nephrol 2008 Mar;69(3):207-212.

Elson RA, Jephcott AE, McGechie DB, Verettas D. Antibiotic-loaded acrylic cement. J Bone Joint Surg Br 1977 May;59(2):200-205.

Hanssen AD. Prophylactic use of antibiotic bone cement: an emerging standard--in opposition. J Arthroplasty 2004 Jun;19(4 Suppl 1):73-77.

Hanssen AD. Local antibiotic delivery vehicles in the treatment of musculoskeletal infection. Clin. Orthop. Relat. Res 2005 Aug;(437):91-96.

Hanssen AD, Spangehl MJ. Practical applications of antibiotic-loaded bone cement for treatment of infected joint replacements. Clin. Orthop. Relat. Res 2004 Oct;(427):79-85.

Henry SL, Ostermann PA, Seligson D. The prophylactic use of antibiotic impregnated beads in open fractures. J Trauma 1990 Oct;30(10):1231-1238.

Henry SL, Ostermann PA, Seligson D. The antibiotic bead pouch technique. The management of severe compound fractures. Clin. Orthop. Relat. Res 1993 Oct;(295):54-62.

Keating JF, Blachut PA, O'Brien PJ, Meek RN, Broekhuyse H. Reamed nailing of open tibial fractures: does the antibiotic bead pouch reduce the deep infection rate? J Orthop Trauma 1996;10(5):298-303.

Madanagopal SG, Seligson D, Roberts CS. The antibiotic cement nail for infection after tibial nailing. Orthopedics 2004 Jul;27(7):709-712.

Marks KE, Nelson CL, Lautenschlager EP. Antibiotic-impregnated acrylic bone cement. J Bone Joint Surg Am 1976 Apr;58(3):358-364.

Masri BA, Duncan CP, Beauchamp CP, Paris NJ, Arntorp J. Effect of varying surface patterns on antibiotic elution from antibiotic-loaded bone cement. J Arthroplasty 1995 Aug;10(4):453-459.

Moehring HD, Gravel C, Chapman MW, Olson SA. Comparison of antibiotic beads and intravenous antibiotics in open fractures. Clin. Orthop. Relat. Res 2000 Mar;(372):254-261.

Nelson CL. The current status of material used for depot delivery of drugs. Clin. Orthop. Relat. Res 2004 Oct;(427):72-78.

Neut D, van de Belt H, van Horn JR, van der Mei HC, Busscher HJ. Residual gentamicin-release from antibiotic-loaded polymethylmethacrylate beads after 5 years of implantation. Biomaterials 2003 May;24(10):1829-1831.

Ostermann PA, Henry SL, Seligson D. [Treatment of 2d and 3d degree complicated tibial shaft fractures with the PMMA bead pouch technic]. Unfallchirurg 1989 Nov;92(11):523-530.

Ostermann PA, Henry SL, Seligson D. The role of local antibiotic therapy in the management of compound fractures. Clin. Orthop. Relat. Res 1993 Oct;(295):102-111.

Ostermann PA, Seligson D, Henry SL. Local antibiotic therapy for severe open fractures. A review of 1085 consecutive cases. J Bone Joint Surg Br 1995 Jan;77(1):93-97.

Patrick BN, Rivey MP, Allington DR. Acute renal failure associated with vancomycin- and tobramycin-laden cement in total hip arthroplasty. Ann Pharmacother 2006 Nov;40(11):2037-2042.

Patzakis MJ, Mazur K, Wilkins J, Sherman R, Holtom P. Septopal beads and autogenous bone grafting for bone defects in patients with chronic osteomyelitis. Clin. Orthop. Relat. Res. 1993 Oct;(295):112-118.

Persson C, Baleani M, Guandalini L, Tigani D, Viceconti M. Mechanical effects of the use of vancomycin and meropenem in acrylic bone cement. Acta Orthop 2006 Aug;77(4):617-621.

van Raaij TM, Visser LE, Vulto AG, Verhaar JAN. Acute renal failure after local gentamicin treatment in an infected total knee arthroplasty. J Arthroplasty 2002 Oct;17(7):948-950.

Samuel S, Ismavel R, Boopalan PRJVC, Matthai T. Practical considerations in the making and use of high-dose antibiotic-loaded bone cement. Acta Orthop Belg 2010 Aug;76(4):543-545.

Schurman DJ, Trindade C, Hirshman HP, Moser K, Kajiyama G, Stevens P. Antibiotic-acrylic bone cement composites. Studies of gentamicin and Palacos. J Bone Joint Surg Am 1978 Oct;60(7):978-984.

Sener M, Kazimoglu C, Karapinar H, Günal I, Afşar I, Karataş Sener AG. Comparison of various surgical methods in the treatment of implant-related infection. Int Orthop 2010 Mar;34(3):419-423.

Shyam AK, Sancheti PK, Patel SK, Rocha S, Pradhan C, Patil A. Use of antibiotic cement-impregnated intramedullary nail in treatment of infected non-union of long bones. Indian J Orthop 2009 Oct;43(4):396-402.

Springer BD, Lee G-C, Osmon D, Haidukewych GJ, Hanssen AD, Jacofsky DJ. Systemic safety of high-dose antibiotic-loaded cement spacers after resection of an infected total knee arthroplasty. Clin. Orthop. Relat. Res 2004 Oct;(427):47-51.

Struijs PAA, Poolman RW, Bhandari M. Infected nonunion of the long bones. J Orthop Trauma 2007 Aug;21(7):507-511.

Thonse R, Conway J. Antibiotic cement-coated interlocking nail for the treatment of infected nonunions and segmental bone defects. J Orthop Trauma 2007 Apr;21(4):258-268.

Ueng SW, Chuang DC, Cheng SL, Shih CH. Management of large infected tibial defects with radical debridement and staged double-rib composite free transfer. J Trauma 1996 Mar;40(3):345-350.

Ueng SW, Wei FC, Shih CH. Management of large infected tibial defects with antibiotic beads local therapy and staged fibular osteoseptocutaneous free transfer. J Trauma 1997 Aug;43(2):268-274.

Ueng SW, Wei FC, Shih CH. Management of femoral diaphyseal infected nonunion with antibiotic beads local therapy, external skeletal fixation, and staged bone grafting. J Trauma 1999 Jan;46(1):97-103.

Wahlig H, Dingeldein E, Bergmann R, Reuss K. The release of gentamicin from polymethylmethacrylate beads. An experimental and pharmacokinetic study. J Bone Joint Surg Br 1978 May;60-B(2):270-275.

Wininger DA, Fass RJ. Antibiotic-impregnated cement and beads for orthopedic infections. Antimicrob. Agents Chemother 1996 Dec;40(12):2675-2679.

Wroblewski BM. Leaching out from acrylic bone cement. Experimental evaluation. Clin. Orthop. Relat. Res 1977 May;(124):311-312.

Zalavras CG, Patzakis MJ, Holtom P. Local antibiotic therapy in the treatment of open fractures and osteomyelitis. Clin. Orthop. Relat. Res. 2004 Oct;(427):86-93.

Zalavras CG, Patzakis MJ, Holtom PD, Sherman R. Management of open fractures. Infect. Dis. Clin. North Am 2005 Dec;19(4):915-929.

7

Management of Bone Bleeding During Surgery and Its Impact on the Incidence of Post-Operative Osteomyelitis

Tadeusz Wellisz
University of Southern California
USA

1. Introduction

1.1 Synopsis

A wide range of orthopedic, cardiothoracic, neurological, and maxillofacial procedures requires that the bone be cut or resected, either to operate on the osseous tissue itself or to gain access to other organs. As any living tissue, bone bleeds when cut or fractured, and to reduce the risk of post-operative complications, bone bleeding needs to be managed during surgery. The present chapter examines the relationship between the management of bleeding and post-operative complications, and, in particular, the impact of bone hemostasis materials on the incidence of post-operative infection of soft tissue and osteomyelitis. Section 2, "Bone Surgery and Management of Bleeding," opens the argument by discussing the increase in the number of procedures involving the bone, the importance of effective bone and soft tissue hemostasis for assuring positive surgical outcome, and the surgeons' reliance on bone wax composed of beeswax, despite serious complications associated with its use. Section 3, "Surgical Site Infections and Osteomyelitis," focuses on the growing incidents of surgical site infections and post-operative osteomyelitis, and the added risk posed by the presence of antibiotic-resistant bacteria. Section 4, "Antibiotic Prophylaxis," discusses systemic SSI prevention and the use and effectiveness of topical antibiotic prophylaxis. "Systemic and Perioperative Risk Factors for Postoperative Osteomyelitis," in Section 5 analyses infection risk factors and predictors of complications following cardiac, orthopedic, and neurosurgical procedures. It focuses on excessive bleeding and subsequent extended duration of surgical procedure as infection risk factors, and the importance of effective bone hemostasis in minimizing the risk. Section 6, "Bone Wax as a Modifiable Risk Factor for Osteomyelitis, Chronic Inflammation, and Inhibited Bone Healing," discusses a body of research linking the use of traditional bone wax, most widely used bone hemostasis material, to inhibition of bone healing, inflammation, and increased soft tissue infection and osteomyelitis rates. The use of bone wax - and the choice of bone hemostasis material in general - remains a largely overlooked modifiable risk factor for osteomyelitis and other post-operative infections. Surgeons are often unaware of the post-operative complications attributed to the use of bone wax and unfamiliar with the range of alternatives available for bone hemostasis. Section 7, "Alternative Bone Hemostasis Materials and Methods," elaborates on a wide range of existing alternatives to bone wax, including synthetic topical bone hemostats which replicate the handling of traditional bone wax without its risks. The section also reviews studies of topical bone hemostasis materials and offers an analysis of existing comparative studies of new bone formation and healing, rate of infection, osteomyelitis, and the materials' effectiveness as bone hemostats, underscoring the role the surgeons' choice of bone hemostasis material can play in the promotion and prevention of post-operative complications. Polymer bone hemostats emerge in the studies as materials that do not inhibit bone healing and do not promote osteomyelitis or inflammation. "Redefining the Management of Bone Bleeding: Osteomyelitis, Bone Healing, and Topical Therapeutics" is the focus of Section 8, which explores the potential of combining topical bone hemostasis materials with therapeutics -- antibiotics or bone grafts – a combination which would make the management of bone bleeding an aspect of a larger surgical procedure and an important step in prevention and treatment of osteomyelitis. Section 9 concludes that a better understanding by the surgeons of the adverse effects of bone wax and of the overall impact bone hemostasis technique and material choice have on the clinical outcome may help reduce infections and the rate of osteomyelitis as well as broaden the repertoire of medical tools available to operating physicians and improve outcomes across surgical procedures.

1.2 Key terms

Osteomyelitis; post-operative infection; bone wax; modifiable risk factor for infection; topical bone hemostasis; topical therapeutics; alternatives to bone wax; bone surgery.

2. Bone surgery and management of bleeding

2.1 Bone bleeding in surgery

Bone, whether sternal, spinal, or any other, is a living tissue, and any invasive procedure involving the cutting of the bone requires management of bone bleeding, both to reduce blood loss and hematoma formation for the patient and to ensure good visibility of the operating site for the surgeon. To optimize surgical success and patient outcome, it is important to maintain a fine balance between bleeding and clotting during surgery, so that blood continues to flow to the tissues at the surgical site, but its loss is not excessive (Samudrala, 2008).[1] Uncontrolled continuous bleeding can obscure the surgical field, prolong operating time, increase the risk of physiologic complications, and expose the patient to additional problems associated with blood transfusion. For patients undergoing elective coronary artery bypass graft surgery, allogeneic blood transfusion has been shown to double the risk of infection (Rogers et al., 2009).[2]

[1] Samudrala, S. "Topical Hemostatic Agents in Surgery: A Surgeon's Perspective." *AORN Journal*, 2008. Supplement: Intraoperative Bleeding and Hemostasis in Surgical Procedures. vol. 88, no 3: p. S2-11

[2] In a cohort study of 24,789 Medicare beneficiaries who received coronary artery bypass graft surgery, allogeneic blood transfusion increased the odds of in-hospital infection 2.0-fold, in-hospital mortality 4.7-fold, 30-day readmission 1.4-fold, and 30-day mortality 2.9-fold. See: Mary AM Rogers, Neil Blumberg, Sanjay Saint, Kenneth M Langa, and Brahmajee K Nallamothu. "Hospital variation in transfusion and infection after cardiac surgery: a cohort study." *BMC Medicine* 2009, 7:37doi:10.1186/1741-7015-7-37

2.2 Growing number of surgeries involving the osseous tissue

Bone tissue is one of the most frequently transplanted tissues, second only to blood (Giannoudis, 2005).[3] It is increasingly needed across surgical fields as bone grafts are used to fill defects caused by trauma, infection of soft tissue and osteomyelitis, tumor resection, reconstruction of congenital malformations, and age-related decrease of bone mass. Over 1.8 million bone graft procedures were reported in 2006, a number that has risen exponentially since 1990 and that continues to grow with the ageing of population (Hladki, 2006).[4]

Other surgical procedures performed on the bone have also been on the rise in the United States. The number of joint arthroplasties currently exceeds 1,000,000 procedures per year (AAOS).[5] According to Centers for Disease Control and Prevention, there were 2,476,000 orthopedic and spinal surgeries in 2007, the last year for which data are available. Spine fusions and excisions of intervertebral discs accounted for 659,000 in-patient operations on the skeletal system while median sternotomies were performed 1,022,000 times in the same period in order to gain access to the heart in angioplasty and coronary artery bypass graft procedures (CDC).[6]

2.3 Management of bleeding and successful surgical outcome

During a surgical procedure involving bone, surgical technique and the management of bone bleeding are important factors in determining a successful outcome. When bone is cut, irrigation is used to prevent heat formation and thermal injury to the bone. Cut surfaces are kept moist to avoid desiccation, and efforts are made to preserve the blood supply. The blood flow through cortical bone occurs through the relatively small vascular channels of the Haversian system. Bone bleeding originates predominantly in the cancellous bone. The hematopoietic elements are contained within a honeycombed network of vascular channels and can be a source of profuse bleeding. Electrocautery, which is useful in soft tissue hemostasis, functions primarily to collapse and seal blood vessels. To be effective in controlling bone bleeding, it would have to generate sufficient heat to create a coagulum that would physically block vascular channels - the thermal injury to the adjacent bone would be of such magnitude, that any hemostatic benefit would be offset by the resultant bone necrosis.

2.4 Effective bone hemostasis

The most immediate and effective way to stem bone bleeding is to physically block the open vascular channels, a process known as tamponade. Until the recent introduction of soluble

---

[3] Giannoudis, P.V., H. Dinopoulos, and E. Tsiridis, "Bone substitutes: an update." *Injury*, 2005. 36 Suppl 3: p. S20-7

[4] Hladki, W., L. Brongel, and J. Lorkowski, "Injuries in the elderly patients." *Przegląd Lekarski*, 2006. 63 Suppl 5: p. 1-4.0

[5] AAOS Medical Letter: "*Antibiotic Prophylaxis for Bacteremia in Patients with Joint Replacements*."February 2009, Revised June 2010. http://www.aaos.org/about/papers/advistmt/1033.asp

[6] Source: National Hospital Discharge Survey: 2007 Summary, table 8. Centers for Disease Control and Prevention http://www.cdc.gov/nchs/fastats/insurg.htm accessed July 31, 2011.

synthetic polymers, the only widely available tamponade material was bone wax, a beeswax based blend. Bone wax sticks to bone blocking the vascular channels, providing immediate bone hemostasis. Although inexpensive and easy to use, bone wax has a number of troublesome side effects. Once applied to bone, bone wax remains at the site indefinitely. Bone wax is known to interfere with bone healing, elicit chronic inflammatory reactions, and increase infection rates (Allison, 1994; Armstrong et al., 2010; Chun, 1988; Finn, 1992; Johnson, 1981; Nelson, 1990; Gibbs, 2004; Sawan et al., 2010; Schonauer et al. 2004; Solheim et al., 1992; Wellisz et al., 2006, 2008a, 2008b).[7] And yet, the use of bone wax remains relatively widespread, and surgeons are often unaware of the complications surrounding its application. In fact, the effect of bone hemostasis materials in general, not just bone wax, on post-operative infection remains largely neglected in the current professional literature. By and large, existing infection studies in orthopedic, cardiac, and neurological surgery do not mention the type of bone hemostasis materials used in any given trial, overlooking the fact that bone hemostasis materials are in themselves modifiable risk factors, both for soft tissue infection and for osteomyelitis.

3. Surgical site infections and osteomyelitis

3.1 Risk of surgical site infection

Surgical site infections (SSI) account for nearly 25% of all hospital infections in the United States. All tissues, soft and osseous, are susceptible to post-operative complications; an increasing number of infections are methicillin-resistant, making treatment more difficult and effective prophylaxis more urgent (Georgia Epidemiology Report, 2004; Kronemyer, 2004; Styers et al, 2006).[8] Although technological advances and focus on prevention lower

---

[7] For detailed discussions of various complications related to the use of bone wax, see: Allison RT. "Foreign body reactions and an associated histological artifact due to bonewax." *Br. J. Biomed. Sci.* 1994; 51:14-17. Armstrong et al. *BMC Surgery* 2010, 10:37 http://www.biomedcentral.com/1471-2482/10/37; Chun PKC, Virmani R, Mason TE, Johnson F. "Bone wax granuloma causing saphenous vein thrombosis." *Am. Heart J.* 1988; 115:1310-1313. Finn MD, Schow SR, Scneiderman ED. "Osseous regeneration in the presence of four common hemostatic agents." *J. Oral Maxillofac. Surg.* 1992;50:608-612. Gibbs L, Kakis A, Weinstein P, Conte J. "Bone wax as a risk factor for surgical site infection following neurospinal surgery." *Infect. Control Hosp. Epidemiol.* 2004; 25:346-348. Johnson P, Fromm D. "Effects of bone wax on bacterial clearance." *Surgery* 1981; 89:206-209. Nelson DR, Buxton TB, Luu QN, Rissing JP. "The promotional effect of bone wax on experimental Staphylococcus Aureus osteomyelitis." *J. Thorac. Cardiovasc. Surg.* 1990; 99:977-980. Sawan A, Elhawary Y, Zaghlool Amer M, & Abdel Rahman M. "Controversial Role of Two Different Local Haemostatic Agents on Bone Healing." *Journal of American Science*, 2010; 6(12):155-163]. (ISSN: 1545-1003); Schonauer, C., E. Tessitore, et al. (2004). "The use of local agents: bone wax, gelatin, collagen, oxidized cellulose." *Eur Spine J* 13 Suppl 1: S89-96. Solheim E, Pinholt EM, Bang G, Sudmann E. "Effect of local hemostatics on bone induction in rats: a comparative study of bone wax, fibrin-collagen paste, and bioerodible polyorthoester with and without gentamicin." *J Biomed Mater Res.* 1992 Jun;26(6):791-800. Wellisz T, Armstrong JK, Cambridge J, Fisher TC: "Ostene, a new water-soluble bone hemostasis agent." *J Craniofac Surg* 17: 420-425, 2006. Wellisz T, An YH, Wen X, Kang Q, Hill CM, Armstrong JK. "Infection rates and healing using bone wax and a soluble polymer material." *Clin Orthop Relat Res* 2008; 466:481-6. Wellisz T, Armstrong JK, Cambridge J, et al. "The effects of a soluble polymer and bone wax on sternal healing in an animal model." *Ann Thorac Surg* 2008; 85:1776-80;

[8] Georgia Epidemiology Report (GER). *Community-associated Methicillin Resistant Staphylococcus aureus (MRSA).* June 2004;20:1-4. Kronemyer B. MRSA incidence on the rise. Infectious Disease News. May 1, 2004. http://www.infectiousdiseasenews.com/article/33489.aspx. Accessed August 5, 2011; Styers D,

the risk of post-operative infection, when the complication does occur, the human and financial cost is extremely high. Patients who develop surgical site infections (SSI) are 60% more likely to spend time in an intensive care unit; they are five times more likely to be readmitted to the hospital; they have three times the length of hospital stay; and their mortality rate is five times that of inpatients without wound infections (CDC, 2011; Noskin et al., 2005).[9] Infections caused by resistant organisms exact an even higher toll on individual patients and healthcare system (Carmeli et al., 1999; Cosgrove et al., 2002; Kronemyer, 2004).[10]

3.2 Risk of bone infection in cardiac, orthopedic, and neurological surgery

In cardiac surgery, infections of median sternotomy wounds are a rare but grave complication. Mediastinitis occurs in 0.3–5% of cases, but it is associated with a mortality rate between 14 and 47% (Losanoff et al., 2002).[11] Left untreated, these infections can extend to aortic and cardiac suture lines, prosthetic grafts, and intracardiac prostheses (Pairolero & Arnold, 1986).[12] The added financial cost of treating mediastinitis to an individual institution has been reported as high as $500,000 USD (Lee et. al, 2009).[13] In orthopedic surgery, approximately 7% of total joint arthroplasties performed annually in the US are revision procedures - the result of deep infections of total joint replacements and the consequent failure of the initial operations (CDC; AAOS, 2010). In neurosurgery, postoperative wound infection following intracranial surgery has a reported incidence ranging from 1% to 8%, with significant geographic variations in Europe and North America, and it carries a high risk of morbidity and mortality if not aggressively treated.[14]

4. Antibiotic prophylaxis

4.1 SSI Prevention

While treatment of Surgical Site Infections (SSI) is essential, the focus in the medical community remains on preventing the complications from occurring. There is much clinical

---

Sheehan DJ, Hogan P, et al. "Laboratory-based surveillance of current antimicrobial resistance patterns and trends among Staphylococcus aureus: 2005 status in the United States." *Ann Clin Microbiol Antimicrob*. 2006. 5:2

[9] Sources: Centers for Disease Control and Prevention (CDC). National Center for Health Statistics. Leading causes of Death. http://www.cdc.gov/nchs/fastats/lcod.htm. Accessed July 30, 2011; for complications and associated cost of infections, see: Gary A Noskin, Robert J. Rubin, et al. "The Burden of Staphylococcus aureus Infections on Hospitals in the United States." *Arch Intern. Med.* 2005;165:1756-1761.

[10] See for example: Carmeli Y, Troillet N, Karchmer AW, et al. "Health and economic outcomes of antibiotic resistance in Pseudomonas aeruginosa." *Arch Intern Med.* 1999;159:1127-1132; Cosgrove SE et al. "Health and economic outcomes of the emergence of third-generation cephalosporin resistance in Enterobacter species." *Arch Intern Med.* 2002. 162:185-190; Kronemyer, 2004

[11] Julian E. Losanoff, Bruce W. Richman, James W. Jones. "Disruption and infection of median sternotomy: a comprehensive review." *Eur J Cardiothorac Surg* 2002;21:831-839

[12] Pairolero PC & Arnold PG "Management of Infected Median Sternotomy Wounds." *Ann Thorac Surg*, 1986; 42:1-2. DOI: 10.1016/S0003-4975(10)61822-X

[13] Lee JC, Raman J, Song DH. "Primary sternal closure with titanium plate fixation: plastic surgery effecting a paradigm shift." *Plast Reconstr Surg* 2010;125:1720-4.

[14] McClelland, S., "Postoperative intracranial neurosurgery infection rates in North America versus Europe: A systematic analysis." *Am J Infect Control* 2008; 36:570-3

evidence that antibiotics used preventively significantly reduce the occurrence of SSI across surgical fields. As a result, antimicrobial prophylaxis is becoming the standard of care. The American Academy of Orthopedic Surgeons (AAOS), the American Academy of Neurosurgeons (AANS), The Society of Thoracic Surgeons (STS), and the North American Spine Society (NASS) currently recommend perioperative use of antibiotics to lower the risk of infection of soft tissue and the incidence of post-operative osteomyelitis in spinal procedures, neurosurgery, orthopedic and cardiac surgery. There is a growing consensus that patients in high-risk groups, those undergoing procedures associated with high infection rates, involving implantation of grafts or prosthetic material, or surgeries in which the consequences of infection are serious, should receive systemic perioperative antibiotics targeting the most likely organisms (AAOS, 2010; Edwards et al., 2006; Engelman et al., 2007; Watters et al., 2007).[15]

4.2 Systemic antibiotic prophylaxis

The value of systemic prophylaxis depends critically upon the activity of the antibiotic towards the causative organisms. In cardiac procedures, peri-operative intravenous antibiotic prophylaxis was shown to reduce the incidence of SWIs by up to 80% compared to placebo (Kreter & Woods, 1992).[16] In neurosurgical and orthopedic procedures, wound infection rates decreased by 63% with IV antibiotic prophylaxis. But IV prophylaxis tends to target infections caused by gram-negative bacteria, and while S. *aureus* and S. *epidermidis* are the most common causes of SSI, they are increasingly methicillin resistant (CDC, 2009).[17] Vancomycin is often the only effective antibiotic available for treatment of surgical site infection caused by methicillin-resistant gram-positive organisms. Since broad systemic use of Vancomycin for prophylaxis is discouraged for epidemiological reasons, local delivery of antibiotic directly to the surgical site may be an alternative or an effective adjunct to systemic SSI prophylaxis.

4.3 Use of topical antibiotic prophylaxis in surgery

While systemic use of antibiotic prophylaxis is generally recommended and practiced, there is evidence that local application directly to the the surgical site is effective at reducing the incidence of post-operative infection of both soft tissue and osteomyelitis in cardiac, spinal, orthopedic and neuro-surgical procedures. Topical application of Vancomycin powder to the sternal edges has been shown to reduce SWI following cardiac surgery (Vander et al.,

[15] For detailed practice guidelines, see: Edwards et al. "The STS Practice Guideline Series: Antibiotic Prophylaxis in Cardiac Surgery, Part I: Duration." *Annals of Thoracic Surgery* 81(1): 397–404 (2006); Engelman R et al. "The STS Practice Guideline Series: Antibiotic Prophylaxis in Cardiac Surgery, Part II: Antibiotic Choice." *Annals of Thoracic Surgery* 2007; 83: 1569-1576; Watters WC III, MD et al. North American Spine Society Evidence-Based Clinical Guidelines for Multidisciplinary Spine Care, 2007. AAOS Information Statement "Antibiotic Prophylaxis for Bacteremia in Patients with Joint Replacements." February 2009, revised June 2010. http://www.aaos.org/about/papers/advistmt/1033.asp retrieved July 30, 2011;

[16] Kreter B, Woods M. "Antibiotic prophylaxis for cardiothoracic operations. Meta-analysis of thirty years of clinical trials." *J Thorac Cardiovasc Surg* 1992;104(3):590-9

[17] Centers for Disease Control and Prevention (CDC). Prevent antimicrobial resistance in healthcare settings. http://www.cdc.gov/drugresistance/healthcare/problem.htm. Accessed September 27, 2009.

1989).[18] There is also anecdotal evidence that cardiothoracic surgeons in the United States commonly consider topical application of Vancomycin to be effective in preventing infection with resistant gram-positive organisms, and that its use is quite widespread.

4.3.1 Effectiveness of topical antibiotic prophylaxis in spinal and cardiac procedures

In one clinical study that highlighted the potential of local antibiotic prophylaxis, Rohde and colleagues reported and analyzed the incidence of spondylodiscitis after lumbar disc surgery in 1642 patients in a German center (Rohde et al., 1999).[19] Postoperative spondylodiscitis is the result of intraoperative contamination and, theoretically, could be prevented with prophylactic antibiotics. The infection is considered rare, but the retrospective design of most existing studies and the scarce use of magnetic resonance imaging for early radiologic diagnosis suggest that the reported incidence rates may be underestimates. Of the 1642 patients, 508 were not given any prophylactic antibiotics, while in 1134 patients a collagenous sponge containing gentamicin was placed in the cleared disc space. In 19 of the 508 patients who were not treated with antibiotic prophylaxis (3.7%), a postoperative spondylodiscitis developed, whereas none of the 1134 patients who received antibiotic prophylaxis became symptomatic, demonstrating that antibiotic-containing sponges placed in the cleared disc space were effective in completely preventing postoperative spondylodiscitis.

Local antibiotic prophylaxis of sternal wound infection was studied in a group of nearly 2000 patients from two cardiothoracic centers in Sweden (Friberg et al., 2005). [20] The control group of 967 patients received routine systemic antibiotic prophylaxis with i.v. isoxazolyl-penicillin. The treatment group of 983, in addition to the same routine intravenous antibiotic prophylaxis, was also treated with a collagen sponge containing 260mg of Gentamicin, which was placed between the sternal halves before closure. The study end-point was any SWI identified at any time over the two-months postoperative follow-up. In total, 129 patients developed a SWI; 42 (4.3%) in the treatment group and more than double -- 87 or 9.0% -- in the control group. In a similar study, 272 patients received a Gentamicin-collagen implant under the sternum before closure and 270 served as controls (Eklund et al., 2005).[21] The incidence of SWI in the control group (5.9%) was 50% higher than in the treatment group (4.0 %).

4.3.2 Infection rate-reducing potential of local antibiotic prophylaxis in cardiac, orthopaedic, and neurological surgery

Because there are relatively few local antibiotic prophylaxis studies, but the results of existing trials are consistently promising, the current North American Spine Society

[18] Vander Salm TJ, Okike ON, Pasque MK, Pezzella AT, Lew R, Traina V, Mathieu R. "Reduction of sternal infection by application of topical vancomycin." *J Thorac Cardiovasc Surg* 1989;98(4):618-22

[19] Rohde et al., "Spondylodiscitis after lumbar discectomy. Incidence and a proposal for prophylaxis." *Spine (Phila Pa 1976)*, 1998 Mar 1;23 (5):615-20.

[20] Friberg O, Svedjeholm R, Soderquist B, Granfeldt H, Vikerfors T, Kallman J. "Local gentamicin reduces sternal wound infections after cardiac surgery: a randomized controlled trial." *Ann Thorac Surg.* 2005;79(1):153-61

[21] Eklund, A.M., M. Valtonen, K.A. "Prophylaxis of sternal wound infections with gentamicin-collagen implant: randomized controlled study in cardiac surgery." *Journal of Hospital Infection* (2005) 59, 108–112.

Guideline, American Academy of Orthopedic Surgeons Recommendations, and Society of Thoracic Surgeons Practice Guidelines suggest further research that would lead to a more thorough and conclusive assessment of the effectiveness of local antibiotic prophylaxis (Watters et al., 2007; AAOS 2010, Edwards et al., 2006; Endelman et al., 2007).

5. Systemic and perioperative risk factors for postoperative osteomyelitis

5.1 Infection risk factors in cardiac surgery

Many systemic factors beyond the surgeon's control increase the patients' risk for soft tissue infection and osteomyelitis. In cardiac surgery, although surgeons vary in their operative treatment of complicated median sternotomy wounds (El Oakley, 1996), there is a considerable consensus, supported by multiple prospective clinical studies, that obesity stands out as one of the main predictors of poststernotomy wound complications and osteomyelitis of the sternum (Milano et al., 1995;[22]; Lamm et al., 1998;[23] Losanoff et al., 2002; Szerafin et al., 1999). Szerafin and colleagues note the need to adjust the dose of antibiotic prophylaxis to the body weight to ensure effectiveness of this infection-preventing measure in obese patients (Szerafin et al., 1999). The incidence of infection of soft or osseous tissue in itself increases risk to patient, regardless of the patient's preoperative condition. Underscoring the importance of effective prophylaxis, Milano and colleagues found that postoperative interval mortality during the first 90 days after surgery for the patients with mediastinitis was double that of the patients without mediastinitis (11.8% compared with 5.5%); between 1 and 2 years after surgery interval mortality in the mediastinitis group was nearly four times the mortality reported for the non-mediastinitis patients (8.1% vs. 2.3%). Having reviewed professional literature and 13 other risk-evaluating studies, Milano prospectively collected data on 20 preoperative and intraoperative variables on 6459 consecutive patients who underwent CABG and identified four highly significant independent predictors for the development of sternal dehiscence and mediastinitis (Milano et al., 1995). Losanoff and colleagues in their comprehensive review also analyzed identifiable risks that may serve as reliable predictors of sternal wound infection (Losanoff et al., 2002).

• Obesity
• Congestive heart failure
• Previous heart surgery
• Duration of the surgical procedure
• Diabetes mellitus
• Chronic obstructive airway disease
• Smoking
• Larger female breast size

Table 1. Predictors of Deep Sternal Wound Infection:

---

[22] Carmelo A. Milano, MD; Karen Kesler, MS; Nancy Archibald, MHA, MBA; Daniel J. Sexton, MD; Robert H. Jones, MD. "Mediastinitis After Coronary Artery Bypass Graft Surgery."*Circulation.* 1995;92:2245-2251 doi: 10.1161/01.CIR.92.8.2245

[23] Lamm P., Gödje O.L., Lange T., Reichart B. "Reduction of wound healing problems after median sternotomy by use of retention sutures." *Ann Thorac Surg* 1998;66:2125-2126

Milano's study and his review of the relevant literature suggest that obesity and duration of surgery are the most important predictors of mediastinitis. Furthermore, his study documents for the first time that post-operative mediastinitis has a significant negative influence on long-term survival independent of the patient's preoperative condition.

5.2 Infection risk factors in orthopedic and neurosurgical procedures

Spinal and orthopedic surgery carries its own systemic risks (Kanafani et al., 2006).[24] There are multiple factors, such as immunodeficiency, immunosuppression, diabetes, existing implants, malnutrition, and others, that may increase arthroplasty patient's risk of bacteremia and hematogenous total join infection following an invasive procedure (AAOS, 2010). A number of factors, including lymphopenia, duration of surgical procedure, and others, increase the risk of infection in spinal surgery patients (Kanafani et al., 2006; Watters et al., 2007). Given the potential adverse outcomes of joint and spinal infections -- both the human toll and the cost of treating spinal complications, infected joint replacements or infections - antibiotic prophylaxis is recommended in combination with patient risk assessment.

• Existing prosthetic joint replacement
• Immunocompromised/immunosuppressed patients
• Inflammatory arthropathies (e.g.: rheumatoid arthritis, systemic lupus erythematosus)
• Drug-induced immunosuppression
• Radiation-induced immunosuppression
• Presence of co-morbidities (e.g.: diabetes, obesity, HIV, smoking)
• Previous prosthetic joint infections
• Malnourishment
• Hemophilia
• HIV infection
• Insulin-dependent (Type 1) diabetes
• Malignancy
• Megaprostheses
• Lymphopenia
• History of chronic infections

Table 2. Risk Factors for Postoperative Hematogeneous or Direct-Inoculation Infection of the Spine or Joints[25]

[24] Kanafani ZA, Dakdouki GK, El-Dbouni O, Bawwab T, Kanj SS. "Surgical site infections following spinal surgery at a tertiary care center in Lebanon: incidence, microbiology, and risk factors." *Scand J Infect Dis.* 2006;38(8):589-592.

[25] Compiled based on Kanafani et al. (2006), AAOS recommendations (revised 2010), and NASS Guidelines (2007)

5.3 Excessive bleeding and duration of surgical procedure as infection risk factors

Although cardiac patient's weight and other health conditions at the time of the operation may be beyond the surgeon's control, the duration of the surgical procedure depends, among other factors, on the management of bone and soft tissue bleeding (Samudrala, 2008). Similarly, in spinal and orthopedic surgery, the myriad systemic risks the patient brings into the operating room cannot be altered by the surgeon, but the duration of each procedure can - it is affected by clear visualization of the site of incision, which in turn depends on the management of bleeding.

Both the spine and the sternum are highly vascular bones. Appropriate hemostasis methods significantly improve the visibility of the surgical site and therefore help shorten the time it takes to perform any given surgical procedure - and reduce the risks associated with the length of spinal or cardiac operations.

6. Bone wax as a modifiable risk factor for osteomyelitis, inflammation, and inhibited bone healing

6.1 Modifiable risk factors

Risk factors for Osteomyelitis include a variety of systemic aspects ranging from cigarette smoking and malnutrition to immunosuppression, and osteoporosis, none of which can be controlled by the surgeon. However, risk factors under the surgeon's control can also predispose a patient to surgical complications and Osteomyelitis. Careful reassessment of all known modifiable risk factors is necessary to help prevent the incidence of post-operative surgical site infections. Prevention is especially important given the prevalence of infections caused by antibiotic-resistant organisms. This reassessment of risk should include a careful look at the management of bone bleeding.

6.2 Role of bone hemostasis materials in preventable complications

Management of bone bleeding involves a decision about what to avoid and what to introduce into the operating site. But the choice of bone hemostasis material may also prove critical in determining the effectiveness of topical antibiotic prophylaxis. Researchers have isolated multiple systemic risk factors contributing to surgical site complications in procedures involving the bone, but the published clinical studies often do not mention the type of bone hemostasis material used in the trials, and consequently exclude them from perioperative risk assesments. And yet, some bone hemostats, such as bone wax, may by virtue of their properties and their very presence in the surgical wound increase the risk of complications (Szerafin et al, 1999).[26] A foreign body introduced into the surgical site can become a nidus of infection, lead to chronic inflammation, and interfere with the bones' reparative processes, thereby undermining any benefit antibiotic prophylaxis, especially topical applications, may have for the clinical outcome.

---

[26] Szerafin and colleagues link the absence of bone wax to reduced instances of mediastinitis: "Nontraumatic surgical techniques, with limited use of electrocautery and without applying bone wax, remain the most important factors in the prevention [of mediastinitis]." In: Szerafin Tamás, MD, Osama Jaber, MD, Árpád Péterffy, MD, PhD. "Reduction of wound healing problems after median sternotomy (letter to the editor)." *Ann Thorac Surg* 1999; 68: 2388.

6.2.1 Bone wax as bone hemostasis material

Bone wax, composed of beeswax and softening agents, has been widely used for over one hundred years. Unadulterated beeswax was used for amputation hemostasis during the US Civil War. The development of modern softened bone wax has been attributed to Victor Horsley in 1892 (Horsley, 1892; Parker, 1892).[27]

In the 1924 edition of Carson's Modern Operative Surgery, the use of bone wax is recommended not for bone hemostasis – the currently prevalent application -- but for preventing bone healing and for the creation of a pseudoarthrosis (Verral, 1924).[28] Since 1924, there has not been a significant change in the formulation of bone wax. The material is still comprised of insoluble and non-resorbable beeswax softened with paraffin and/or isopropyl palmitate (Schonauer et al., 2004).[29] Bone wax has no inherent hemostatic quality, and its effect on the bone remains consistent with Carson's description.

The material's appeal is in its ease of use and its ability to effectively tamponade the vascular spaces in the bone, stopping bleeding immediately. Contrary to Carson's recommendation, it is being used in procedures such as median sternotomy or spinal fusion, in which bone fusion and healing are required -- and in which pseudoarthrosis, or a failure of callus formation resulting in a non-osseous union of bone fragments, is the precise opposite of the desired surgical outcome.

Although effective in stopping bone bleeding, bone wax has troublesome adverse effects. Once applied to the bone, the material remains at the surgical site indefinitely. It may become a nidus of infection and if contaminated, it may cause infection of the soft tissue or osteomyelitis (Allison, 1994; Chun et al., 1988; Finn et al., 1992; Gibbs et al., 2004; Johnson et al., 1981; Nelson et al., 1990; Wellisz et al., 2006, 2008a, 2008b).

6.2.2 Inflammation and bone wax

Bone wax remains at the site of application indefinitely and can cause giant cell formation as well as local inflammation of the surrounding tissue (Allison, 1994).[30] Sorrenti et al. evaluated the reactions to bone wax in human tibias in 12 patients who had undergone tibial tubercle elevation. The patients underwent re-operation after 5 to 13 months, and bone biopsies were performed. A progressive reaction was described that began with a foreign body giant cell reaction with giant cells containing vacuoles filled with bone wax, to the formation of mature fibrous tissue. Reactions to bone wax consisted mainly of pain and swelling, often exacerbated by infection (Sorrenti, 1984).[31] Alberius et al. utilized a rat

[27] Horsley, V. (1892). "Antiseptic wax [Letter]." *Br Med J* **1**: 1165. Parker, R. (1892). "Aural pyaemia siccessfully treated by removing putrid thrombus of jugular vein and lateral sinus." *The British Medical Journal* 1: 1076-1077

[28] Verrall, P. J. (1924). "Operation on Joints." *Modern Operative Surgery*. H. W. Carson. London, Cassell & Co. . **1:** 69.

[29] Schonauer C, Tessitore E, Barbagallo G, Albanese V, Moraci A. "The use of local agents: bone wax, gelatin, collagen, oxidized cellulose." *Eur Spine J*. 2004;13 (suppl 1):S89–S96.

[30] Allison RT. "Foreign body reactions and an associated histological artefact due to bone wax." *Br J Biomed Sci* 1994;51:14-7.

[31] Sorrenti SJ, Cumming WJ, Miller D. "Reaction of the human tibia to bone wax." *Clin Orthop Relat Res* 1984:293-6.

calvarial bone model to identify the three stages of inflammatory reaction to bone wax: 1) a nonspecific inflammatory response; 2) a foreign body reaction; and 3) a marked fibrous reaction (Alberius et al., 1987).[32] The observation is consistent with histologic findings associated with the implantation of bone wax in a rat tibia model, which typically include foreign-body reactions characterized by giant cells, plasma cells, fibrous tissue, and a lack of bone formation (Howard & Kelley, 1969). [33]

The inflammatory reactions to bone wax may also be a source of post-operative pain. A report from Norway described seven patients with intractable pain following the use of bone wax in foot surgery (Anfinsen et al., 1993).[34] Five of the patients were pain-free after the bone containing the inflamed bone wax was resected. Anecdotal reports describing adverse inflammatory reactions to bone wax are also common (Allison 1994; Anfinsen et al. 1993; Angelini et al., 1987; Ates et al., 2004; Aurelio et al., 1984; Bolger et al., 2005; Chun, et al., 1988; Cirak & Unal 2000; Hadeishi et al., 1995; Julsrud, 1980; Katz& Rootman, 1996; Kothbauer et al., 2001; Low & Sim 2002; Patel et al., 2000; Verborg et al., 2000; Wolvius & van der Wal 2003;).[35] Reactions consist mainly of pain and swelling, often exacerbated by infection.

6.2.3 Infection and bone wax

There is evidence that bone wax not only remains at the surgical site indefinitely but also actually increases infection rates. Researchers Johnson and Fromm found that in a rabbit iliac crest defect model bone wax decreases the natural ability of bone to clear bacteria

[32] Alberius, P., B. Klinge, et al. (1987). "Effects of bone wax on rabbit cranial bone lesions." *J Craniomaxillofac Surg* 15(2): 63-67.

[33] Howard TC, Kelley RR. "The effect of bone wax on the healing of experimental rat tibial lesions." *Clin Orthop Relat Res* 1969; 63:226 –32.

[34] Anfinsen, O. G., B. Sudmann, et al. (1993). "Complications secondary to the use of standard bone wax in seven patients." *J Foot Ankle Surg* 32(5): 505-508.

[35] See: Allison, 1994; Anfinsen et al. 1993; Angelini, el-Ghamari, et al. "Poststernotomy pseudo-arthrosis due to foreign body reaction to bone wax." *Eur J Cardiothorac Surg* 1987; 1(2): 129-130.et al., 1987; Ates, O., S. R. Cayli, et al. 2004. "Bone wax can cause foreign body granuloma in the medulla oblongata." *Br J Neurosurg* 2004; 18(5): 538-540. Aurelio, J., B. Chenail, et al. "Foreign-body reaction to bone wax. Report of a case." *Oral Surg Oral Med Oral Pathol* 1984; 58(1): 98-100. Bolger WE, Tadros M, et al. "Endoscopic management of cerebrospinal fluid leak associated with the use of bone wax in skull-base surgery." *Otolaryngol Head Neck Surg* 2005; 132(3): 418-420. Chun PK, Virmani R, et al. "Bone wax granuloma causing saphenous vein graft thrombosis." *Am Heart J* 1988; 115(6): 1310-1313. et al., 1988; Cirak B & Unal O. "Iatrogenic quadriplegia and bone wax. Case illustration." *J Neurosurg* 2000; 92(2 Suppl): 248.; Hadeishi H., N. Yasui, et al. (1995). "Mastoid canal and migrated bone wax in the sigmoid sinus: technical report." *Nurosurgery* 1995; 36(6): 1220-1223; discussion 1223-1224;. Julsrud, ME (1980). "A surgical complication: allergic reaction to bone wax." *J Foot Surg* 1980; 19(3): 152-154.Katz SE & Rootman J. "Adverse effects of bone wax in surgery of the orbit." *Ophthal Plast Reconstr Surg* 1996; 12(2): 121-126., 1996; Kothbauer KF, Jallo GI, et al. "Foreign body reaction to hemostatic materials mimicking recurrent brain tumor. Report of three cases." *J Neurosurg* 2001; 95(3): 503-506.; Low WK & Sim CS. "Bone wax foreign body granuloma in the mastoid." *ORL J Otorhinolaryngol Relat Spec* 2002; 64(1): 38-40.; Patel RB et al. "Bone wax as a cause of foreign body granuloma in the cerebellopontine angle. Case illustration." *J Neurosurg* 2000; 92(2): 362.; VerborgOK et al. "A retroperitoneal tumor a. s a late complication of the use of bone wax." *Acta Orthop Belg2000*; 66(4): 389-391.; Wolvius EB & van der Wal KG "Bone wax as a cause of a foreign body granuloma in a cranial defect: a case report." *Int J Oral Maxillofac Surg* 2003; 32(6): 656-658.;

(Johnson & Fromm, 1981).[36] In a rat tibia model, Nelson and colleagues observed that the presence of bone wax reduced the amount of *Staphylococcus aureus* needed to produce osteomyelitis by a factor of 10,000 (Nelson et al., 1990), a finding that is particularly alarming given the growing prevalence of the methicillin-resistant *Staph. aureus*. In a clinical study of spinal procedures conducted by Gibbs and colleagues, infection rates following spinal surgery increased ten-fold – 1 in 7 vs. 1 in 72 infections -- when bone wax was used for bone hemostasis (Gibbs et al., 2004).[37] Similarly, researchers observed that bone wax increased the risk of mediastinitis following sternotomies performed during cardiac procedures (El Oakley, 1996; Fynn-Thompson et. al., 2004; Hollenbeak et. al., 2000; Losanoff et al., 2002; Szerafin et al., 1999).[38]

6.2.4 Bone wax and bone healing

The healing potential of bone, whether subject to trauma or surgery, is influenced by a variety of biochemical, biomechanical, cellular, hormonal, and pathological processes. The cellular components of bone consist of osteogenic precursor cells, osteoblasts, osteoclasts, osteocytes, and the hematopoietic elements of bone marrow, all of which are integral to new bone formation and regeneration. When applied to the cut or resected surface of the bone, whether sternal, vertebral, cranial, or other, traditional bone wax inhibits bone healing by interfering with the formation of new bone (osteogenesis).

6.2.4.1 Bone wax and inhibition of new bone formation

Living bone is in a constant state of bone deposition, resorption, and remodeling. This continuously occurring natural cycle of creation, destruction, and re-shaping of the osseous tissue is what facilitates the bone healing process (Kalfas, 2001).[39] Bone wax not only compromises the bone's ability to heal by increasing the risk of osteomyelitis (Gibbs et al., 2004), but it also interferes with healing directly by disrupting the regenerative processes necessary to achieve an osseous fusion after surgery.

Bone healing occurs in three distinct but overlapping stages: 1) the early inflammatory stage, when hematoma forms and granulation occurs; 2) the repair stage, in which cartilage and callus replace hematoma; and 3) the late remodeling stage, in which the bone regains its shape, circulation improves, and mechanical strength returns (Kalfas, 2001).

The first 1 to 2 weeks are a period in which inflammation and revascularization occur. During the first few hours and days, inflammatory cells and fibroblasts infiltrate the bone, which results in the formation of granulation tissue, ingrowth of vascular tissue, and migration of mesenchymal cells. The mesenchymal cells then differentiate into osteoblasts and osteoclasts.

---

[36] Johnson P, Fromm D. "Effects of bone wax on bacterial clearance." *Surgery* 1981;89:206- 209

[37] Gibbs L, Kakis A, Weinstein P, et al. "Bone wax as a risk factor for surgical-site infection following neurospinal surgery." *Infect Control Hosp Epidemiol* 2004; 25:346Y348

[38] El Oakley RM, Wright JE. "Postoperative mediastinitis: classification and management." *Ann Thorac Surg* 1996;61:1030-6. Fynn-Thompson F, Vander Salm TJ. "Methods for reduction of sternal wound infection." *Semin Thorac Cardiovasc Surg* 2004;16:77-80. Hollenbeak CS, Murphy DM, Koenig S, Woodward RS, Dunagan WC, Fraser VJ. "The clinical and economic impact of deep chest surgical site infections following coronary artery bypass graft surgery." *Chest* 2000;118:397-402.

[39] Kalfas, I.H., MD. "Principles of Bone Healing." *Neurosurg Focus* 2001; 10 (4):Article 1, p. 7-10

Osteoblasts are mature, metabolically active bone forming cells, which arise from osteoprogenitor cells located in the deeper layer of periosteum and the bone marrow. They secrete osteoid, the unmineralized organic matrix that subsequently undergoes mineralization, giving the bone its strength and rigidity. As their bone forming activity nears completion, some osteoblasts are converted into osteocytes whereas others remain on the periosteal or endosteal surfaces of bone as lining cells. Osteoblasts also play a role in the activation of bone resorption by osteoclasts, setting the stage for later bone remodeling.[40]

6.2.4.2 Bone wax and inhibition of bone fusion

With the application of a thin layer of bone wax on a cut surface of the bone, even if bone wax has been applied and then scraped off, interference with bone healing occurs. A group of researchers demonstrated in 1969 that bone wax prevents bone healing in an animal model and concluded that bone wax is contraindicated in areas where bone fusion is desired (Howard & Kelley, 1969).[41] In the clinical setting, autopsy studies have demonstrated persistent sternal nonunion attributed to the presence of bone wax (Sudman et al., 2006).[42] Sternal bone nonunion after cardiac surgery is almost always associated with concomitant mediastinitis (Losanoff et al., 2002; El Oakley & Wright, 1996).

Sternal nonunion observed by Sudman and colleagues was accompanied by chronic inflammatory reactions with the presence of residual bone wax up to 10 years after median sternotomy procedure (Sudman et al., 2006).

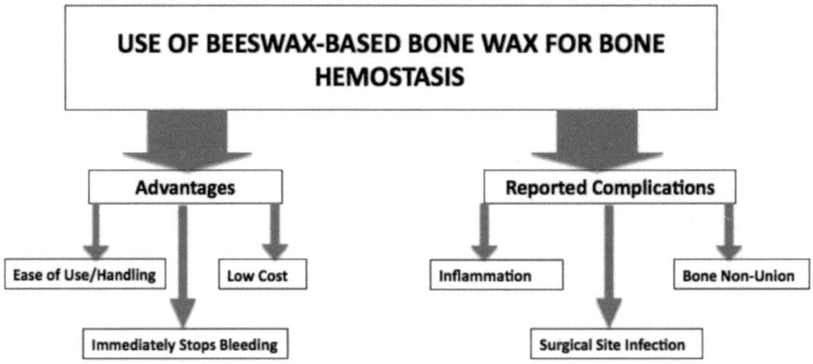

Fig. 1. Bone Wax Advantages and Complications

Solheim and colleagues examined the properties of local hemostats for osseous tissue, assuming that, to be effective, the materials should be absorbable, biocompatible and should not inhibit osteogenesis. They evaluated different local hemostats by observing tissue response and effect on demineralized bone-induced heterotopic osteogenesis in the abdominal muscle of 120 rats. Non-absorbable bone wax of 88% beeswax and absorbable

---

[40] See: Copenhaver WM, Kelly DE, Wood RL: "The connective tissues: cartilage and bone," in Copenhaver WM, Kelly DE, Wood RL (eds): *Bailey's Textbook of Histology, ed 17.* Baltimore: Williams & Wilkins, 1978, pp 170–205; Recker RR: "Embryology, anatomy, and microstructure of bone," in Coe FL, Favus MJ (eds): *Disorders of Bone and Mineral Metabolism*. New York: Raven, 1992, pp 219–240.

[41] Howard TC, Kelley RR. "The effect of bone wax on the healing of experimental rat tibial lesions." *Clin Orthop Relat Res* 1969; 63:226 –32.

[42] Sudmann B, Bang G, Sudmann E. "Histologically verified bone wax (beeswax) granuloma after median sternotomy in 17 of 18 autopsy cases." *Pathology* 2006; 38:138–41.

bovine fibrin-collagen paste both significantly inhibited osteoinduction, whereas a bioerodible polyorthoester drug delivery system with or without 4% gentamicin did not. Bone wax was not absorbed and induced a chronic foreign body reaction. Fibrin-collagen paste induced less inflammation with numerous monocytes and macrophages with engulfed material. Bioerodible polyorthoester caused a very moderate tissue reaction and was mostly resorbed after four weeks (Solheim et al., 1992).[43]

Despite its good handling and effectiveness in stopping bone bleeding instantly, the long-term complications associated with the use of traditional bone wax far outweigh its usefulness as a bone hemostasis material. Although for its ease of use and effectiveness in surgery it remains the most commonly used bone hemostasis material, given its ties to widely reported complications, a variety of alternative bone bleeding management methods have been developed.

7. Alternative bone hemostasis materials and methods

7.1 Surgical technique and management of bone bleeding

Management of bleeding is an integral aspect of the surgical technique. One of the options available to the surgeon operating on the osseous tissue is a mechanical barrier, such as that created by bone wax, which works to occlude bleeding from the open channels of the bone. In soft tissue hemostasis, surgeons most frequently chose electrocautery, a technique in which heat causes capillaries and small blood vessels to collapse and seal. Cushing first reported the use of this technique in 1921, after he used it in neurosurgical procedures. Electrocautery has since become a common hemostatic tool in modern surgery across all specialties, becoming a soft tissue corollary to bone wax.

7.1.1 Electrocautery and bone hemostasis

Electrocautery works through a pulsating (or intermittent) wave delivered to the surgical site by a unipolar device causing tissue dehydration and vessel thrombosis (Neumayer, 2008).[44] Despite the structural differences between soft tissue and cut bone surfaces, electrocautery is commonly used for both. The thermal settings used to seal bleeding vessels are generally ineffective in stemming bleeding from open vascular channels in the bone. Higher heat settings can stop bone bleeding, but burning tissue to the sufficient degree for a charred coagulum physically to block blood flow damages osseous tissue, interferes with bone healing, and increases the incidence of postoperative infection. Excessive use of this technique for bone should be avoided. (El Oakley et al., 1996; Tang et al., 2004; Nelson et. al., 1990; Nishida et al., 1991).[45]

---

[43] Solheim E, Pinholt EM, Bang G, Sudmann E. "Effect of local hemostatics on bone induction in rats: a comparative study of bone wax, fibrin-collagen paste, and bioerodible polyorthoester with and without gentamicin." *J Biomed Mater Res*. 1992 Jun;26(6):791-800.

[44] Neumayer, L., Vargo, D. (2008) "Principles of Preoperative and Operative Surgery", In: *Townsend: Sabiston Textbook of Surgery, 18th ed.* Courtney M. Townsend Jr. R. Daniel Beauchamp B. Mark Evers, Kenneth L. Mattox, pp. (251-279), Saunders Elsevier, 978-1-4160-3675-3, Philadelphia, PA

[45] El Oakley RM, Wright JE. "Postoperative mediastinitis: classification and management." *Ann Thorac Surg* 1996;61:1030-6.

7.1.2 Hemostasis through natural clotting

Another approach to bone Hemostasis is to let the bone bleed throughout the surgery. In this way, the surgeon does not introduce any foreign materials into the site and allows the bleeding bone to clot naturally. However, research has shown that the risks of unnecessary bleeding include increased blood loss and the costs and multiple risks associated with blood transfusions (Rogers et al, 2009).[46] Median sternotomies cause heavy bleeding, and complex spinal reconstructive procedures are invariably associated with excessive intraoperative blood loss, which significantly increases the risk of severe perioperative complications (Block, 2005).[47] Samudrala summarizes the benefits of effective hemostasis, which include decreased morbidity and mortality, fewer transfusions, reduced surgical time, better visualization of the surgical field - and, above all, better surgical outcome (Samudrala, 2008).[48]

7.2 Topical bone hemostats

7.2.1 Mechanical barrier

Topical hemostatic agents are mechanical barriers routinely used to achieve hemostasis of cancellous bone surfaces during neurological, cardio-thoracic, orthopedic, maxillofacial, and a variety of other surgical procedures, including procurement of bone graft material from the iliac crest. A mechanical barrier works to occlude bleeding from the open channels of the bone, the way bone wax does. The topical hemostatic agents developed as an alternative to bone wax have various active ingredients and mechanisms of actions, thus affecting hemostasis and bone healing differently.

7.2.2 Synthetic tamponade

A common method of occluding bleeding used strictly for the vascular surface of cut or resected bone is a tamponade, which creates a physical barrier that stops blood flow by blocking osseous blood channels, the way bone wax does. Tamponade materials are beneficial to the surgeon by providing hemostasis that is both immediate and easy to apply. Products in this group are direct alternatives to bone wax and offer many of the same benefits, but not the risks. Physical barriers are applied directly to the bone, can be shaped to the surgeon's needs and work immediately. While bone wax remains at the site of application indefinitely creating a host of problems, newer products made of water-soluble

Nelson DR, Buxton TB, Luu QN, Rissing JP. "The promotional effect of bone wax on experimental Staphylococcus aureus osteomyelitis." *J Thorac Cardiovasc Surg* 1990;99:977-80.

Nishida H, Grooters RK, Soltanzadeh H, Thieman KC, Schneider RF, Kim WP. "Discriminate use of electrocautery on the median sternotomy incision. A 0.16% wound infection rate." *J Thorac Cardiovasc Surg* 1991;101:488-94.

Tang GH, Maganti M, Weisel RD, Borger MA. "Prevention and management of deep sternal wound infection." *Semin Thorac Cardiovasc Surg* 2004;16:62-9.

[46] Rogers MA, Blumberg N, Saint S, Langa KM, Nallamothu BK. "Hospital variation in transfusion and infection after cardiac surgery: a cohort study." *BMC Med* 2009;7:37.

[47] Block JE.. "Severe blood loss during spinal reconstructive procedures: the potential usefulness of topical hemostatic agents." *Med Hypotheses.* 2005; 65(3):617-21

[48] Samudrala, S.. "Topical Hem static Agents in Surgery: A Surgeon's Perspective." *AORN Journal*, 2008. Supplement: Intraoperative Bleeding and Hemostasis in Surgical Procedures. vol. 88, no 3: p. S2-11

alkylene oxide copolymers (AOC) provide immediate hemostasis but remain at the site for less than 48 hours (Magyar et. al., 2008).[49] These copolymers are inert, and they are eliminated from the body unmetabolized via the kidneys and liver. Recent research in animal models has shown that AOC based product does not increase infection rates, does not promote inflammation, and does not interfere with bone healing (Armstrong, 2010; Magyar et al., 2008; Sawan et al., 2010; Wellisz et al. 2006, 2008a, 2008b).[50] An AOC based bone hemostasis material (Ostene®) has been available since 2006 and is currently distributed by Baxter International, Inc.

7.3 Soft tissue hemostats

Bleeding from bone can also be controlled with soft tissue hemostats. Soft tissue hemostasis materials can aid in the activation of the body's natural clotting mechanism. Unlike bone wax, soft tissue hemostats are made from a range of resorbable ingredients. These ingredients, discussed more fully below, take anywhere from days to months to resorb.

7.3.1 Gelatin

Gelatin based agents are generally made from animal skin gelatin mixed and baked into a sponge, powder, or a film. These materials work by creating a physical matrix followed by swelling of the material to control bleeding. Gelatin sponges are non-absorbable and can expand up to 200% of their initial volume. If left in the wound, they may act as a nidus for infection and abscess formation (Lindstrom, 1956).[51] Gelatin-based agents have also been reported to delay bone healing (Schonauer *et al*, 2004).[52]

7.3.2 Thrombin

Thrombin is derived from either bovine or human sources. It provides hemostasis in soft tissue by converting fibrinogen to fibrin to form clots and activate clotting factors. Thrombin

---

[49] Magyar CE, Aghaloo TL, Atti E, Tetradis S." Ostene, a new alkylene oxide copolymer bone hemostatic material, does not inhibit bone healing." *Neurosurgery* 2008;63:373-8; discussion 8.

[50] Armstrong et al. BMC Surgery 2010, 10:37 http://www.biomedcentral.com/1471-2482/10/37., Magyar CE, Aghaloo TL, Atti E, Tetradis S. "Ostene, a new alkylene oxide copolymer bone hemostatic material, does not inhibit bone healing." *Neurosurgery* 2008;63:373-8; discussion 8., Sawan A, Elhawary Y, Zaghlool Amer M, & Abdel Rahman M. "Controversial Role of Two Different Local Haemostatic Agents on Bone Healing." *Journal of American Science*, 2010; 6(12):155-163]. (ISSN: 1545-1003., Wellisz T, Armstrong JK, Cambridge J, Fisher TC: "Ostene, a new water-soluble bone hemostasis agent." *J Craniofac Surg* 17: 420-425, 2006. Wellisz T, An YH, Wen X, Kang Q, Hill CM, Armstrong JK. "Infection rates and healing using bone wax and a soluble polymer material." *Clin Orthop Relat Res* 2008; 466:481-6. Wellisz T, Armstrong JK, Cambridge J, et al. "The effects of a soluble polymer and bone wax on sternal healing in an animal model." *Ann Thorac Surg* 2008; 85:1776-80;

[51] Lindstrom, P.A., "Complications from the use of absorbable hemostatic sponges." *AMA Arch Surg.* 1956; Iss. 73, pp. 133-141

[52] Schonauer C, Tessitore E, Barbagallo G, Albanese V, Moraci A. "The use of local agents: bone wax, gelatin, collagen, oxidized cellulose." *Eur Spine J.* 2004;13 (suppl 1):S89–S96.Shearwood McClelland III, "Postoperative intracranial neurosurgery infection rates in North America versus Europe: A systematic analysis." *Am J Infect Control* 2008; 36:570-3

works quickly and is easy to use. However, bovine thrombin has been known to trigger immunologic reactions (Achneck et. al., 2010).[53]

Thrombin is commonly mixed with a gelatin sponge for areas with heavier bleeding. This product is effective because the gelatin ingredient works as a physical matrix while the thrombin works within the clotting cascade. The issues associated with this product include swelling, and it needs contact with fibrinogen in order to work (Achneck et. al., 2010).

7.3.3 Oxidized Regenerated Cellulose (ORC)

Oxidized regenerated cellulose-based products are sold in sheets and act as a physical matrix that promotes the initiation of clotting. ORC also works by swelling and gel formation, as well as surface interactions with proteins, platelets and intrinsic and extrinsic pathway activation (Schonauer, 2004). The low PH of this product is shown to have an antimicrobial effect. However, the acidity may cause inflammation of surrounding tissue and interfere with healing (Tomizawa, 2005).[54] ORC has also been shown to promote a foreign body reaction and reduce bone repair in rat studies (Geary & Frantz, 1950; Ibarrola *et al.*, 1985).[55]

7.3.4 Collagen

Microfibrillar Collagen is derived from bovine corium. It is available as flour, foam, and in sheets. These products work by initiating platelet adherence and activation of the clotting cascade. Though some proved promising in their ability to promote clotting in reconstructive spinal surgery (Block, 2005)[56], collagen-based products are associated with infection and delayed bone healing (Armstrong et al., 2008). Inflammation and residual material upon resection at up to 90 days have been found by Barbolt et al. (2001)[57] and Ereth et al. (2008).[58]

7.3.5 Fibrin

Fibrin sealants are made up of two parts, thrombin (human) and fibrinogen, that are combined at the time of surgery. They work by inducing platelet aggregation and initiating the clotting cascade when applied directly to bleeding bony sites. The fibrinogen determines

[53]Achneck HE, Sileshi B, Jamiolkowski RM, Albala DM, Shapiro ML, Lawson JH. "A comprehensive review of topical hemostatic agents: efficacy and recommendations for use." *Ann Surg* 2010;251:217-28.

[54] Tomizawa Y. "Clinical benefits and risk analysis of topical hemostats: a review." *J Artif Organs* 2005;8:137-42.

[55] Geary JR, Kneeland Frantz V. "New absorbable hemostatic bone wax; experimental and clinical studies." *Ann Surg* 1950;132:1128-37., Ibarrola JL, Bjorenson JE, Austin BP, Gerstein H. "Osseous reactions to three hemostatic agents." *J Endod* 1985;11:75-83.

[56] Block JE.."Severe blood loss during spinal reconstructive procedures: the potential usefulness of topical hemostatic agents." *Med Hypotheses.* 2005; 65(3):617-21

[57] Barbolt TA, Odin M, Leger M, Kangas L. "Pre-clinical subdural tissue reaction and absorption study of absorbable hemostatic devices." *Neurol Res* 2001;23:537-42.

[58] Ereth MH, Schaff M, Ericson EF, Wetjen NM, Nuttall GA, Oliver WC, Jr. "Comparative safety and efficacy of topical hemostatic agents in a rat neurosurgical model." *Neurosurgery* 2008;63:369-72; discussion 72.

the mechanical strength of the sealant, while the thrombin concentration determines the rapidity of the clot (Achneck et al., 2010).[59] Fibrin sealants are most frequently used for soft tissue hemostasis, but they have also been used for bone bleeding control during osseous tissue repair. Fibrin sealants are often used as an adjunct to other hemostasis materials.

7.3.6 Platelet Rich Plasma (PRP)

Platelet rich plasma (PRP) that is derived from the patient is also used in surgery for bone hemostasis. PRP is derived from the patient's own blood by separating red blood cells from the fibrin and plasma in a centrifuge. The plasma, which forms a gel, is applied where hemostasis is needed. This technique relies on growth factors that trigger early wound healing said to be present in the PRP. The true benefit for PRP in bone hemostasis has yet to be demonstrated (Griffin et al. 2008)[60], and the technique has shown to be a markedly expensive bone hemostasis alternative. Moreover, like all the other soft tissue hemostats, platelet rich plasma cannot replicate the handling and immediate hemostasis effect of bone wax, which many topical bone hemostasis materials seek to offer.

7.4 Topical bone hemostats – towards a comparative analysis

Few comparative studies of topical bone hemostasis materials have been published to date. Although more research and clinical data would help the surgeons navigate the field of available alternatives to bone wax more effectively and assess their merits more thoroughly, a comparative analysis is beginning to emerge. Because bone healing and the risk of infection are the main complications associated with bone wax, in their comparative studies of management of bone bleeding alternatives, the researchers tend to focus on new bone formation and osteomyelitis without losing sight of the materials' effectiveness as hemostats.

7.4.1 Studies of new bone formation and healing with topical bone hemostats

In 1992, Solheim and colleagues examined traditional bone wax, absorbable bovine fibrin-collagen paste, and a bioerodible polyorthoester drug delivery system. They concluded that, of the three bone hemostatics under scrutiny, polyorthoester alone did not significantly inhibit osteoinduction and, after causing a very moderate tissue reaction, was mostly resorbed at the end of week four of the study (Solheim et al., 1992).

In a 1992 comparative study, Finn and colleagues evaluated the potential for bone regeneration in the presence of four common hemostatic materials in a dog model in a manner that parallels iliac bone procurement in humans in oral and maxillofacial surgery. The agents compared were Avitene (microfibrillar collagen; Medchem Products, Inc, Woburn, MA); bone wax (beeswax with isopropyl palmitate; Ethicon, Inc, Somerville, NJ); Gelfoam (absorbable gelatin sponge; The Upjohn Company, Kalamazoo, MI); and Surgicel (oxidized regenerated cellulose; Johnson & Johnson Products, Inc, Patient Care Division, New Brunswick, NJ). Five surgical defects were created in each dog for placement of the

[60] Griffin XL, Smith CM, Costa ML. "The clinical use of platelet-rich plasma in the promotion of bone healing: a systematic review." *Injury* 2009;40:158-62.

Principal Agent	ALKYLENE OXIDE COPOLYMERS	MICROFIBRILLAR COLLAGEN	GELATIN	THROMBIN	GELATIN GRANULES THROMBIN	OXIDIZED REGENERATED CELLULOSE	BEESWAX
Supplied	1g, 2.5g, 3.5g Bars	Sponge/flour	Sponge	Powder /Solution	Gel in Syringe	Pad/ Sponge	2.5g Bar
Price+	2	Flour 3 Foam 4	2	Powder 2 Solution 3	2mL 2to3 5mL 4	2	1
Ingredients	Water Soluble Synthetic Copolymers	Bovine Corium Collagen	Animal Gelatin	Bovine Thrombin	Bovine Gelatin Bovine Thrombin	Wood pulp	Beeswax, Vaseline, Isopropyl palmitate
Hemostatic Action	Mechanical occlusion	Platelet release stimulation	Mechanical occlusion swells, gel formation	Activates Fibrin	Mechanical + Activates Fibrin	Mechanical occlusion swells, gel formation	Mechanical occlusion
Time to Hemostasis	Immediate	< 10 Minutes	2 + Minutes	2+ Minutes	1.5 + minutes	2+ Minutes	Immediate
Remains at Site	24-48 hours	<12 weeks	4 - 6 weeks	minutes	6 - 8 weeks	7-14 days	Indefinitely
Advantages	• Immediate hemostasis • Ease of use • Adheres to wet surfaces • Dissolves	• Immediate hemostasis • Binds to surfaces • Does not swell	• Binds to surfaces	• Improves gelatin sponge performance	• Syringe delivery system	• Bacteriostatic	• Immediate hemostasis • Ease of use
Adverse Effects		• Interferes with healing • Allergic reactions • Infection • Adhesion formation	• Interferes with healing • Swelling • Encapsulation of fluid • Foreign body reactions • Nidus for infection	• Allergic reactions • Antibody formation	• Interferes with healing • Swelling • Foreign body reactions • Nidus for infection • Antibody formation	• Interferes with healing • Swelling • Foreign body reactions	• Inhibits bone formation • Allergic reactions • Giant cell granulomas • Nidus for infection • Inflammation

Table 3. Bone Hemostasis Materials Comparison Chart.

+ *The prices are relative. The cost is estimated at price per application. Prices can vary based on institution and geographic location. The price ranges from $0-$300. 1 – under $50; 2- $50-$100; 3- $101-$200; 4 – Above $200

four materials; one defect served as an empty control site. After two month healing, radiographic and histologic examination showed new bone formation in the presence of Avitene, Surgicel, and Gelfoam. Residual material incorporated in bone, without foreign-body response, was noted in the Avitene and Gelfoam sites. Bone wax, however, showed an intense foreign-body reaction, characterized by giant cells, plasma cells, fibrous granulation tissue, and lack of bone reformation. On the basis of these initial findings, it was concluded that Surgicel, Avitene, and Gelfoam might be adequate hemostatic agents for use in iliac bone procurement, whereas the use of bone wax appears to be contraindicated (Finn et al, 1992).[61]

In 2010, Sawan and colleagues compared the effect of bone wax and a water-soluble alkylene oxide copolymer (AOC) material on mandibular bone healing in a rabbit model. Sawan's comparative study of 45 rabits was designed to assess the role of bone wax and the effectiveness of a new synthetic alternative bone hemostat in the context of oral and maxillofacial surgery. The animals were divided into three groups: bone wax and polymer groups and a hemostat-free group, which served as a control. A surgical bone defect was created in the anterior mandibular area. Alkylene oxide copolymer (AOC) hemostat-treated defects showed faster healing rate at the end of the first and second weeks than defects left untreated. The copolymer (AOC) disappeared from the surgical defect by the end of week one without any presence of inflammatory cells in the defect. In the bone wax group, the defects showed large empty vacuoles, representing bone wax remnants with inflammatory cells infiltration that interfered with bone healing. Study results showed that water soluble alkylene copolymer is a biodegradable material and that it does not interfere with bone healing. In contrast, bone wax proved to cause foreign body reaction, inhibiting bone healing (Sawan et al., 2010).

Two studies of topical bone hemostats conducted by Wellisz and colleagues in 2006 and 2008 compared the effect of non-resorbable traditional bone wax and water-soluble alkylene oxide copolymer (AOC) on sternal bone healing and cranial bone healing respectively in an animal model. After six weeks, the results of the sternal healing study involving 20 rabbits showed normal bone healing in the polymer-treated group and nonunion with fibrotic scar tissue and the absence of new bone formation in the bone wax group. While the bone hemostasis was immediate and comparable for both materials, the application of the polymer hemostatic material to the sternum resulted in significantly stronger union compared with the use of bone wax. Comparative cranial bone healing by Wellisz and colleagues assessing bone healing with bone wax and AOC in a group of 24 rabbits produced similar results (Wellisz et al., 2006, 2008a).

In a recent study, Armstrong and colleagues compared the effect of a water-soluble alkylene oxide copolymer (AOC) to oxidized regenerated cellulose (ORC) and microfibrillar collagen (MFC) on early bone healing in a rabbit tibia model with 12 animals. A group with no hemostatic material at all served as the control. Hemostasis was immediate after application of MFC and AOC, after 1-2 minutes with ORC, and >5 minutes for control. At 17 days post-surgery, micro-CT analysis showed near-complete healing in control and AOC groups, partial healing in the ORC group, and minimal healing in the MFC group. Fractional bone

[61] Finn, M. D., S. R. Schow, et al. "Osseous regeneration in the presence of four common hemostatic agents." *J Oral Maxillofac Surg*, 1992; 50(6): 608-612.

volume was 8 fold greater in the control and AOC groups than in the MFC group and over 1.5-fold greater than in the ORC group. MFC remained at the application site with minimal healing at the defect margins and early fibrotic tissue within the defect. ORC-treated defects showed partial healing but with early fibrotic tissue in the marrow space. Conversely, control and AOC treated defects demonstrated newly formed woven bone rich in cellular activity with no evidence of AOC remaining at the application site. Armstrong and colleagues concluded that early healing appeared to be impaired by the presence of MFC and impeded by the presence of ORC. In contrast, AOC did not inhibit bone healing and may be a better bone hemostatic material for procedures where bony fusion is critical and immediate bone hemostasis required (Armstrong et al., 2010).

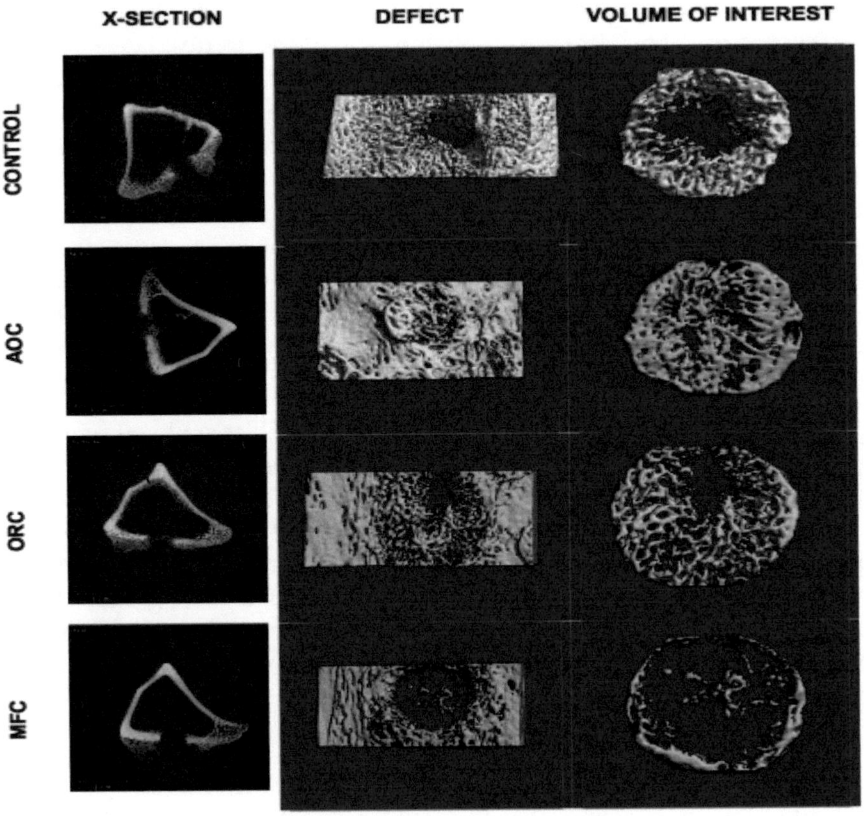

Fig. 2. Representative micro-CT images of excised rabbit tibiae at 17 days post-surgery. *Left column*: Cross-section views through the center of the defect showing newly formed bone as slightly opaque in untreated (control), alkylene oxide copolymer- and oxidized regenerated cellulose-treated defects, and an absence of opacity in microfibrillar collagen-treated defects (bar = 5.0 mm). *Center and right columns*: micro-CT generated binarized images of mineralized tissue of the defect area (center) and area analyzed within the defect (right). AOC-treated and untreated (control) defects show substantial, well developed mineralized tissue, ORC-treated defect shows a more diffuse structure of mineralized tissue, and minimal mineralized tissue is observed within the MFC-treated defect. (Armstrong et al., 2010)

7.4.2 Studies of osteomyelitis with topical bone hemostats

A 2008 comparative study assessing infection rates and healing in bone wax and AOC polymer treated bones with no treatment group as a control was designed to compare the two materials in a contaminated environment in a rabbit tibia defect model involving 24 animals. Bone defects were treated with the two topical bone hemostasis materials and then subject to a bacterial challenge by inoculation with Staphylococcus *aureus*. After 4 weeks, 100% of defects in the bone wax group became infected and developed osteomyelitis; none had evidence of bone healing. In the AOC polymer group and control group, 25% of defects developed osteomyelitis. The remaining 75% of defects in the polymer and control groups cleared the bacteria, showed no signs of osteomyelitis, and exhibited normal bone healing. The polymer-treated defects had a considerably lower rate of post-operative osteomyelitis and positive bone cultures compared with the bone wax-treated group. Wellisz and colleagues determined that there were no differences between the AOC polymer-treated group and control group in the rates of osteomyelitis, positive cultures, or bone healing, concluding that AOC may be a good alternative to bone wax when the risk of infection and bone healing are a concern (Wellisz et al., 2008b).

7.4.3 Studies of effective bleeding management with topical bone hemostats

In 2005, Block assessed the clinical effectiveness of several approaches to bone bleeding management in the context of complex spinal reconstructive procedures associated with excessive blood loss – the perioperative hemorrhage may be equivalent to estimated total blood volume, which significantly increases the risk of severe post-operative complications. Since highly vascular and widely exposed bony surfaces are not amenable to standard hemostatic maneuvers effective during soft tissue surgery, Block hypothesizes that underappreciated topical hemostatic agents may provide benefit by reducing the need for autologous predonation, banked donor blood, or antifibrinolytic agents. Topical agents Block evaluated -- combining collagen, thrombin and fibrin -- have demonstrated initial promise by inducing platelet aggregation and initiating the clotting cascade when applied directly to bleeding bony sites. Block's conclusion: clinical studies are clearly warranted (Block, 2005).

8. Redefining the management of bone bleeding: osteomyelitis, bone healing, and topical therapeutics

More clinical studies evaluating the merits of next generation bone hemostasis materials – their handling, biocompatibility, safety, and effectiveness – are indeed warranted. Further research of the effectiveness of a wide range of existing alternatives to bone wax would help surgeons assess the properties and best use of all the available bone hemostasis options. It would open the way to using the management of bone bleeding as a tool to control blood loss and, at the same time, reduce the risk of post-operative infection, both of the soft tissue and osteomyelitis.

8.1 Management of bone bleeding and topical therapeutics

Topical use of anti-microbial agents applied to the cut sternum or vertebrae during surgery already shows promise in helping lower the incidence of post-operative osteomyelitis and soft tissue infection (Eklund, 2005; Friberg, 2005; Rohde, 1999).

Some of the newly available synthetic materials designed to control bone bleeding in surgery may be able to expand the repertoire of choices available to surgeons during various surgical procedures without increasing risk to patients. Topical bone hemostasis agents in particular have the potential to redefine the management of bone bleeding and reduce the risk of post-operative complications, including osteomyelitis, by combining the application of bone hemostats with the delivery of therapeutics directly to the cut bone.

8.2 Osteomyelitis prevention and topical bone hemostasis with antibiotics

A soluble bone hemostasis material that is easy to handle, stops bleeding by mechanical occlusion, and does not inhibit osteogenesis or increase the risk of infection, may be mixed with antibiotics and used for local prophylaxis during and immediately after surgery. Such a formulation would retain the carrier's hemostatic properties to help manage bone bleeding and also allow for a controlled release of antibiotic of choice into the wound to prevent post-operative infection of the bone (osteomyelitis) or the surrounding tissue. The compound could be used during any surgical procedure - orthopedic, maxillofacial, neurological, or cardiac -- that involves the cutting of bone. If the existing studies of local antibiotic prophylaxis are any guide, antimicrobial bone hemostats used as an adjunct to systemic infection-preventing measures could reduce the risk of osteomyelitis at least by half.

8.3 Bone healing and topical bone hemostasis with bone growth factors

An analogous formulation combining bone hemostatic properties with bone growth factors could be used to deliver bone graft material to resected bone, whether in spinal fusion, repair of infected arthroplasty, or in the course of major reconstructive procedure following sternal wound debridement and removal of foreign materials during the treatment of deep mediastinitis. Bone graft delivered to the surgical site with topical bone hemostasis material as a carrier would be both osteoinductive and hemostatic, osteoconductive and easily moldable. Management of bone bleeding which incorporates bone hemostasis into the larger surgical procedure could simplify the operation, help reduce risk, and improve clinical outcome.

9. Conclusion

The choice of bone hemostasis material is a modifiable but widely overlooked post-operative infection risk factor, and proper management of bone bleeding may help reduce that risk. As a foreign body introduced during surgery into the wound, the bone hemostasis material can become a nidus of a surgical site infection. Traditional bone wax, in particular, illustrates this point. Despite its good handling and proven effectiveness, it inhibits bone healing and increases the risk of osteomyelitis across surgical procedures. Although great advances have been made in the use of antibiotic prophylaxis to reduce surgical wound complications, a better understanding of the impact of bone hemostasis technique and material choice on healing may help reduce infections and the rate of osteomyelitis even further, improving clinical outcomes. The possibility of combining topical bone hemostasis materials with therapeutics, such as antibiotics or bone grafts, may in the future broaden the repertoire of medical tools available to surgeons and redefine the role the management of bone bleeding could play in the prevention and treatment of osteomyelitis.

10. Acknowledgments

The author would like to thank Anna Chodakiewicz and Kimberly Nolan for their invaluable assistance in preparing this manuscript.

11. References

AAOS Medical Letter: "*Antibiotic Prophylaxis for Bacteremia in Patients with Joint Replacements*." February 2009, Revised June 2010. http://www.aaos.org/about/papers/advistmt/1033.asp

Allison RT. Foreign body reactions and an associated histological artifact due to bone wax. *Br. J. Biomed. Sci.* 1994;51 : 14-17.

Anfinsen, O. G., B. Sudmann, et al. (1993). "Complications secondary to the use of standard bone wax in seven patients." J Foot Ankle Surg 32(5): 505-508.

Armstrong et al. "The effect of three hemostatic agents on early bone healing in an animal model." BMC Surgery 2010, 10:37 http://www.biomedcentral.com/1471-2482/10/37

Block JE.Severe blood loss during spinal reconstructive procedures: the potential usefulness of topical hemostatic agents. Med Hypotheses. 2005; 65(3):617-21

Brightmore T. G., P. Hayes, et al. (1975). "Haemostasis and healing following median sternotomy." Langenbecks Arch Chir Suppl: 39-41

Carmeli Y, Troillet N, Karchmer AW, et al. Health and economic outcomes of antibiotic resistance in Pseudomonas aeruginosa. Arch Intern Med. 1999;159:1127-1132

Centers for Disease Control and Prevention (CDC). Prevent antimicrobial resistance in healthcare settings. http://www.cdc.gov/drugresistance/healthcare/problem.htm. Accessed September 27, 2009.

Centers for Disease Control and Prevention (CDC). National Center for Health Statistics. Leading causes of Death. http://www.cdc.gov/nchs/fastats/lcod.htm. Accessed July 30, 2011

Chun PKC, Virmani R, Mason TE, Johnson F. Bone wax granuloma causing saphenous vein thrombosis. *Am. Heart J.* 1988; 115:1310-1313.

Copenhaver WM, Kelly DE, Wood RL: The connective tissues: cartilage and bone, in Copenhaver WM, Kelly DE, Wood RL (eds): Bailey's Textbook of Histology, ed 17. Baltimore: Williams & Wilkins, 1978, pp 170–205

Cosgrove SE et al. Health and economic outcomes of the emergence of third-generation cephalosporin resistance in Enterobacter species. Arch Intern Med. 2002. 162: 185-190

Edwards et al. The STS Practice Guideline Series: Antibiotic Prophylaxis in Cardiac Surgery, Part I: Duration. Annals of Thoracic Surgery 81(1): 397–404 (2006); Engelman R et al. The STS Practice Guideline Series: Antibiotic Prophylaxis in Cardiac Surgery, Part II: Antibiotic Choice. Annals of Thoracic Surgery 2007; 83: 1569-1576

Finn MD, Schow SR, Scneiderman ED. Osseous regeneration in the presence of four common hemostatic agents. *J. Oral Maxillofac. Surg.* 1992;50:608-612.

Friberg O, Svedjeholm R, Soderquist B, Granfeldt H, Vikerfors T, Kallman J. Local gentamicin reduces sternal wound infections after cardiac surgery: a randomized controlled trial. Ann Thorac Surg. 2005;79(1):153-61

Geary JR, Kneeland Frantz V. New absorbable hemostatic bone wax; experimental and clinical studies. Ann Surg 1950;132:1128-37.

Georgia Epidemiology Report (GER). *Community-associated Methicillin Resistant Staphylococcus aureus (MRSA).* June 2004; 20:1-4.

Giannoudis, P.V., H. Dinopoulos, and E. Tsiridis, Bone substitutes: an update. *Injury,* 2005. 36 Suppl 3: p. S20-7

Gibbs L, Kakis A, Weinstein P, et al. Bone wax as a risk factor for surgical-site infection following neurospinal surgery. Infect Control Hosp Epidemiol 2004; 25:346Y348

Griffin XL, Smith CM, Costa ML. The clinical use of platelet-rich plasma in the promotion of bone healing: a systematic review. Injury 2009;40:158-62.

Hladki, W., L. Brongel, and J. Lorkowski, [Injuries in the elderly patients]. *Przegl Lek,* 2006. 63 Suppl 5: p. 1-4.0

Horsley V. Antiseptic wax. *Br. Med. J.* 1892; 1:1165 (letter)

Howard TC, Kelley RR. The effect of bone wax on the healing of experimental rat tibial lesions. Clin Orthop Relat Res 1969; 63:226 –32.

Ibarrola JL, Bjorenson JE, Austin BP, Gerstein H. Osseous reactions to three hemostatic agents. J Endod 1985;11:75-83.Johnson P, Fromm D. Effects of bone wax on bacterial clearance. Surgery 1981; 89:206-209.

Kalfas, IH., MD. Principles of Bone Healing. Neurosurg Focus 2001; 10 (4):Article 1, p. 7-10 From: http://pathwiki.pbworks.com/w/page/14673867/Bone23-27 (Accessed 7/31/2011)

Kanafani ZA, Dakdouki GK, El-Dbouni O, Bawwab T, Kanj SS. Surgical site infections following spinal surgery at a tertiary care center in Lebanon: incidence, microbiology, and risk factors. *Scand J Infect Dis.* 2006;38(8):589-592.

Kreter B, Woods M. Antibiotic prophylaxis for cardiothoracic operations. Meta-analysis of thirty years of clinical trials. J Thorac Cardiovasc Surg 1992;104(3):590-9

Kronemyer B. MRSA incidence on the rise. Infectious Disease News. May 1, 2004. http://www.infectiousdiseasenews.com/article/33489.aspx. Accessed August 5, 2011

Lamm P., Gödje O.L., Lange T., Reichart B. Reduction of wound healing problems after median sternotomy by use of retention sutures. Ann Thorac Surg 1998; 66:2125-2126

Losanoff, J.E., Richman, B.W., Jones, J.W., Disruption and infection of median sternotomy: a comprehensive review *Eur J Cardiothorac Surg* 2002;21:831-839

Mary AM Rogers, Neil Blumberg, Sanjay Saint, Kenneth M Langa, and Brahmajee K Nallamothu. Hospital variation in transfusion and infection after cardiac surgery: a cohort study. *BMC Medicine* 2009, 7:37doi:10.1186/1741-7015-7-37

Mclelland, S., Postoperative intracranial neurosurgery infection rates in North America versus Europe: A systematic analysis. Am J Infect Control 2008; 36:570-3Nelson DR, Buxton TB, Luu QN, Rissing JP. The promotional effect of bone wax on experimental Staphylococcus Aureus osteomyelitis. *J. Thorac. Cardiovasc. Surg.* 1990; 99:977-980.

Milano, A. Carmelo MD; Karen Kesler, MS; Nancy Archibald, MHA, MBA; Daniel J. Sexton, MD; Robert H. Jones,

MD Mediastinitis After Coronary Artery Bypass Graft Surgery.Circulation. 1995;92:2245 2251 doi:10.1161/01.CIR.92.8.2245

National Hospital Discharge Survey: 2007 Summary, table 8. Centers for Disease Control and Prevention
http://www.cdc.gov/nchs/fastats/insurg.htm accessed July 31, 2011.

Nelson DR, Buxton TB, Luu QN, Rissing JP. The promotional effect of bone wax on experimental Staphylococcus aureus osteomyelitis. J Thorac Cardiovasc Surg 1990;99:977-80.

Neumayer, L., Vargo, D. (2008) Principles of Preoperative and Operative Surgery, In: *Townsend: Sabiston Textbook of Surgery, 18th ed.* Courtney M. Townsend Jr. R. Daniel Beauchamp B. Mark Evers, Kenneth L. Mattox, pp. (251-279), Saunders Elsevier, 978-1-4160-3675-3, Philadelphia, PA Rohde et al., "Spondylodiscitis after lumbar discectomy. Incidence and a proposal for prophylaxis." Spine (Phila Pa 1976), 1998 Mar 1;23 (5):615-20.

Nishida H, Grooters RK, Soltanzadeh H, Thieman KC, Schneider RF, Kim WP. Discriminate use of electrocautery on the median sternotomy incision. A 0.16% wound infection rate. J Thorac Cardiovasc Surg 1991;101:488-94.

Noskin G.A., Robert J. Rubin, et al. "The Burden of Staphylococcus aureus Infections on Hospitals in the United States." Arch Intern. Med. 2005;165:1756-1761.

Parker, R. (1892). "Aural pyaemia siccessfully treated by removing putrid thrombus of jugular vein and lateral sinus." The British Medical Journal 1: 1076-1077

Pairolero PC & Arnold PG. Management of Infected Median Sternotomy Wounds Ann Thorac Surg, 1986; 42:1-2. DOI: 10.1016/S0003-4975(10)61822-X

Recker RR: Embryology, anatomy, and microstructure of bone, in Coe FL, Favus MJ (eds): Disorders of Bone and Mineral Metabolism. New York: Raven, 1992, pp 219–240.

Rogers MA, Blumberg N, Saint S, Langa KM, Nallamothu BK. Hospital variation in transfusion and infection after cardiac surgery: a cohort study. BMC Med 2009;7:37.

Sawan A, Elhawary Y, Zaghlool Amer M, & Abdel Rahman M. "Controversial Role of Two Different Local Haemostatic Agents on Bone Healing." Journal of American Science, 2010; 6(12):155-163]. (ISSN: 1545-1003).

Schonauer C, Tessitore E, Barbagallo G, Albanese V, Moraci A. The use of local agents: bone wax, gelatin, collagen, oxidized cellulose. Eur Spine J. 2004;13 (suppl 1):S89–S96.Shearwood McClelland III, Postoperative intracranial neurosurgery infection rates in North America versus Europe: A systematic analysis. Am J Infect Control 2008; 36:570-3

Solheim E, Pinholt EM, Bang G, Sudmann E. Effect of local hemostatics on bone induction in rats: a comparative study of bone wax, fibrin-collagen paste, and bioerodible polyorthoester with and without gentamicin. J Biomed Mater Res. 1992 Jun;26(6):791-800.

Sorrenti SJ, Cumming WJ, Miller D. Reaction of the human tibia to bone wax. Clin Orthop Relat Res 1984:293– 6.

Samudrala, S.. "Topical Hemostatic Agents in Surgery: A Surgeon's Perspective." *AORN Journal*, 2008. Supplement: Intraoperative Bleeding and Hemostasis in Surgical Procedures. vol. 88, no 3: p. S2-11

Styers D, Sheehan DJ, Hogan P, et al. Laboratory-based surveillance of current antimicrobial resistance patterns and trends among Staphylococcus aureus: 2005 status in the United States. *Ann Clin Microbiol Antimicrob.* 2006. 5:2

Sudmann B, Bang G, Sudmann E. Histologically verified bone wax (beeswax) granuloma after median sternotomy in 17 of 18 autopsy cases. Pathology 2006; 38:138–41.

Szerafin Tamás, MD, Osama Jaber, MD, Árpád Péterffy, MD, PhD. Reduction of wound healing problems after median sternotomy (letter to the editor). *Ann Thorac Surg* 1999; 68: 2388.

Tang GH, Maganti M, Weisel RD, Borger MA. Prevention and management of deep sternal wound infection. Semin Thorac Cardiovasc Surg 2004;16:62-9.

Tomizawa Y. Clinical benefits and risk analysis of topical hemostats: a review. *J Artif Organs* 2005;8:137-42.

Eklund A.M. , M. Valtonen, K.A. Werkkala: Prophylaxis of sternal wound infections with gentamicin-collagen implant: randomized controlled study in cardiac surgery. Journal of Hospital Infection (2005) 59, 108–112.

Vander Salm TJ, Okike ON, Pasque MK, Pezzella AT, Lew R, Traina V, Mathieu R. Reduction of sternal infection by application of topical vancomycin. J Thorac Cardiovasc Surg 1989;98(4):618-22.

Verrall, P. J. (1924). Operation on Joints. Modern Operative Surgery. H. W. Carson. London, Cassell & Co. 1: 69.

Watters WC III, MD et al. North American Spine Society Evidence-Based Clinical Guidelines for Multidisciplinary Spine Care, 2007.

Wellisz T, Armstrong JK, Cambridge J, Fisher TC: Ostene, a new water-soluble bone hemostasis agent. J Craniofac Surg 17: 420-425, 2006.

Wellisz T, An YH, Wen X, Kang Q, Hill CM, Armstrong JK. *Infection rates and healing using bone wax and a soluble polymer material.* Clin Orthop Relat Res 2008; 466:481-6.

Wellisz T, Armstrong JK, Cambridge J, et al. The effects of a soluble polymer and bone wax on sternal healing in an animal model. Ann Thorac Surg 2008; 85:1776-80.